The
Hepatitis C
Handbook

The
Hepatitis C
Handbook

Matthew Dolan

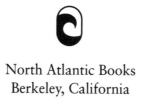

North Atlantic Books
Berkeley, California

The Hepatitis C Handbook

Published by
North Atlantic Books
P.O. Box 12327
Berkeley, California 94712

First published in the U.K. by Catalyst Press, 1996, 1998
P.O. Box 13036, London NW1 3WG, United Kingdom

Cover image of HCV based on electron micrograph
Book design by Paula Morrison

Printed in the United States of America

The Hepatitis C Handbook is sponsored by the Society for the Study of Native Arts and Sciences, a nonprofit educational corporation whose goals are to develop an educational and cross-cultural perspective linking various scientific, social, and artistic fields; to nurture a holistic view of arts, sciences, humanities, and healing; and to publish and distribute literature on the relationship of mind, body, and nature.

Library of Congress Cataloging-in-Publication Data
Dolan, Matthew
    The hepatitis C handbook / by Matthew Dolan ; foreword by Iain Murray-Lyon and John Tindall.—Rev. ed.
        p. cm.
    Previously published by Catalyst Press, 1997.
    Includes bibliographical references and index.
    ISBN 1-55643-313-1 (alk. paper)
    1. Hepatitis C—Handbooks, manuals, etc.   I. Title
RC848.H425D65   1999
616.3'623—dc21   98-52148
                                                                             CIP

3 4 5 6 7 8 9 / 03 02 01

To Doreen Billings,
mother, wife, friend, hepatitis C patient,
liver transplant recipient

Died October 13, 1997

Acknowledgments and Thanks

I could not have produced this book without the help of innumerable individuals and institutions. Some of those to whom I owe a debt of thanks include the hepatitis C support group based at Mainliners in London, especially Leena, Bob, Grant, Kathy, Francesca, Sue, and Soledad; John Tindall and the staff of the Gateway Clinic; Iain M. Murray-Lyon; Jason McClure and friends; Andrea Efthimiou-Mordaunt; Geoff Dusheiko; Giorgina Mieli-Vergani; Christopher Tibbs; Graham Alexander; Graham Foster; Robert Batey; Christine Beveridge; Jill Smith; John Babish; Berwyn Clarke; Alex Wodak; Elizabeth Webb; Quing Cai Zhang; Lucy McGrath; Lynn and the "infobabes"; Crina Dimitriou and the HEPC list; Janet Piesold; Brendan Duffy; Jose Luiz Garcia; the British Liver Trust; the American Liver Foundation; the HCV Global Foundation, especially Ron Duffy and Joey Tranchina; the Mainliners Agency; the Children's Liver Disease Foundation; the Hemophilia Society; and the Lindesmith Center.

Important Note to Patients

The medical information contained in this book does not represent my advice. It is simply a selection of pertinent information from divergent sources, which will hopefully enable patients to make sense of their situation and to make informed decisions regarding treatments and lifestyle. Doctors must be consulted before taking treatment. The author disclaims any responsibility for patients acting without formal medical advice.

A Note about Spelling

This book combines American and British spelling protocols. In some cases this reflects the origin of documents quoted in the text. I hope readers will be tolerant of the inconsistencies.

A Note about References

Because this book is designed for lay use as well as for medically qualified professionals, I have generally confined the use of references to substantiate key findings; I did not want to fill the book with too much text that might be superfluous to many readers. However, suggestions for further reading have been included in hope that these will be adequate for medical professional readers.

Contents

Part 3: Treatment Options

Part 4: Lifestyle Issues

Part 5: Notes, Afterword, Resources, and Index

Foreword

by Dr. Iain M. Murray-Lyon, MD, FRCP, FRCPE (Ed)
Consultant Physician and Gastroenterologist
Charing Cross, Chelsea and Westminster Hospitals

Hepatitis C is a common, recently discovered viral infection usually contracted from the use of intravenous drugs, often decades previously, or less commonly blood or blood products prior to the introduction of screening by the Blood Transfusion Services. Sexual transmission is rare, and in some cases the origin of the infection is obscure. The majority of individuals chronically infected with this virus feel entirely well, and the diagnosis comes as a total and devastating surprise. Others suffer from a range of symptoms including disabling fatigue.

This fully updated new second edition of Matthew Dolan's very successful handbook gives a clear factual account of hepatitis C and constructively addresses the significance of the diagnosis and lifestyle changes that may be helpful. It guides the patient to an informed and balanced choice between the currently available range of treatment options including interferon and other antiviral agents as well as Chinese herbal remedies. It aims to disempower the virus and to hand back control and well-being to the individual. I am sure that sufferers will greatly benefit from reading it.

Foreword

by John Tindall, MCSP, SRP, BAc, MRTCM
Manager of the Gateway Clinic and Chinese medicine specialist

The medical profession and general public are now becoming aware of the prevalence of HCV in the population, and even at this early stage it appears that a considerable number of people are affected throughout the world. This will have immense health implications.

The Western medical system has responded with a strong pharmaceutical approach, and yet this does not necessarily yield a high level of success. There are many unanswered questions. It is not by accident that this book, which has been well researched throughout, is written and constructed by someone with HCV.

Through the many natural health care systems that have been used over the centuries and have lasted the test of time, there are many suitable remedies for the problems that emerge related to HCV. As holistic health care has grown in popularity over the last fifteen years, it is understandable that clients would seek options outside the Western medical model.

This book presents a fair appraisal of the varied approaches one could take. This may permit clients to make an informed decision and expend their freedom of choice. For anyone interested in the issues of HCV, be they health professionals or not, this text is exceptionally informative and appropriate for our present times. The whole world is having to respond to this health concern, and this book will be among those that contribute to a greater understanding of the possible directions that are available for people to maintain optimum health.

Foreword

by Jason Scott McClure
Medical writer, Quantum Media, *Focus on Hepatitis C
International Newsletter*

Hepatitis C is no longer someone else's problem. The viral liver disease remains incurable, continues to resist drug treatments, causes suffering and death within the rank and file of all societal, economic global communities while the number of those infected shows no signs of leveling off.

Those diagnosed with hepatitis C represent only the tip of the iceberg. This enigmatic disease is an accelerating worldwide disaster, and this book gives us the whole truth about hepatitis C and the specter of its insidious influence on our bodies and our lives.

Matthew Dolan sounded the alarm with his first informative and comprehensive book, *The Hepatitis C Handbook*. Now in his latest project, Matthew Dolan has accurately compiled a vast amount of research on HCV drawn from quality medical sources. It is extraordinarily informative and draws attention to important issues which need to be addressed. Both Western and non-Western medical regimes and thoughts are to be found within the pages of this book.

One thing is certain: the Hepatitis C epidemic is not simply going to go away. Considering the enormous magnitude of this epidemic, the information presented in this book needs to reach as broad an audience as possible. Both medical professionals, HCV individuals, and the general public will benefit from considering the facts and thoughts it presents.

Prologue

I found out that I had antibodies to hepatitis C on August 6, 1993. Although I had met someone who had mentioned that he had "Hep C" a few months earlier, he knew nothing about it, and it did not occur to me that I might have been at risk. The only information I had was in the letter that informed me of the diagnosis. Despite the reassuring tone—"in the normal healthy person this infection is usually extremely mild ... you should NOT be unduly worried"—I received the impression that they were not entirely sure. The letter went on to say, "I would strongly advise you to talk to your own doctor about this in further detail ... he will be able to refer you a specialist."

For the next two months I chose to ignore the diagnosis, preferring to believe that the condition was trivial to the point of being irrelevant, as implied in the first section of the letter. During this period I met a retired general practitioner of medicine and raised the subject with him. He told me that hepatitis "non A non B," as it was then generally known, was no more serious than "a touch of food poisoning." This led me to adopt an even more dismissive attitude.

It was not until I met a number of other people who had been diagnosed with HCV antibodies and began to listen to their stories that I began to realize that what I had been told had no basis in fact and that hepatitis C was indeed a serious illness. What struck me in particular were the differing, sometimes alarming fragments of information that they had been given. Several mentioned that they had heard that HCV infection led to liver cancer; others stressed the more subtle symptoms such as tiredness and adverse reactions to alcohol; a few linked HCV to seemingly unrelated conditions such as depression or kidney disease.

As I became increasingly aware of the poverty of the information available regarding prognosis and treatment, I resolved to see my doctor and obtain a referral to a specialist. I also decided to become involved in the formation of a support group and to commence a systematic program of research into the virus and available treatments. It quickly became apparent that there was an urgent need for a book to assist the rapidly increasing numbers of people diagnosed with HCV in the process of coming to terms with their condition and in seeking treatment appropriate to their individual situation and disposition. The process of accepting the diagnosis, absorbing the implications, learning how to live with the virus, assessing the strengths and weaknesses of various treatment options and making lifestyle changes reflecting what is now known about hepatitis C has been very challenging for me and the other patients who have helped me with this book. It is an ongoing process; personal change has been gradual, and the continuous emergence of new information about HCV sometimes means that new adjustments need to be made.

Since the central objective of this book is to empower hepatitis C patients to make appropriate decisions about treatment and lifestyle following diagnosis, I have included extensive factual and scientific information. Some will find this superfluous. However, I was so frustrated by the poor factual quality of the information given to me that I decided to include a high level of scientific detail here. I now realize that much of the necessary information simply wasn't available at that time.

A good knowledge of the current thinking about the virus has proved useful in making decisions about treatment and lifestyle. As I became familiar with some of the real symptoms, often unmentioned by my doctors, and was able to identify some of them in myself, I became convinced that it was unlikely that I would be able to obtain a full picture from them. Their knowledge was incomplete, their focus was narrow, they seemed reluctant to acknowledge the wider pattern of problems experienced by patients, they persistently sought to minimize the seriousness of HCV, and they were dismissive of alternative treatments despite persistent positive reports from those who had tried them. In the light of all this I felt that I needed to explore patients' experiences of alternative and complementary medicines, and to look at HCV from some different perspectives.

This book represents the results of my researches—thousands of hours of reading, on-line database searches, and interviews. More importantly it contains the accumulated experience of many people living with hepatitis C—the people who have accompanied me on my journey from ignorance through anxiety towards a confident and informed basis of living with this virus and, perhaps, eventually overcoming it. What has emerged is a fascinating picture of a wider pattern of HCV symptoms together with a great variety of treatments and lifestyle choices that can address these problems.

None of the treatment systems described in this book represent a complete answer to HCV. However, I hope that readers will be able to see what each of them has to offer and then be able to make an informed choice about his or her own treatment. I hope that the juxtaposition of these treatments, along with information about lifestyle, will enable readers to see how they might be able to achieve an improved prognosis and a better quality of life. Unlike a couple of the recent hepatitis C books that have appeared since the first edition, this work has emphatically not been subsidized, commissioned, or in any way helped by any of the pharmaceutical companies active in the production of hepatitis C treatments; it is an independently produced piece of work, primarily aligned with, and informed by, patients and their experiences.

Introduction to the Revised Edition

I decided to write a second edition of this book largely because of the positive response to the first. I also wished to take the opportunity to update and expand the contents to reflect wider readership, recent research findings, and specific areas of interest requested by patients and professionals; for instance this is reflected by the addition of chapters on children and Ayurvedic medicine and the inclusion of information from and pertaining to the U.S. and Canada. I have consulted many more leading experts in relevant fields and their work. My feeling is that we now have a clearer understanding of hepatitis C and an improved basis for delineating appropriate responses.

As before this book is primarily aimed at people who have hepatitis C. It will also appeal to health workers, medical practitioners, people with related conditions such as chronic fatigue syndrome, and the families of patients. The purpose of the book is fivefold:

1. To explain as clearly as is currently possible what hepatitis C is and how it affects exposed individuals

2. To describe the scale and pattern of its presence in the human population and how it may manifest itself

3. To identify the broad treatment options available and enable the reader to "get a feel" for which of these may be suitable for them as an individual and to enable them to get their preferred treatment needs met

4. To empower the readership with the ability to adjust their lifestyles in such a way so as to minimize the impact of hepatitis C on their quality of life and longevity

5. To assist health professionals in the process of making decisions relating to hepatitis C in general and patients in particular

Unlike the glossy pamphlets on hepatitis C, which are often handed out to patients, this book does go into the medical details. It does not attempt to patronize; most people will be capable of grasping the details covered here. The reason for this is that hepatitis C is a multifaceted subject; any attempt to reduce it to a few paragraphs of simplistic text will inevitably mislead or fail to cover the requisite range of information. It is also sometimes necessary for patients to have a good understanding of the subject in order to get their treatment needs met; unfortunately there are a lot of uninformed medical practitioners who will fail to treat hepatitis C patients appropriately.

The text covers the physical, mental, and emotional aspects of the illness and the corresponding experiences of patients. The structure of the book reflects the stories of patients themselves and mirrors their varied experiences and perspectives. I hope that readers will be able to adopt a positive approach to the condition as well as obtaining effective treatment.

I hope that doctors and other medical professionals will also read this book, and thereby be better able to recognize, prevent, and treat this prevalent, frequently debilitating, and sometimes life-threatening condition. It is currently a fact that rates of diagnosis are extremely low in Europe and North America, that misdiagnosis is commonplace, and also that poorly thought out treatment prescriptions can precipitate adverse effects in people with hepatitis C. The text is intended to help doctors to be able to identify such problems in individual patients, become aware of varied clinical presentations and predispositions, and to respond appropriately.

Because hepatitis C is usually a chronic condition, there is normally plenty of time to absorb the implications of the diagnosis and to become informed about lifestyle changes and treatment options. It is the experience of a number of patients that their hepatitis C diagnosis has prompted them to review their lives and make a number of positive ongoing changes. Combined with the support of treatment options outlined in the text, some patients now feel that their current level of health is better than if they had never contracted the hepatitis C virus (HCV). Thus, for some patients at least, it seems that hepatitis C can be highly responsive to lifestyle adjustments and various treatments.

The Structure of This Book

This book opens with facts and figures about the virus and its prevalence. Transmission, epidemiology, and the origins of the virus are discussed in chapter 2, together with professional briefings regarding the prevention of the further proliferation of HCV. Information regarding the various tests that patients are likely to encounter are covered in detail in chapter 3, together with a discussion of the implications of a diagnosis and whether or not to get tested. I have also included information on the implications of coinfection with HIV, hepatitis B, and hepatitis G, which is common in some sections of the patient population. Chapters on children, hemophilia, and Cooley's anemia have been added in order to address issues specific to these groups. Because there is so much confusion and downright ignorance regarding HCV, this section may help the reader to understand what it is he or she is dealing with.

The second part concentrates on the response to having HCV. This section is designed to enable the reader go through the process of coming to terms with their condition and to begin to operate from a position of strength and confidence. I have included some practical advice on how to deal with members of the medical profession because this has proved to be a problematic area for many.

The third part summarizes the main treatment options open to HCV patients. Some of these approaches are complementary and may therefore be used in conjunction with each other. It is important to read this section carefully in order to avoid potentially hazardous combinations of treatments. Prognosis data is included where possible, although we are in the early days regarding the quantification of success rates. The options listed here are not exhaustive, but they do encompass the broad types of approach available and the ones most commonly used by patients I have met.

Although the book examines and discusses the intricacies of the various treatments available for hepatitis C, it is not prescriptive. Each treatment option is outlined in a way that reflects my understanding of its workings based upon interviews with practitioners backed up by research. I have tried to present each one in an objective manner that does not reflect my own personal choice of approach. I believe that no single doctor could achieve this because he or she would inevitably be biased in favor of their "native" methodology.

The fourth part covers the lifestyle adjustment choices open to patients. This section is very important for all HCV+ people and vital for those who decide not to take treatment. The aim of this section is to give readers the best possible chance of living with HCV without inadvertently contributing to a worse prognosis.

The fifth part of this book contains additional technical information, a glossary, a comprehensive list of resources to help readers locate future support and information, and the index.

Part
1

Background Facts, Figures, and Theories

1

The Virus:
Symptoms and Natural History

HEPATITIS C IS BAFFLING. Doctors, when they are not pondering the latest enigmatic research finding, or yet another associated medical condition, can become excited about the intellectual challenge it presents. Though more is being discovered, findings sometimes raise at least as many new questions as they answer. Replete with instances of widespread "black holes" in medical knowledge, theoretical paradoxes, "mind boggling" statistics, and factual gaps, the subject is both fascinating and frightening.

The Nature and Characteristics
of the Hepatitis C Virus (HCV)

Viruses are the most basic living organisms. They are simply pieces of protein and nucleic acid encoding replication information encased in an envelope. In HCV this envelope is composed of lipids, fatty tissues common in animal chemistry. Viruses appear to have no purpose other than to propagate themselves. They are entirely dependent on "host" cells for this.

HCV infects the liver. Until recently almost all research into HCV concentrated upon this organ. More recent investigations have revealed that HCV infects other cells, notably a category of white blood cells scientifically termed *peripheral blood mononuclear cells* (PBMCs) and the lymphatic system as a whole; this is thought to make the condition more difficult to treat. It has also been found to

3

affect (not necessary infect) a number of other parts of the body, and many experts now regard this as a systemic condition (see below).

Viruses generally cause damage to human beings in one of two ways: either they damage cells directly by invading them or replicating in a way that damages their hosts, thus destroying the structure or undermining their function—known as *cytopathic*—or they provoke an immune system response, which in turn destroys surrounding cells or causes chemical imbalances that induce malign biochemical processes—known as *immunopathic.*

Initially most specialists believed that HCV belonged to the cytopathic category and that damage was confined to the liver. This was significant because it provided the basis for determining treatment strategy; for instance this inference meant that immune response inducing drugs such as interferon could be used without fear of provoking immunopathic injury. However, it is now clear that HCV also causes injury through immunopathic mechanisms, and that in many cases the degree of tissue damage—usually a kind of hardening and scarring process called *fibrogenesis*—can only be explained by some kind of immune response. The puzzlement of doctors is well illustrated by the following quote:

> The exact mechanisms by which this virus causes hepatitis are not known. For several reasons the predominant mechanism for injury has been thought to be direct hypertoxicity … clinical observations in treated patients are most consistent with a cytopathic form of liver injury…. Despite this compelling circumstantial evidence, there is also reason to suspect noncytopathic mechanisms for hepatic injury. First not all individuals infected with HCV have liver injury. Second, the presence in liver biopsies of inflammation, lymphoid follicles and lymphatic bile duct injury suggests an immune-mediated attack.[1]

If it is the case that liver cells are in fact damaged by some kind of immune-mediated self-destruct mechanism, then treatment and damage limitation needs to follow that particular logic (for instance, there are drugs and natural medicines that can inhibit the production of substances linked to this pattern of damage). A clear majority of hepatologists now lean toward the immunopathic mechanism of injury and point to cases of patients with very high viral loads and nonexistent liver disease to illustrate their point. Experts in extra-hepatic symptoms, such as lymphoma and chronic fatigue, also tend to conclude that disease and debilitation is caused by the body's reaction to the presence of HCV. However, this has not yet been proven beyond doubt.

The dynamics of disease progression are still poorly understood; the immunopathic mechanisms behind some forms of injury are obscure. It seems that sometimes the immune system reacts to the presence of the virus by sending out many different chemical messengers, which "instruct" surrounding cells to take certain types of action that may include self-destruction or making abnormal biochemical changes.

Some people with chronic HCV experience a range of associated symptoms, most of which are usually classified as "autoimmune." Research is only now beginning to be able to reveal links between the existence of immunopathic problems and other factors, such as the strain of hepatitis C virus, the level of infection, the genetic makeup of individual patients, or lifestyle factors. The situation is not helped by the fact that some of these conditions may be exacerbated by impaired liver function. Thus there is often a strong case for a complex combination of causes for some of these conditions.

HCV is frequently described as an indolent virus. Just as the word suggests, this means that it is thought to be slow to proliferate in the infected individual and usually takes a long time to cause serious clinical disease. This is very important information for the patient and is the main reason why infection is more likely to be debilitating than fatal, why symptoms can take a long time to progress, and, most importantly, why a cure or effective countermeasures might be found before the damage becomes irreversible.

This indolence is not properly understood. Some research suggests that HCV naturally replicates itself slowly, and that this is related to the longevity of the cells it usually inhabits. Another potential reason for this indolence is that HCV is so genetically unstable that it makes many "unviable" copies of itself that simply don't survive. Certainly the liver tissue of infected patients reveals the presence of many virus particles (virions) with different RNA structures.

Over a long period of time several different viable HCV RNA patterns emerge, but this process is slowed by the predominantly faulty reproduction process.

On the other hand it may be the case that many HCV virions are effectively neutralized by other parts of the immune system, but that the rate at which this occurs is lower than that of viral replication. The phagocytosis process, detailed in the chapter on the immune system, does eliminate cells infected by HCV. However, it seems that some virions replicate in sites beyond the reach of antibodies. The debate is similar to that which surrounds HIV and is discussed in the section on models of viral persistence.

HCV is exceptionally tiny, even by the standards of viruses, which also helps to explain how it escaped detection for so long. Using the very latest technology—a high-power electron micrograph—doctors at the Nihon University of Medicine in Tokyo have been able to produce a picture of the virus. However, this is described as "putative" (meaning "supposedly") in some Western medical literature, indicating a degree of skepticism.

It circulates in extremely low concentrations in the blood of most infected patients, which is one of the reasons why tests for the presence of HCV are expensive and difficult to perform (see tests section). However, it is extremely virulent, which means that infection with only tiny amounts of HCV can cause significant illness. It is extremely infectious, meaning that it is easily passed from a carrier to a new host where there is the opportunity via blood-to-blood contact, and it is also extremely resilient, meaning that it is hard to kill.

Hepatitis C is classified as an RNA virus. This means that its genetic material is made up of ribonucleic acid, as opposed to DNA, deoxyribonucleic acid. RNA viruses are less genetically stable than DNA viruses. The structure of DNA can be visualized as two rings with interlocking teeth. This means that when reproduction takes place the genetic code of the "parent" is imposed correctly on the "child." However, the genetic structure of RNA is visualized as a series of linked strands. This reflects the fact that viruses such as HCV are quite unstable and prone to rapid mutation. (A technical description of the virus is on pages 437–445.)

Because of this, HCV has evolved into different strains that are largely, but not exclusively, linked to various parts of the world. The various types are distinguished by variations in their genetic maps. The following list shows the system developed by Dr. Peter Simmonds of Edinburgh University and is the most widely used:

Type 1a: Predominates in the U.S.; common in the U.K. and Europe

Type 1b: Found mainly in Japan and Europe; significant in the U.S.

Type 2: Common in Japan, also found in China

Type 3: Prevalent in Scotland, common in Europe and the U.K., less in the U.S.

Type 4: Predominates in the Middle East and Africa

Type 5: Mainly found in South Africa.

Type 6: Found in the restricted regions of Hong Kong and Macao

The existence of these types may be important to patients because most hepatitis specialists now suspect that they may influence prognosis, clinical disease profile, and response rates to drug therapy (see pages 197–199 for details). Their behavior is broadly similar, despite variations in genetic makeup. The same goes for the subtypes of these strains, of which there are now at least eighty. The full significance of these types is still not known.

HCV is a fragile virus, which continues to mutate while present in individual patients. This results in a high degree of genetic variation, or heterogeneity, which is associated with greater resistance to antiviral therapy. Therefore patients are likely to have minor variations of these broad categories of HCV; the longer the persistence of the infection in the body, the more quasi species are likely to be present. Quasi species in particular sites, such as the liver, may diversify from those in other body parts. These quasi species present a more complex problem to the immune system. The likelihood of successful antiviral therapy can be reduced by this continuing evolution of genetically divergent versions of HCV. One of the arguments in favor of taking drug therapy is that even if it doesn't effect a sustained response, there is evidence to suggest that it may eliminate variants of the virus. This is discussed in the section on conventional treatment.

HCV may be distantly related to the pestiviridae, which cause conditions that affect livestock such as bovine viral diarrhea and hog cholera. It bears greater resemblance to the flaviviridae group, and is now usually classified as a flavivirus; this group includes viruses that cause conditions such as yellow fever and dengue fever. The closest known relative is the recently discovered GBV group of viruses, also referred to as hepatitis G, although the exact nature of the relationship is not yet known.

A Note about Retroviruses

Unlike hepatitis B and HIV, HCV is not a retrovirus, although at one time some virologists suspected that it might be. Retroviruses are DNA types and characterized by the fact that not only do they invade host cells but that they also attempt to integrate their own genetic structure into that of the host cell. This causes additional disruption and has the effect of corrupting the healthy DNA and using the infected cells to further the proliferation process.

The Course and Symptoms of Hepatitis C

The first questions in the minds of many newly diagnosed patients are along the lines of "How serious is this?" "How is it going to affect me in my everyday life?" "How is it going to impact on my life expectancy?"

This section of the book will help to provide answers to these questions, although much may also depend upon how you respond to information in the later chapters. It is important to appreciate that hepatitis C is a long-term condition; as emphasized above symptoms and disease often evolve over a long period of time, and no single patient is likely to experience them all. It may also be useful to note that the degree of symptoms very often bear little relationship to the degree of injury found in the liver.

Symptoms Reported by Patients

The following is a list of common symptoms reported by patients. This list might be used to characterize a "hepatitis C syndrome." Very few people experience all of these, and some of them seem to come and go:

- Flulike illness; alternate chills and fever
- Stabbing pains in the liver region
- Indigestion
- Irritable bowel syndrome
- Joint pains
- Vivid dreams, night sweats
- Depression, mood swings, seasonal affective disorder
- Chronic fatigue or sudden attacks of exhaustion
- Adverse reactions to alcohol
- Abdominal bloating
- Frequent urination, often during the night
- Loss of appetite
- Aversion to fatty foods
- Itchy skin
- Diarrhea
- Mental fatigue, frequent or continuous headache
- Cognitive dysfunction, attention deficit disorder, "brain fog"
- Irregular or poor sleep quality, not feeling rested after sleep
- Chest pains, palpitations
- Pronounced fluid retention
- Puffy face
- Swellings under armpits, in the groin area, and around the neck
- Blood sugar disorders
- Dizziness and peripheral vision problems, such as "floaters"

- Sleep dust in the eyes, eyesight difficulties
- Small red patterns of inflamed blood vessels known as "spider naevi"
- Numbness in peripheral regions of the body

Women report particular additional symptoms:

- Irregular menses
- Severe premenstrual tension
- Additional menopause-related problems
- Lower libido

Some people with hepatitis C conclude that they must have chronic fatigue syndrome (CFS), otherwise known as "yuppie flu" or "M.E." (myalgic encephalomyelitis). This is an important overlapping factor for many HCV+ individuals and a section on CFS/M.E. has been included to address a number of issues arising from this (see pages 31–37).

Clinical Symptoms

It is now apparent that HCV is best viewed as a systemic condition. Clinical symptomatic profiles can be grouped as follows.

The first category is disease caused by the presence of the virus in the liver and lymphatic system. HCV is described as both hepatotropic and lymphatotropic. Hepatotropic infection can cause progressive liver disease; lymphatic infection can cause lymphatic disorders.

The second category embraces disease caused by the disordered response of the body to these infections. There are two general types of disordered response:

The first of these are various distinct autoimmune conditions, which are brought about by the immune system attacking body tissues. These are relatively easy to diagnose.

The second are various CFS/M.E.–like syndromes, which tend to be more difficult to pin down and are not well understood.

On this basis some doctors are now attempting to define several emerging models of disease, which relate to the processes that are dominant in an individual patient. Distinct patterns of progression may correspond to the differing "host factors."

These types are speculative, but may help in the development of more flexible models of treatment. For convenience I have labeled these profiles as type A and type B. These types correspond to a perception of predisposition and do not account for patterns of disease progression caused by lifestyle or environmental factors, which are discussed later in the book.

Type A is more prone to gradual liver disease progression. Patients will also experience secondary and immunopathic symptoms, but disease may be more logically (though subtly) linked to impaired liver function. Progression rates will vary wildly, perhaps relating to factors such as age of exposure, but also may be related to some hitherto undetected genetic component. This seems to be the largest group, encompassing perhaps 70% of patients.

Type B, or the M.E. type, appears to be unlikely to develop significant liver disease, but is predisposed to marked symptoms of a particular type, typically including aching joints, brain fog, and fatigue. Viral load may be very low, even undetectable, or very high. Perhaps 20% of patients fall into this category, which looks very likely to be related to identifiable genetic factors. Disease may be less life threatening but can be severely debilitating. See pages 31–33 for further details of the type B profile.

In addition there appear to be two other, less numerous presenting profiles:

Type C is particularly vulnerable to the development of severe lymphatic disease. However, this may be linked to cofactors such as lifestyle or environment, and also the strain of HCV and possible coinfection with hepatitis G, rather than inherent host characteristics, such as genetic inheritance.

Type D is predisposed to rapid liver disease progression. A few cases of patients becoming cirrhotic after less than five years of infection have been reported. Again it may be that a combination of genetic and extraneous factors influence this profile. The inability to present an effective immune response to HCV may be treatable (see augmentative immunotherapy, page 212).

The complex matrix of factors which are thought to influence progression are discussed further later in this chapter.

It is also worth noting that no one has yet established the physical extent of HCV infection and the indirect impact throughout the body. In a few years' time we may well be discussing additional categories of symptoms.

Liver Disease and Types A and D Patients

Although a number of people have put forward figures claiming to show the numbers of patients who are likely to progress to various stages of liver disease, the reality is that the data is not yet good enough to fully support these claims. Until recently estimates were based upon current cross sections of the HCV+ population as opposed to long-term retrospective studies of large numbers of patients. True long-term studies will only be available in the long term.

The following section describes notable stages of progression, along with some "markers," and discusses prognostic factors.

The Acute Phase

Very few people with HCV realize that anything is wrong with them at or around the time they contract the virus; less than 5% suffer the classic acute symptoms of hepatitis infection such as jaundice, diarrhea, and nausea. When these symptoms do appear they are usually no more serious than those of hepatitis A (see below). Some doctors believe that such an acute reaction is a sign of effective immune response, and an indicator of the type B disease profile. There have been a few reports of death occurring during this phase—the November 1993 issue of *Canadian Nurse* carried the following report.

> On September 30, 1991, registered nurse Bev Holmwood sustained a needlestick injury while working in a Vancouver Island operating room. Just over two months later she died, the result of hepatitis C she contracted during the accident. Her story is a sad reminder of what research has already shown: Sharps injuries are the single greatest cause of serious, and often deadly, infection among nurses and other health care personnel.

The "invisibility" of the massive scale of hepatitis C infection to public health authorities owes a lot to the fact that it is overwhelmingly a chronic condition. This means that its effects are slow to manifest themselves and are often quite subtle, being open to misinterpretation by patients and misdiagnosis by doctors.

The Chronic Phase

Although it was once thought that 50% of patients exposed to HCV cleared the virus naturally, most specialists now accept that very few people achieve such a "spontaneous" clearance. In adults the rate has been estimated to be 1% per year (see page 102 for details about children and their higher rates). Some of those that have apparently "cleared" the virus or have very low levels of viremia actually fall into the second category of patient, type B, described in the section on M.E. below. Initial optimism was partly due to the inaccuracy of early tests for hepatitis C.

The rate at which infected patients go on to experience symptoms and the severity of these symptoms varies wildly. Some develop serious problems within five years while others are in passable shape after twenty years or more. It seems that people infected in later life are likely to deteriorate more rapidly than those infected in their youth. People infected when they are young might be expected to have a greater likelihood of developing liver disease over the next four to six decades or so because their normal life expectancy is much greater. However, it is thought that the immune system response in younger patients may be more comprehensive, resulting in a more effective long-term management of HCV (see pages 101–112).

Few, if any, escape symptoms altogether; it is not yet known whether the "asymptomatic carrier state" described by some specialists is a long-term reality for some patients, or merely a period of time prior to the onset of symptoms. It does seem to be the case that for some the condition is mildly irritating, while for others it is life threatening. It is also apparent that the rate of progression can vary wildly from one patient to another. Some doctors think that the patient's genetic makeup may also have some bearing on the rate of progression; others believe that viral genotype may influence the course of the illness, and still more feel that lifestyle factors have a strong bearing.

One recent attempt to summarize the situation was made in a

letter written by Jules L. Dienstag, MD, of the gastroenterology unit of Massachusetts General Hospital to *Gastroenterology*, the professional journal. [*Gastroenterology*, 112(2):651–655, Feb 1997]. In the letter he wrote:

> In fact, little controversy exists over one inescapable conclusion: progression of hepatitis C occurs gradually and inexorably over time; in point-prevalence studies, the clinical severity of chronic hepatitis C increases from mild to moderate, to severe, and ultimately to hepatic decompensation and even hepatocellular carcinoma with increasing years of infection.... Liver biopsy studies at this two decade milestone unearthed moderate to severe chronic hepatitis in 68% and cirrhosis in 21%; only 10% had mild histological lesions....[2,3]

This is one view. Doctors do not yet possess a comprehensive understanding of the natural history of hepatitis C, a point acknowledged by Dienstag. His analysis focuses on people infected by blood transfusion, a group thought to have a slightly worse prognosis when compared to some other sections of the patient population. Dr. Graham Alexander of Cambridge University thinks that for at least 80% of patients clinical progression in terms of liver disease is likely to be countered by natural immune response. Hence he sees a picture where a certain amount of liver disease progression occurs for a few years after infection, but that this is arrested when the immune system manages to learn how to cope with HCV. Thus there is a plateau effect in the dynamics of the disease. This view has been reinforced by Dr. Leonard Seef, whose presentation at the second HCV Global Conference (Oakland Marriott Hotel, August 1998) made a strong case for the slow progression and low mortality of HCV-related liver disease.

Patients with chronic hepatitis are sometimes classified according to the degree and type of injury found in their livers. (This is known as histology.) In the case of hepatitis C it is very difficult to ascertain the health of the liver without a biopsy; unlike hepatitis B, blood test results are poor indicators of histological health. Biopsy results have been traditionally classified as follows:

- **Chronic persistent hepatitis:** The liver has not suffered significant structural distortion; minor inflammation confined to the portal tract; no evidence of scarring.

- **Chronic active hepatitis:** More inflammation spreading to other parts of the liver and not confined to portal tracts. A few early signs of scarring may be present.

- **Cirrhosis:** See below.

- **Lobular hepatitis:** Also known as protracted hepatitis, this condition is characterized by patterns of inflammation or necrosis in the lobules, often unrelated to the progression described above. This term is no longer used.

These classifications have proved to be of limited use in hepatitis C patients because the severity of symptoms are often unrelated to the degree of liver damage and also because they are sometimes too loose to provide meaningful comparisons. In any case these terms of classification are now being superseded by a numerate scoring system, which offers a more precise basis for meaningful comparison (a discussion of liver disease is included in the chapter on tests, pages 79–90).

A recent study in Italy revealed that 0.9% of the entire population has chronic active hepatitis, indicating a probability of significant numbers of people becoming cirrhotic in the future. Since hepatitis C is by far the biggest cause of this figure, it lends credence to the notion that a degree of progression is likely in the majority of patients and that the clinically asymptomatic phase is unlikely to persist.

Hepatitis C is a serious chronic illness. In clinical terms overall mortality of patients from HCV-related liver failure has been estimated at between 5 and 10% among transfused patients.[4] However, this group often has a higher viral load than the average, and this is thought to adversely influence prognosis. The New South Wales, Australia, hepatitis C support group cites a figure of 7% as the overall premature death rate from HCV.

People who have been infected early in life, such as children who have contracted the virus at birth or hemophiliacs, infected through tainted blood products in infancy, face the theoretical prospect of developing more severe problems at an earlier age. In reality the quality of information is not yet good enough to give accurate long-term prognosis expectations. As well as a lack of long-term patient data, there are also a number of variables that are thought to influence prognosis that are difficult to measure; lifestyle factors such as diet and exercise are difficult to factor into the equation, although some work has been done on the influence of alcohol consumption.

In clinical terms HCV infection usually begins to cause problems in the livers of vulnerable patients between five to ten years after infection. This corresponds to the anecdotal evidence above and the subjective symptoms of deteriorating well-being reported by patients. Sometimes these do not become severe for twenty or thirty years. However, a few patients, speculatively classed as type Ds, can progress to cirrhosis within five years. There is some evidence to suggest that people who are infected in later life are more prone to rapid deterioration. Because the majority of patients in the U.S., Canada, Australasia, and Western Europe have been infected in their twenties or thirties, the average profile is one of more serious symptoms not appearing until the forties, fifties, or sixties.

Chronic inflammation can lead to the alteration of liver structure, impairment of blood circulation, and the death of liver cells—necrosis. The key process is called fibrosis; as liver cells die, fibrous tissue is deposited. This fibrous tissue disturbs the portal circulation of blood through the liver. The destruction of liver cells impairs the liver's ability to store nutrients and to detoxify chemicals produced by the body or coming in from outside.

The majority of patients with chronic hepatitis C infection experience fluctuations in their sense of well-being. This is reflected in the results of various biochemical tests, which often demonstrate a classic pattern of sharply fluctuating liver enzyme levels that probably correspond to ongoing damage to liver cells. This is discussed in the section on tests. However, these disturbances do not necessarily correlate with the severity of symptoms, and they are far from being a conclusive indicator of significant liver damage.

Cirrhosis

It is currently said that 20% of patients with the "polyphasic" pattern of symptoms progress to cirrhosis of the liver, which is currently the eighth leading overall cause of death in the United States. Again the data is not yet good enough to accept this as statistical fact—figures from Italy seem to suggest that a higher proportion progress to cirrhosis. This means that the liver itself becomes scarred. Nodules of regenerated liver cells are an invariable feature, resulting in the usually smooth surface of the liver becoming nodular or lumpy. The implications of this are quite well described in a Roche Products patient information booklet on hepatitis C:

> Cirrhosis can lead to problems because blood is unable to flow freely through the liver and becomes diverted around it. The first symptom is ascites, which is a swelling of the abdomen with fluid. This needs to be treated with a low salt diet, and possibly a diuretic to help the kidneys excrete more salt and water. The second problem is distended blood vessels around the stomach and gullet (called varices) that enlarge because the blood is trying to find a way around the scarred liver. These blood vessels can bleed into the stomach, which may need urgent treatment. The third problem, which is fortunately rare, is the development of liver cancer hepatocellular carcinoma (HCC) in patients with cirrhosis.... Once cirrhosis has developed, it cannot get better again, even if the liver inflammation which caused it improves.

There is a pattern of differing natural history according to the sex of the patient—males have been observed to suffer from more severe liver disease and faster progression. The slower progression of females has been logically linked to menstruation and the resultant reduced level of iron in hepatocytes (liver cells)—higher levels being linked to disease progression. Patients with cirrhosis may also start to experience some additional symptoms associated with liver disease. According to Dr. David Patch, these may include the following:

Circulatory changes. Because the liver doesn't break down certain blood chemicals as efficiently, blood vessels can become dilated, leading to the heart having to work harder (portal hypertension).

Encephalopathy. This is an extremely alarming condition. Patients may experience impaired mental function because the liver is not breaking down waste products in the blood as efficiently as it should or because blood is bypassing the liver. (Laxatives are sometimes used to treat this. Note that many HCV patients with symptoms of mental dysfunction do not have cirrhosis; there are other mechanisms at work.)

Bleeding varices. This is a medical emergency that requires skilled treatment. The symptoms are vomiting up blood and/or passing black bowel motions (stools). Varices are swollen blood vessels, especially in the esophagus, which are caused by blood bypassing the liver. Sometimes these vessels can burst. If varices burst immediate hospital treatment is vital. Effective treatments are well established for this condition.

In the later stages of cirrhosis, jaundice (yellow skin) may occur, caused by the buildup of bile pigment that is usually passed by the liver into the intestines. Some people with cirrhosis experience intense itching due to bile products that are deposited in the skin. Gallstones often form in persons with cirrhosis. The liver also has trouble removing toxins, which may build up in the blood. These toxins can dull mental function and lead to personality changes and even coma (encephalopathy). Early signs of toxin accumulation in the brain may include neglect of personal appearance, unresponsiveness, forgetfulness, trouble concentrating, or changes in sleeping habits. Drugs are usually filtered out by the liver, and this cleansing process also is slowed down by cirrhosis. The liver does not remove the drugs from the blood at the usual rate, so the drugs act longer than expected, building up in the body. People with cirrhosis are often very sensitive to medications and their side effects. Processing of nutrients and hormones is also impaired, as is the production of proteins.

Advanced liver disease can play an influential role in the development of a number of other medical conditions that are sometimes used as "markers" for progression. For instance, thrombocytopenia (a decrease in circulating blood platelets) is often diagnosed in the later stages of progression. One major report from Italy analyzed survival for hepatitis C patients diagnosed with cirrhosis:

> ... a total of 405 cirrhotic patients were evaluated: these patients had a cumulative survival rate of 99.1% at five, 76.8% at ten and 49.4% at fifteen years. Comparing the age-adjusted death rate of our patients with the general Italian population, we observed that in patients with liver cirrhosis it was 3.14 and 2.84 times higher in men and women, respectively. Bilirubin was an independent indicator of survival. Several complications, such as oesophageal varices, ascites, jaundice, hemorrhage, hepatic encephalopathy and hepatocellular carcinoma significantly reduced the survival rate and were indicated as major complications, while thrombocytopenia, cholelithiasis (gall stones), and diabetes did not affect survival and thus were called minor complications. Incidence of hepatocellular carcinoma was very high especially in males, without correlation with etiology. In conclusion, the progression of virus-induced chronic active hepatitis to cirrhosis is not influenced by sex and etiology. Similarly, the different etiology does not modify the natural history of cirrhosis while the occurrence of one or more major complications significantly shortens survival. The longer survival rate observed in patients with cirrhosis included in this study is probably due to the selective inclusion of patients with early disease and no evidence of portal hypertension.[5]

While some patients with cirrhosis go on to develop liver failure or cancer, the report demonstrates that half of patients with HCV-related cirrhosis were without signs of end stage liver disease fifteen years after their diagnosis of cirrhosis. The report also shows the link between the development of more serious secondary clinical conditions and liver failure. Much of the information in the treatment and lifestyle sections of this book is included with a view to increasing the chances of patients slowing or arresting this progression.

Liver Cancer—Also Known as Hepatocellular Carcinoma (HCC)

Anyone who has had cancer themselves or has friends or relatives diagnosed with this condition will know what a formidable threat it is. In essence cancer is the accumulation, concentration, and proliferation of abnormal cells. Such cells fail to carry out the functions of their healthy neighbors and expand at their expense, eventually threatening the function of the affected tissue. Such cells do not follow "normal" instructions and behave anarchically.

HCV can cause primary liver cancer. In this instance clusters of abnormal liver cells develop, which multiply unchecked and replace the functioning liver cells; moreover they tend to spread (metastasize) outside the liver. Malignant liver cancer is a very serious condition that is also difficult to treat; liver transplantation usually offers the best chance of a cure.

By contrast most types of secondary liver cancer, or metastatic liver cancer, meaning that cancer has spread from another site to affect the liver, are seldom curable. Secondary liver cancer is often associated with rapid deterioration and extreme resistance to treatment. The recent death of Linda McCartney demonstrates the malignancy of secondary HCC; in her case primary breast cancer had eventually spread to the liver.

Patients with primary liver cancer seldom survive for more than two years; much depends upon the type and extent of the tumor as well as the patient. Although treatment is difficult, there are some more promising approaches currently being developed; these are covered in the chapters on treatment.

In the case of HCV patients it is still unknown what percentage of those with cirrhosis progress to HCC. One recent Italian study found that 22/163 cirrhotic patients progressed to HCC over the subsequent five to seven years, meaning a 13.5% chance of progression. The same study concluded that patients with genotype 1b were at a higher risk.[6] Noncirrhotic patients have occasionally been known to develop HCC as well, an alarming finding.[7] As many as 5% of HCV+ HCC patients may "skip" the cirrhotic phase.

It is extremely difficult to accurately estimate the probability of HCC incidence for all HCV+ people. Methods used, such as incidence per year, are misleading because the time period from exposure and a number of other controlling variables are often not identifiable or are not included in statistics. However, it seems that if 20% progress to cirrhosis and 13.5% of these progress to HCC within ten years, and an additional number progress without cirrhosis, an overall figure of 3% would appear to be a conservative estimate of lifetime probability. This compares to a background HCC average incidence of about 0.05% in Western countries. (Rates in Eastern countries such as Japan and China are much higher.) Thus HCV significantly increases the likelihood of developing HCC. It is important to stress that there are not yet enough data to provide exhaustive figures on this; some specialists believe that some HCV strains are more pernicious than others, particularly type 1b. However, others argue that this is because type 1b has been around longer and therefore that liver disease is more likely to have progressed further in infected patients.

Hepatologists do not yet understand precisely how HCV causes liver cancer. The cancer-causing properties of hepatitis B have been attributed to its retroviral qualities. HCV is not a retrovirus but is still a significant risk factor—again it appears that hepatitis C breaks the established rules and that further research is urgently needed. Early work by Duke researchers (a specialist cancer unit) suggests that a tumor suppressor gene, called M6P/IGF2R, may be damaged by HCV infection, favoring the survival of liver cells lacking this anticancer gene. Such an insight, if it is proved correct, may form the basis of effective antiprogression therapy (see pages 215–216 for details of therapies to retard progression from cirrhosis to HCC.)

What is known is that HCV is now the leading cause of HCC in Japan and is looking like becoming the number 1 cause in the U.S. Although lifestyle factors are generally underresearched in HCV, alcohol intake has been studied, and it is definitely a contributory factor in the development of HCC, especially in patients with cirrhosis (see chapter 22). Japanese research suggests that patients with cirrhosis are five times more likely to develop HCC than noncirrhotic patients, that patients coinfected with hepatitis B have double the risk, and that patients who are "heavy smokers" have 2.5 times the risk of progression to liver cancer.

There is also a correlation between the level of iron deposition in liver cells and the incidence of HCC (discussed in chapter 18). The pieces of the jigsaw have yet to fall fully into place, but some patterns are emerging.

Aflatoxins are also known to be a cofactor—these substances are produced by fungi that grow on certain foods, particularly nuts, stored in hot and humid conditions. This is one reason why some nutritionists advise hepatitis patients to avoid all nuts (see the chapter on diet for more information).

The genetic predisposition of patients is also thought to be an influence on the likelihood of HCC developing, just as it is thought to influence the probability of other types of cancer occurring.

An excellent and frank account of cancer and the difficulties of its treatment is included in the book *How We Die* by Sherwin B. Nuland. The relevant chapter is called "The Malevolence of Cancer."

Summary of Factors That Influence
Clinical Liver Disease Progression

Virus factors

- Duration of infection
- Genotype
- Viral load
- Degree of heterogeneity
- Coinfection HBV or HIV
- Single strain infection

Patient factors

- Age and age at infection
- Lifestyle, especially alcohol consumption
- Genetic makeup—HLA type
- Immunological health
- Sex—males progress faster

Environmental factors are currently emerging as a possible third category; this aspect is discussed in chapter 22.

Lymphatic Disease and Non-Hodgkin's Lymphomas

Non-Hodgkin's lymphomas (NHLs) are cancers located in the lymphatic drainage network, which can be seen as part of the body's immune defense and elimination system. The network consists of vessels running throughout the body, and the nodes are the centers of activity. Lymphatic fluid circulates through the system; this fluid contains cells known as lymphocytes (see pages 427–432 for details) which act as a defense against infection. Swellings in the nodes are often a normal sign that the body is engaged in fighting off an infection. HCV inhabits this system in very low concentrations.

It is possible that the widely reported recent dramatic increases in the numbers of people diagnosed with NHL—typically a rise of 75% over the past twenty years—is linked to the hepatitis C pandemic (though other viruses such as HIV, and environmental factors have also been implicated). This aspect of hepatitis C has been consistently underreported. This may be partly due to the overwhelmingly "hepatocentric" view of HCV in the medical profession, but also relates to the generally low level of HCV awareness and its "silent killer" status.

From the patients' perspective lymphoma can be as life threatening as liver disease. Because mainstream treatments for this condition are relatively effective if an early diagnosis is made, it is important to be particularly aware of this dimension.

Although HCV almost always infects the lymphatic system, most lymphatic disease is regarded as subclinical; in other words it is not diagnosed and therefore remains untreated. Until recently lymphoma was not thought to cause many instances of serious illness in hepatitis C patients. It seems that occasionally this "benign" infection can switch to malign B cell NHL. Research in Italy has revealed that 34% of patients presenting with non-Hodgkin's lymphoma have hepatitis C.

Overall prevalence rates of lymphatic cancer in HCV patients are hard to come by and have to be inferred. Lymphoma can strike at any age, and symptoms are insidious because they are reported in varying degrees by so many hepatitis C patients.

Classic Symptoms of Lymphatic Disease

- Painless swellings, usually in the neck, armpits, or groin
- Excessive sweating or fever, especially at night
- Persistent itch all over the body (known as pruritis)
- Loss of appetite
- Weight loss
- Tiredness

Scans can detect enlarged lymph nodes in the abdomen in some patients with chronic hepatitis C. Many experience occasional subclinical symptoms of lymphatic infection and enlarged glands; sarcoidosis and granuloma may also be diagnosed, although these are less common. Some reports indicate that lymphatic abnormalities in hepatitis C patients may be "pseudolymphomas," effectively suggesting a new class of disorder specific to HCV. Lymphoma may also play a role in the progression of liver disease and the appearance of symptoms such as cognitive dysfunction. The diagnosis of lymphoma, which is described as a "malignant proliferation of lymphoid tissue" in *Black's Medical Dictionary,* is usually made by taking a biopsy of a cell sample from a suspect node.

A number of other reports have confirmed the very high prevalence of HCV among NHL patients; development of this condition may be linked to coinfection with yet another virus such as hepatitis G. Some researchers believe that there is a strong link to environmental factors such as radiation and pesticides. These may well act as cofactors with HCV in causing these increased rates of NHL. More research needs to be carried out into the implications of lymphatic infection, and improved awareness is necessary for early diagnosis; because hepatitis C patients are at additional risk, regular diagnostic checks are advisable if any of the above symptoms persist. The treatments and lifestyle sections contain further information on lymphoma.

Autoimmune and Other Extrahepatic Diseases Linked to HCV

A number of autoimmune diseases are linked to hepatitis C, although it should be stressed that apart from autoimmune thyroid disease, their occurrence is quite sporadic, and of clinical relevance in no more than 10% of patients at any one time; the majority of these will be female. Their occurrence may owe at least as much to the presence of HCV in the lymphatic system as to the liver.

Autoimmune diseases occur as a direct result of the immune system attacking the patient's organs. Different conditions correspond to differing parts of the body being attacked. These can manifest at any time. An article entitled "Viral Hepatitis and Autoimmunity: Chicken or Egg?" by Christian Strassburg and Michael Manns appeared in the June 1995 edition of *Viral Hepatitis Review*. It concluded that:

> Chronic hepatitis C infection has been found to be associated with an array of autoimmune disease including cryoglobulinemia, autoimmune thyroid disease, autoimmune hepatitis, membrano proliferative glomerulonephritis, polyarthritis, porphyria cutanea tarda, Sjögren's syndrome, etc. which can affect virtually all organs. . . . This means that immune stimulants such as interferon may cause more problems in patients with autoimmune symptoms.

(This may also help to explain the wider pattern of symptoms experienced by many patients.)

Another report echoed these findings and gave figures for the presence of some of these immune disturbances: cryoglobulinemia (36%), rheumatoid factor (70%), antitissue antibodies (41%), salivary gland lesions (49%), lichen planus (5%), Sjögren's disease (57%). The paper went on to stress the vital importance of thorough patient testing before the prescription of interferon: "Interferon is known to induce and or aggravate autoimmune thyroid disease. . . . Check for serological markers of autoimmune thyroid disease."[8]

Blood and lymph system. Cryoglobulinemia is a disorder in which abnormal proteins within the blood may cause damage to the skin, nervous system, and kidneys. Mixed cryoglobulinemia (MC) affects the lymphatic system as well as the blood. Some experts believe that MC is linked to the development of lymphatic cancer:

> These data suggest that HCV infection is involved in the pathogenesis of MC through both direct participation in the immune complex related vasculitis and by triggering the lymphoproliferative disorder underlying the disease. This latter disorder seems to be related to HCV lymphotropism which could also be responsible for the evolution of MC to malignant lymphoma.[9]

Peripheral symptoms. MC is linked to a number of other secondary symptoms including Raynaud's disease, also known as "red hands." This is characterized by poor peripheral blood flow to the hands and feet, leading to sudden feelings of coldness in these extremities. (Note that smoking with Raynaud's is considered by doctors to be extremely hazardous.)

Poor blood flow to parts of the brain might also be linked to depression and "brain fog."

Kidneys. Membrano proliferative glomerulonephritis is a form of immune-mediated kidney disease; immune complexes are deposited in the glomeruli, the parts of the kidney responsible for filtering the blood. Kidney disease is thought to be linked to mixed cryoglobulinemia in many cases. Symptoms are uncomfortable and debilitating, including edema (swelling and fluid retention) and a loss of blood protein via the urine, known as proteinuria (urine tests reveal the presence of albumin).

High rates of HCV prevalence have been detected among patients attending renal dialysis units and in kidney transplant programs. Focal glomerulosclerosis, a related disorder, has also been found in significant numbers in this group of HCV patients.[10] Again it is likely that many more patients have subclinical kidney dysfunction.

Bones and joints. Blood test results from HCV+ people often find elevated levels of rheumatoid factor; this may be associated with the development of rheumatoid arthritis (RA), a debilitating condition involving painful, swollen joints, which is usually associated with middle-aged and elderly people living in damp climates. The association with and causal links to HCV were explored in a recent letter to the *Lancet,* the mainstream U.K. medical journal:

> Our findings indicate that increased HCV-RNA concentrations are associated with Rheumatoid Factor in patients who are persistently infected with HCV ... we found that the immunopathogenic mechanisms of autoimmune disease with appearance of rheumatoid factors do require the continuing presence of the triggering virus....[11]

This means that RA in hepatitis C patients may be much more closely linked to liver disease progression than previously thought. At first RA was presumed to be an immunopathic manifestation of hep C. Thus this extrahepatic symptom will be found in many "type A" patients and may not be primarily related to immune reaction. Viral hepatitis C seems to cause symptoms which overlap with classic signs of autoimmune hepatitis. In Traditional Chinese Medicine liver disease is classically linked to joint and ligament problems, so this conclusion looks to be shared by specialists from differing perspectives.

Bodywide. Antitissue antibodies indicate an immunological disorder where the immune system is reacting to a particular organ or piece of tissue. The discovery of a variety of these markers in a significant proportion of patients indicates a status of widespread, low-level, generalized autoimmune disease.

Mouth. Lichen planus (LP) is a skin disease that shows up in blotches and can also occur in the mouth. The saliva glands can also be affected. Oral LP may indicate an increased risk of mouth cancer. Bleeding gums can be a sign of liver dysfunction.

Eyes. Sjögren's syndrome manifests as dryness and grittiness in the eyes and is often associated with autoimmune destruction of tear glands. Mooren's ulcer and acute retinal pigment epithelitis are other eye conditions that have been diagnosed in HCV+ patients. Additionally the collagen disorder scleroderma, which is directly related to liver dysfunction, can affect the eyes.

Stroke. A Spanish report has linked HCV to the presence of anti-cardiolipin antibodies,[12] which are associated with thrombosis. (Thrombosis is a dangerous condition where the blood clots in arteries and veins, causing swellings and sometimes strokes.) The report found that 22% of patients had these antibodies.

Pancreas/blood sugar. A number of reports have found high rates of HCV in patients diagnosed with diabetes type II mellitus and have suggested a causal link. The following is a typical conclusion:

> A high prevalence of HCV infection was detected in diabetic patients, and most of anti-HCV positive patients presented with abnormal LFTs. Therefore, testing for HCV infection of diabetic patients with abnormal LFTs is mandatory. The lack of any particular epidemiological factor for HCV infection in our diabetic population suggests that HCV may have a direct role in the development of diabetes.[13]

Important note to HCV patients diagnosed as diabetic: The diabetes treatment called Rezulin has been reported as being linked to a number of cases of liver failure.

Liver—immunopathic. Research has indicated that HCV is a major cause of type II autoimmune hepatitis, a relatively rare condition that is characterized by the presence of antibodies to the liver/kidney microsomes (anti-LKM1). This is a very serious condition that, if untreated, progresses to cirrhosis within three years in over 80% of patients. Interestingly some of these patients have been successfully treated with interferon, despite the apparent contraindication. This association is particularly common in Italy.

Lungs. Abnormal infiltrates have been reported to be linked to hepatitis C in some patients. This factor may underlie reports of lung disease antagonized by interferon in combination with the Japanese herbal medicine Sho Saiko To (see chapter 15), as well as intermittent reports of lung disease.

Skin. Porphyria cutanea tarda is a blistering disease of the skin affecting light-exposed areas. It may be triggered by HCV infection. Systemic lupus erythematosus—commonly known as lupus—occurs suspiciously frequently in populations that are known to have high incidences of HCV—for instance, black females in the U.S. aged thirty to fifty. Diagnoses of psoriasis are also sometimes linked to hepatitis C. Skin problems may be related to mixed cryoglobulinemia, though they are associated with vasculitis.

Blood vessels. Vasculitis—a painful, debilitating condition characterized by inflamed blood vessels—is also common in HCV patients.[14] It is likely that the list of associated conditions will grow as more research is carried out.

Thyroid abnormalities are quite common; it can become either overactive (hyperthyroidism) or underactive (hypothyroidism). Because this gland regulates a number of metabolic processes, malfunction causes debility. Hyperthyroidism causes insomnia, weight loss, palpitations, and ankle swelling. Hypothyroidism causes physical and mental sluggishness. Both conditions are treatable. However, because these are common symptoms of hep C, and overlap with other related difficulties, diagnosis can be difficult.

Bowel conditions such as Crohn's disease, which is an inflammatory condition, or the common "irritable bowel syndrome" may be associated with HCV. Such conditions are not thought to be secondary to chronic liver disease, but may contribute to overall clinical complexity. Stomach and digestion problems are common and may often be linked to dietary issues. More serious stomach problems, such as the appearance of ulcers or cancerous growths, may be linked to the presence of the notorious *Heliobacter pylori,* apparently a common cofactor in the development of stomach disease in the general population. This condition is treatable—do consult a gastroenterologist.

In general it may be that undetected HCV actually helps to explain the increasing worldwide frequency of some of these conditions and represents a kind of "missing link" in epidemiologists' understanding of patterns of disease presentation. The colossal global prevalence of hepatitis C detailed in chapter 2 certainly demonstrates adequate scale. Some clinicians have tried to piece together the process by which autoimmune diseases develop; possible mechanisms for this are discussed in the chapters on diet and treatments.

One of the more alarming aspects is that patients presenting with signs of autoimmune disease are understandably often prescribed immunosuppressant drugs—however some clinicians think that these may be hazardous for hepatitis C patients (see note on corticosteroids on page 218 in the chapter on conventional medicine).

Having said all this it is important to stress the point made earlier—patients will often find that they are experiencing symptoms that specialists would not normally expect given a particular set of liver function test results. While many specialists are reluctant to admit that they could be mistaken, some leading experts frankly admit that they do not have all the answers. Speaking at the first international hepatitis C conference held in London in 1995 Professor Robert Batey, director of the gastroenterology department at the John Hunter Hospital in New South Wales, had the following to say about HCV symptoms: "It's a very confusing area. We do not yet know how hepatitis C affects the whole body of patients."

This is a refreshing admission, and it has been echoed by Professor Geoffrey Dusheiko, of the Royal Free Hospital in London. Hepatitis C is a frustrating subject to get to grips with. Some paradigms appear to cast a great deal of light on the subject and offer a basis for interpretation and treatment. However, no single one of them seems to have all of the answers. Hepatitis C cannot be seen exclusively as a liver disease. Its symptoms vary from one patient to another, as does its pathology. What it does over a long period of time is not yet clear. Given this situation of inconclusive evidence, it is important for patients to take a degree of responsibility for themselves in asserting what their symptoms are and selecting appropriate courses of action. No one has all the answers; no one is even sure exactly what questions should be posed.

HCV and Myalgic Encephalomyelitis (M.E.)
or Chronic Fatigue Syndrome (CFS)

It is not uncommon for hepatitis C patients to have been previously diagnosed as having M.E. Research from Australia suggests that 40% of patients previously diagnosed as suffering from M.E. are HCV+.[15] This does not necessarily mean that they have been misdiagnosed since the two conditions are not mutually exclusive. According to a leading hepatitis C specialist based in London a significant number of patients present with symptoms that are consistent with chronic fatigue syndrome.

Similarities in the Response of the Medical Establishment

The term M.E. describes a symptom complex with varied patterns of presentation and a variety of causes. It is now usually called chronic fatigue syndrome. Other terms sometimes used include "post viral fatigue syndrome," "post infectious fatigue syndrome," and "chronic fatigue immune deficiency syndrome." The word "syndrome" conveys the central problem of M.E. campaigners; it means "a characteristic pattern of symptoms" and has to be used because there is, as yet, no identified and widely agreed cause of M.E. Since Western medicine is unused to accepting the existence of illnesses on the basis of symptoms alone, it has proved difficult to get M.E. taken seriously by some parts of the medical establishment. This means that patients have to spend a lot of time convincing doctors that they genuinely have a severe debilitating condition and fending off accusations of malingering or mental instability.

Type B patients. Although many patients are vulnerable to aspects of M.E. syndrome, some appear to be particularly susceptible to this form of illness, and simultaneously unlikely to develop advanced liver disease; I have tentatively classed these as "type B" (see page 11).

It is now thought that perhaps 20% at most of those exposed to HCV have the genetically acquired ability to engage the virus "naturally" although many of these will fail to actually clear it. Such patients may have "occult" infection despite having no detectable virus in their blood. Younger patients and "responders" to antiviral therapy may also more likely to fall into this category (see sections on children and treatment for further information).

According to Dr. Christopher Tibbs, consultant physician and gastroenterologist, studies of people who are antibody positive but PCR negative (i.e., individuals who have been exposed to HCV but are not apparently currently infected) suggest that the human leucocyte antigen profile of patients determines the likelihood of their being able to mount a "detectable T-cell mediated response to the virus."

Not all patients with a favorable HLA type manage to do this, and it seems that very few patients, if any, actually clear the virus spontaneously once they have become chronically infected.

There is now quite a lot of evidence to support this view that stresses the powerful predisposing role of the patients' genetic inheritance. For instance, a study from Japan examining the relationship between HLA type and the severity of liver disease concluded:

> These results demonstrate that the cellular immune response of the asymptomatic carrier group is less activated than the response of the chronic active hepatitis group, and that HLA DR13 may be closely associated with this low activity of hepatitis among HCV carriers.[16]

Another report from Italy found a strong likelihood of an association between the HLA type of patients repeatedly exposed to HCV infected blood, their apparently negative HCV status, their HLA type, and the occurrence of immunological abnormalities correlating with those found in M.E. patients:

> Our results represent clear evidence for a relationship between HCV infection and immune extrahepatic abnormalities ...[17]

Most significantly of all a recent Italian study concluded:

> Presence of HLA-DR5 antigen appears as a protective factor against a severe outcome of chronic infection, being correlated with a benign evolution of the infection, often asymptomatic, or a less severe chronic liver disease.[18]

Patients who present without clear signs of liver disease and with low or undetectable virus can experience problems; doctors may often be unwilling to accept that such patients are experiencing debilitating symptoms. An example of this comes from the experience of Christine, who had recently been diagnosed HCV antibody positive and HCV PCR negative:

> For years I have had debilitating bouts of a wide range of things from depression to tiredness, palpitations, disorientation, forgetfulness, looking out of my eyes and not being able to see through the cloudiness of my mind.... Yesterday, three months after my diagnosis, I received confirmation that my PCR test is negative. Now I am confused. Do I run down the street naked screaming with joy or do I hold my breath and wait? My gastroenterologist is of the opinion that if your LFTs are fine, then so are you.

This scenario will be familiar to some HCV patients. Despite the fact that hepatitis C is a definite viral infection, most medical practitioners assume an "asymptomatic" status unless liver function tests are seriously abnormal. (As chapter 3 demonstrates there are serious problems with reliance on such indicators.) Both conditions have been labeled "benign" by certain members of the medical establishment who seem to be more concerned with suppressing public fears than with taking patients' complaints at face value.

M.E. campaigners have taken a number of steps to have the condition taken seriously. As well as forming patient support groups and bringing pressure to bear on health policy makers, they have conducted some in-depth research into the symptoms and developed coherent theories regarding their origin. Some of these are very relevant to HCV patients.

Mental Symptoms, Possible Causes, and HCV

Although isolated instances of M.E.-like outbreaks can be found throughout the twentiethth century, it was during the 1980s that it became recognized throughout the industrialized world. *Newsweek* called it "yuppie flu"; both the name and the connotations stuck. Unlike HCV, which has "junkie" associations, M.E. conjured up images of ambitious clean-cut young people in business suits being struck down by fatigue as a result of overworking and stress. Although stress was always acknowledged as a powerful factor, the more scientifically minded researchers realized that there was a strong possibility of a specific cause, most probably an elusive, as-yet-unidentified virus. Abnormal ratios of T helper to killer cells also tended to indicate that the immune system was trying to respond to some unidentified pathogen. (Note that recent research indicates that people who have been exposed to HCV, but have apparently fought it off, continue to have high T helper to killer ratios; this provides another potential "missing link" between HCV and M.E.) Human herpes viruses were considered as culprits, and HTLV, cytomegalovirus, Epstein-Barr, and Coxsackie were all carefully scrutinized; although their possible past or present occurrence could help to explain some of the symptoms, none was adequate to explain the whole syndrome.

If the Australian figures are correct, then HCV may be the cause of symptoms in a high proportion of M.E. patients. Since it was effectively invisible until 1991, it qualifies as the missing virus in the post viral fatigue syndrome hypothesis and is accepted as one cause by the M.E. association. The simple conclusion from this information would be to test all M.E. patients for HCV, reclassify those who are positive, and dismiss the validity of M.E. hypotheses as explanations for illness in these patients. However, it may be the case that M.E. hypotheses remain true for these patients and are equally valid for other HCV patients. In other words, HCV patients suffer from current and post virus fatigue syndromes. While what is known about HCV explains commonplace basic issues such as physical tiredness, autoimmune disorders, and liver disease, it does not do a very good job with more subtle problems such as poor concentration.

Hepatologists would suspect that mental dysfunction in HCV patients was caused by encephalopathy, the condition where the liver fails to clear the blood of toxins to the extent that brain function becomes impaired. However, encephalopathy is a condition that is usually associated with cirrhosis; many HCV patients who are not cirrhotic and have few signs of serious liver disease complain of regularly experiencing periods where mental function is impaired. Perhaps the M.E. theory explains the symptom better than the hepatological one.

In the book *Recovering from M.E.* by William Collinge (Souvenir Press, 1993) cognitive problems are described as the primary symptom of M.E. Common impairments are listed as follows:

> Problems with memory sequencing, spatial disorganization, trouble giving and following directions, difficulty processing problems, slow intellectual speed, difficulty processing visual and auditory information, forgetfulness, irritability, mental confusion, inability to concentrate, impairment of speech and/or reasoning, light headedness, or feeling in a fog, word finding problems, distractibility, difficulty processing more than one thing at a time, inability to perform simple math functions, problems with verbal recall, related motor problems, disturbances in abstract reasoning, sequencing problems, memory consolidation, short-term memories being easily distorted or perturbed.

These symptoms ring bells with many HCV patients. Some M.E. commentators suspect that they are caused by the direct action of an unknown virus on brain tissue; no one has yet established whether or not HCV actually infects the brain.

Given the characteristics of HCV, it may well be able to cross the blood-brain barrier. Recent research into HIV patients coinfected with HCV shows that the latter virus is present in cerebrospinal fluids (CSF) and that HCV may therefore replicate in this medium:

> This report shows the presence of HCV in CSF and raises the possibility that the CNS may act as a reservoir site for HCV.[19]

Other M.E. experts suspect that mental symptoms may be linked to the overactive response of the immune system. It is suggested that the overproduction of various cytokines (immunological chemical messengers) might be enough to disrupt brain function; perhaps interferons can cross from the blood into the brain and disrupt mental process.

There has been little research into the direct impact of HCV on the brain, the immunological status of hepatitis C patients, or the possibility of overproduction of cytokines disrupting mental function. HCV is known to infect certain blood cells and would therefore be expected to reach the brain. Whether it causes damage there is not known and needs to be researched; the results may cast a great deal of light on both conditions.

Another common symptom is depression. Dr. Charles Shephard, author of *Living with M.E.*, hypothesizes that this may be linked to virally caused disruption of serotonin production. Serotonin is vital in the regulation of mood, sleep, and appetite. Researchers have also speculated that fatigue, depression, and mental dysfunction may be caused by poor cerebral blood circulation. HCV patients undergoing interferon therapy and complaining of depression have been shown to suffer from altered cerebral blood circulation. Depression is also linked to poor sleep quality, a symptom reported by both groups of patients.

Others have pointed out that depression is quite a reasonable response to the symptoms of M.E. and hepatitis C, particularly the restrictions these conditions exert on the lives of patients.

Physical Symptoms, Observations, and HCV

As well as the major symptoms of fatigue and general debilitation, there are a number of more obscure diagnoses and observations that suggest physiological links between the two conditions in some patients. The following are a selection of these.

According to figures from the U.S., 80% of patients with chronic fatigue immune deficiency syndrome have elevated levels of serum angiotensin-converting enzyme, known as SACE. High SACE scores are associated with sarcoidosis, a disorder that is often found in lymphoma patients; lymphoma is sometimes linked to hep C (see above).

Both groups report autonomic overactivity as a common symptom. This means that some biological processes become overactive, typically manifesting as overfrequent urination or palpitations. In the case of HCV frequent urination may also be caused by autoimmune kidney disease.

Until recently no one had linked cardiac disorders directly to HCV; however, research at the university of Kyoto in Japan has now found a correlation with hypertropic cardiomyopathy. M.E.

researchers have discovered abnormal heart rhythms and hypotension in some of their patients, making it even more likely that there is a link between these two conditions in many cases.

Both groups of patients report that the severity of symptoms fluctuates and suspect that stress is a major precipitating factor in the onset of an "attack." The role of stress is discussed in chapter 24.

There are many other areas of mutual interest; M.E. patients and literature can provide a useful source of information, particularly on the practicalities of living with illness.

Impact on the Quality of Life

It has been consistently reported that HCV causes debilitation out of all proportion to currently detectable signs of clinical liver disease. There have been a number of surveys into the impact of HCV on the quality of life of patients. These have demonstrated that hepatitis C causes significant deterioration in a number of key areas including physical well-being, levels of pain, general health, vitality, social functioning, ability to work, and emotional and mental well-being. Hepatitis C has been shown to have a more severe impact than type II diabetes and chronic hepatitis B.

Research carried out recently at St. Mary's School of Medicine in London confirms these findings and concludes that the significant reduction in patients' quality of life is caused by the virus and definitely not by surrogate lifestyle factors such as drug use. Importantly the report also stresses that debilitation is significant even in the absence of cirrhosis.[20]

Research conducted by Veterans Affairs Medical Center, Pittsburgh, concluded that "patients are uniquely vulnerable to depression and psychological stress."

The report found abnormally high levels of emotional stress, tension and anxiety, confusion and bewilderment, depression, sleep disturbance, fatigue, and sleep disturbance regardless of background factors such as income, religion, and other objective parameters. Another recent study of HCV patients with advanced liver disease concluded:

Total mood disturbance (p = 0.038), tension and anxiety (0.047), confusion and bewilderment (p = 0.035) and depression and dejection (p = 0.035), as assessed by Profile of Mood States Scale were significantly higher in patients with HCV than other patients. Patients with HCV were significantly more depressed as assessed by Beck Inventory scores (p = 0.014).[21]

Overall Impact on Life Expectancy

While some speculative figures on the likelihood of death from liver disease are included above, the overall impact of HCV on patients' longevity is still a matter of guesswork. It seems likely that some of the less immediately life-threatening secondary conditions will lead to deterioration in the overall level of health. Left untreated these are quite likely to contribute to a diminished life expectancy as well.

Conclusion

HCV is a relentless and baffling pathogen that frequently defies classification. On the whole it currently seems to be more likely to be debilitating then fatal. However, we are definitely suffering from a serious, unpredictable, and poorly understood illness whose consequences can no longer be minimized. The fact that the symptoms vary from one patient to the next, that they can take decades to emerge, and the increasing evidence of a sinister but unpredictable pattern of related illness and debilitation means that it is difficult to face the future without a feeling of apprehension. The good news is that HCV is responsive to treatment and informed lifestyle adjustments, which are detailed in the later parts of the book.

Patients' Experiences of HCV Symptoms

Thanks to Mandy Cheetham, former research officer of the Hemophilia Society, for researching and collating some of these stories.

Mrs. J. has been infected with HCV for at least ten years. She has cirrhosis, varices, arthritis, lupus, and diabetes. She has had to give up work. She feels that her relationship with her husband and children has suffered badly. Some days she has to stay in bed. If it wasn't for her family she thinks she might commit suicide.

Peter is thirty-four. "I had my diagnosis in October 1995. For two years previously I had been feeling very unwell—upset stomachs, extreme tiredness, I was losing a lot of weight, and I had an almost continuous headache. I decided to get it checked out. They tested me for everything and came up with nothing. A short while later I bumped into a friend who was looking very worried. He told me that he had been diagnosed with hepatitis C and his symptoms were very similar to mine. By this time I was wondering whether I was being hypochondriac. Anyway I got it checked out, and the test revealed that I had it.

"I think that I've had a jaundiced outlook on life—very pessimistic, very down, a great deal of mental fatigue. This means that I can be doing something and that halfway through the task I loose concentration. Combined with physical tiredness this is extremely debilitating. My head seems to be stuffed with cotton wool; none of my cognitive functions work properly. My intellectual wherewithal seems to take a huge nosedive; I become a dullard for a little while and then it wears off. The mental aspect is pretty horrendous; I often feel extremely confused, as though I am loosing the plot. My sleep patterns have been very disrupted with lots of nightmares accompanied by night sweats which don't help. I have had all of these symptoms to a greater or lesser degree over the past ten years."

Mrs. F.'s HCV diagnosis has had a devastating effect on her family and her employment. Over six years her health became progressively worse due to HCV. She didn't know from day to day how she was going to feel. Her doctor advised her to cut down on the number of hours worked, but her employers refused to have her back on that basis. Mrs. F. feels that this was due to her diagnosis of hepatitis C.

G. is an ex-IVDU in his mid-thirties who reckons he has had hepatitis C for about fifteen years. He stopped drinking and taking drugs three years previously, largely because he had begun to feel extremely ill after each binge, particularly where drinking was concerned. He went for a test after some friends mentioned hep C to him and he realized that he had been at risk. Although his liver enzymes were mildly elevated, his tiredness started to lift very quickly after he started to take herbs and food supplements and managed to give up smoking as well. He is currently able to pursue a new career on the stage.

"I just don't leave the house from Friday night to Monday morning. I've never been lazy, but I just can't do the things I used to. I rarely go out socially any more either. I'll often fall asleep after work. Doctors and nurses tell me I'm pushing myself too hard, but I know it's my health."—Mr. I.

"My general health has rapidly deteriorated over the past four years. I suffer from chronic fatigue and am unable to finish a full day's work. Joint aches, pains, decreased appetite and weight loss, itching, the need for nine hours sleep a night. I feel that in the last four years my physical stamina has aged by about fifteen years. I've grown old before my time. Due to all the above my general confidence has been reduced."—Mr. A.

"I have extremely debilitating abdominal pain constantly. I feel sick after every meal. I am tired from a few hours after waking, and I suffer crushing bouts of depression. The thought of taking my own life is a daily event."—Mr. C.

One recently diagnosed sufferer, Tony, a Londoner in his mid-thirties, stated: "I thought I was just getting old. When I was working I would get sudden attacks of total exhaustion and I'd just have to go home. I felt like a car that had run out of petrol."

"I've been living with hep C for years, although I only began to understand what was going on very recently, after attending meetings of a support group. Having given up alcohol and drugs years ago, I couldn't understand why I was feeling like death for long periods of time, when all my peers seemed to be experiencing ever better states of physical and mental health. I was diagnosed as being clinically depressed and as having M.E., before I got the hep C diagnosis.

"What I think now is that these bouts of depression and exhaustion were caused by my immune system going into overdrive, in a vain attempt to purge the virus. They would come on seemingly unpredictably and last for between two weeks and three months. Typically I would try to make up for lost time when I wasn't feeling ill. This often led to me taking on too much, becoming stressed and overstretched; I believe that this "overbusy" behavior had a lot to do with my relapses, that my immune system went out of balance as a result of these bouts of overactivity. Now I try to smooth out my life and not take things too seriously."—David

"In 1987 I went to see my GP as I was generally tired and unwell, especially in the mornings when I woke up feeling really horrible. Routine blood tests were performed and I was told that everything was fine. But I did not feel fine.

"After a couple of months I began to get visible symptoms—severe rashes on my arms and legs and joint pains in my arms and legs. During the next two years I was supplied with numerous diagnoses: rheumatoid arthritis, lupus, mixed connective tissue disorder (and a few others with complicated names I can't remember.)

"In 1991 I received a final diagnosis—cryoglobulinemia—I was also told that I had hepatitis C. No one explained the connection between the two illnesses; I just thought I was unlucky to have managed to get two diseases at once.

"I became more and more ill; I now had kidney disease associated with the cryo which (I now realized) was in turn, related to hep C. Finally I was admitted to hospital with severe fluid retention and hypertension. My hemoglobin levels were also dangerously low. My hospital notes said that I was suffering from membrano-proliferative glomerulonephritis and nephritic syndrome.

"I received a plasma exchange and was treated with drugs and corticosteroids. The steroids seemed to help, but I was later disturbed to discover that they might have been inadvisable for hep C.

"At present my cryo symptoms are well under control; however, my liver symptoms are worsening and my biopsy results were not good. My hepatologist thinks that I should be receiving interferon/ribavirin treatment. My nephrologist disagrees. Meanwhile I take Chinese herbs, swim regularly, and feel reasonably well."—Kathy

A List of Conditions Linked to Hepatitis C

Clinically linked

- Arthritis, polyarthritis and rheumatoid
- Autoimmune hepatitis
- Blood circulation disorders
- Chronic hepatitis/liver disease
- Chronic fatigue syndrome
- Cirrhosis
- Cognitive dysfunction
- Cryoglobulinemia, mixed cryoglobulinemia
- Depression
- Diabetes (mellitus type II), blood sugar disorders
- Glomerulonephritis
- Hypertropic cardiomyopathy
- Indigestion
- Ischaemia (cerebral and renal)
- Kidney disease
- Lichen planus
- Liver cancer
- Lymphoma (non-Hodgkin's B-cell and Burkitts)
- Porphyria cutanea tarda
- Raynaud's disease
- Sjogren's syndrome
- Spider naevi
- Thrombosis
- Thyroid disease—autoimmune hyper- and hypothyroidism
- Vasculitis

Suspected or possible

- Alcohol intolerance
- Aplastic anemia
- Autonomic overactivity
- Crohn's disease, irritable bowel syndrome
- Emotional lability
- Post viral fatigue syndrome and M.E.
- Psoriasis, systemic lupus erythematosus

In addition a range of conditions generally linked to advanced liver disease may be diagnosed in seriously ill patients. Doctors should note that the milder conditions, such as those involving joint pains and skin complaints, often present as subclinical symptoms.

References

1. Therapy for chronic hepatitis C. Davis GL et al. *Viral Hepatitis,* 23(3), Sept 1994.

2. Mortality and morbidity of transfusion-associated type C hepatitis: an NHLBI multi-center study. Seef LB et al. *Hepatology,* 20, A204, 1994.

3. Natural history of viral hepatitis type C. Seef LB. *Semin Gastrointestinal Dis,* 6, 20–27, 1995.

4. Long term mortality after transfusion related NANB hepatitis. Seef LB et al. *New England Journal,* 327, 1906–11, 1992.

5. Viral liver cirrhosis: natural course, pathogenesis and clinical implications of the complications. Gentilini P, Laffi G, La Villa G, Casini-Raggi V, Romanelli RG, Buzzelli G, Mazzanti R, Marra F, Pinzani M, Zignego AL. *Ann Ital Med Int,* 11 (Suppl 2):23S–29S, Oct 1996.

6. Hepatitis C virus genotypes and risk of hepatocellular carcinoma in cirrhosis: a prospective study. Bruno S, Silini E, Crosignani A, Borzio F, Leandro G, Bono F, Asti M, Rossi S, Larghi A, Cerino A, Podda M, Mondelli MU. *Hepatology* 25:754–758, 1997.

7. HCV-associated hepatocellular carcinoma without cirrhosis. el-Refaie et al. *Journal of Hepatology,* 24(3):277–85, March 1996.

8. Immunological disorders in C virus chronic active hepatitis. Pawlotsky et al. *Hepatology,* 19:841–8, 1994.

9. Hepatitis C virus infection in mixed cryoglobulinemia and B-cell non-Hodgkin's lymphoma: evidence for a pathogenetic role. Zignego AL, Ferri

C, Giannini C, La Civita L, Careccia G, Longombardo G, Bellesi G, Caracciolo F, Thiers V, Gentilini P. *Arch Virol,* 142(3):545–555, 1997.

10. Prevalence of hepatitis C in patients with idiopathic glomerulopathies in native and transplant kidneys. Cosio FG, Roche Z, Agarwal A, Falkenhain ME, Sedmak DD, Ferguson RM. *Am J Kidney Dis,* 28(5):752–5758, Nov 1996.

11. Letter from Department of Medical Virology and Epidemiology of Viral Diseases, University of Tubingen. Jahn G et al. *The Lancet,* 351, Jan 24, 1998.

12. Detection of anticardiolipin antibodies and b-2-GPI in cryoprecipitate of patients with chronic hepatitis C and cryoglobulinemia. Rodriguez-Rosado R et al. *J Hepatology,* 23 (Suppl):95, 1995.

13. High prevalence of hepatitis C virus infection in diabetic patients. Simo R, Hernandez C, Genesca J, Jardi R, Mesa J. *Diabetes Care,* 19(9):998–51000, Sept 1996.

14. Cryoglobulinemia with vasculitis ass. with HCV. Marcellin P et al. *Gastroenterology,* 104, 272–77, 1993.

15. Dr. Robert Batey (Gastroenterologist, Hunter Hospital, NSW, Australia), speaking at the first International Conference on Hepatitis C. Regents Park College, 1994.

16. Increased frequency of HLA DR.13 in hepatitis C virus carriers with persistently normal ALT levels. Kuzushita N et al. *J Med Virol,* 48(1):1–7, Jan 1996.

17. HLA class II genes in chronic hepatitis C virus—infection and associated immunological disorders. Congia M et al. Presented at the American Association for the Study of Liver Diseases, 1996.

18. HLA-DR.5 antigen. A genetic factor influencing the outcome of hepatitis C virus infection? Peano G, Menardi G, Ponzetto A, Fenoglio LM. *Arch Intern Med,* 154(23):2733–52736, Dec 12, 1994.

19. Detection of hepatitis C virus genomic sequences in the cerebrospinal fluid of HIV-infected patients. Morsica G, Bernardi MT, Novati R, Uberti Foppa C, Castagna A, Lazzarin A. *Journal of Medical Virology,* 53(3):252–54, Nov 1997.

20. Chronic hepatitis C infection causes a significant reduction in quality of life in the absence of cirrhosis. Foster G et al. *Hepatology,* 27 (1):209–5212, 1998.

21. Vulnerability to psychologic distress and depression in patients with end-stage liver disease due to hepatitis C virus. Singh N, Gayowski T, Wagener MM, Marino IR. *Clinical Transplantation,* (5 Pt 1):406–11, Oct 11, 1997.

2

The Epidemiology of Hepatitis C

The information in this chapter is intended to provide a framework for the understanding of HCV transmission. The intention is to develop understanding of HCV and reduce rates of transmission. The information provided here is not intended for use in the attachment of blame or guilt.

The Discovery of Hepatitis C

JAPANESE DOCTORS WERE probably the first to appreciate the nature and novelty of the threat to public health posed by hepatitis C. In the 1970s they realized that there must be some hitherto unknown pathogen at work while trying to establish the cause of abnormally high rates of chronic liver disease apparent in certain parts of that country. They were particularly concerned by the high incidence of cirrhosis and liver cancer normally only associated with heavy, long-term alcohol abuse or exposure to hepatitis B.

At this time there were two known viruses associated with hepatitis, which literally means inflammation of the liver: hepatitis A, which causes acute but relatively short-lived illness, and hepatitis B, which has similar but more severe jaundicelike symptoms but disappears in all but about 7% of those infected in adulthood. It was felt that neither of these could explain the picture of long-term disease that was becoming apparent. Doctors in Europe and North America soon began to notice the sporadic appearance of patients with a similar clinical profile. In particular, hemophiliacs began to present with symptoms of liver disease that could not be attributed to hepatitis A or B. Specialists in tropical medicine also began to realize that they were looking at a new condition.

The new condition was simply called "Non-A Non-B" (NANB) hepatitis, but its presence was clearly linked to long-term liver disease. For many years patients with the various symptoms of hepatitis who couldn't be diagnosed as having A or B were simply diagnosed as having NANB type. Most doctors felt that the NANB condition was not serious, and the development of this attitude underlies many of the current problems patients have when dealing with nonspecialist practitioners. This view persists.

It was not until 1989 that the suspicions of the Japanese and Western specialists were confirmed. The hepatitis C virus was explicitly identified and genetically mapped by the Chiron Corporation in the U.S. using recombinant molecular technology, a new methodology dependent on the latest advances in immunology, cloning, genetic engineering, and microbiology. For those who are interested, this is an outline of the process Chiron Corporation undertook.

The characteristics of HCV RNA were identified by first extracting infected blood from a chimpanzee that had been injected with infected human blood. Chimps are the only other animals that had been found to be susceptible to this NANB form of hepatitis.

This plasma sample was then centrifuged to form a recoverable chunk of the infectious material. Nucleic acid, the genetic material of HCV, was extracted from it and then cloned. The resulting genetic profile sample was then compared to samples of blood from patients presumed to be infected. After one million tests one of these sequences was found to react with antibodies in the infected serum. The original clone was then amplified.

It was only at this stage that the scientists were in a position to identify hepatitis C. The resulting clone was then used to express this antigen and form the basis for an antibody test (see chapter 3). This test for the presence of HCV antibodies, known as ELISA I (indicating exposure to the virus), was quickly marketed, and the extent of the problem began to become apparent.

The Worldwide Distribution
and Prevalence of Hepatitis C

Using the new test, blood transfusion services and government agencies across the globe began to screen their populations for HCV antibodies. The results clearly demonstrated the result of five decades of global intermixing of blood; hepatitis C was present in every population that was tested, although there were great variations in the rate from one population to another. However, a good overview was provided by the findings of a Roche Biocare report into HCV prevalence in 1994. According to this report, which is based on the results of surveys by public health bodies of their blood donor populations, the figures are cited in the table on page 48.

One problem with these figures is that they are based upon surveys of blood donors who have been prescreened for known virus exposure risk factors, and therefore exclude many likely carriers. This section of the population consistently demonstrates lower prevalence rates than the population as a whole. Other sources have produced more alarming figures. Here are some other reports that reflect the extent and seriousness of the problem.

"Worldwide 500 million people suffer from hep C.... In Europe as a whole it is estimated that 16 million people have the virus. In the U.K. there are no prevalence data; the size of the problem is simply not known," according to the British Liver Trust supplement "C Positive" (Spring 1995).

In the U.S. prevalence is very likely to be significantly higher than in the blood donor figure provided above. The Center for Disease Control (CDC) currently cites the figure of 5.5 million as a good median estimate. Prevalence range is frequently cited as being between 0.7 and 2.5%; in general the broader, and therefore more representative the sample base, the more likely a higher figure is to be found. Figures of 7 million and above have also been suggested.

One survey suggested a much higher prevalence; the September 1993 edition of the *American Journal of Obstetrics and Gynecology* featured a report that found that 4.3% of 599 pregnant women had antibodies to HCV. The survey was conducted in an inner city,

Worldwide Prevalence of HCV Antibodies in Blood Donors

United States	0.6–1.5%
Canada	0.3–1.2%
Western Europe	
France	0.7%
Germany	0.13–0.83%
Greece	0.56%
Italy (north)	1.3%
Italy (south)	2.9%
The Netherlands	0.7%
Spain	1.2–2.2%
United Kingdom	0.5–1.0%
Eastern Europe	
Hungary	1.6%
Poland	2% (4.5% south)
Latin America	
Argentina	1.5%
Brazil	1.4–3.1%
Cuba	1.6%
Africa	6%
Cameroon	14.5%
Far East	
Hong Kong	0.5%
Japan	1.5%
Korea	1.3%
Singapore	1.7%
Taiwan	0.95%

and it was inferred that the infection rate would be lower in suburban and rural populations.

The ongoing rate of infection is suggested by the following: A report by the Baltimore College of Dental Surgery in the June 1993 edition of the U.S. dental magazine *Oral Surgery and Medical Oral Pathology* stated, "Hepatitis C accounts for 20% to 40% of all viral hepatitis, with between 150,000 and 170,000 new cases reported in the United States each year."

In general the overall prevalence rates in the U.S. and Canada are of the same order as in northwestern Europe, being significantly less than in middle prevalence regions such as Eastern Europe and well below the colossal figures cited in some developing countries. However, there are three factors that mean that prevalence in certain parts of the U.S. population will be higher:

- The relatively heavy involvement in military conflicts, particularly in East Asia

- The presence of relatively high numbers of immigrants from regions with high background prevalence

- The earlier occurrence of significant levels of IV drug use in certain sections of the U.S. population

Further details and explanation is provided in the "Transmission" section below.

Although there has been no systematic prevalence analysis of the U.K., there have been a number of smaller-scale ad hoc investigations that provide the basis for accurate estimates. Leading hepatologists often put the figure at around 600,000.

However, Graham Alexander, consultant hepatologist at Addenbrooke's hospital in Cambridge, who has performed the only truly random survey—based upon sampling of organ donors in East Anglia—has found that prevalence is very close to 2%. This would equate to 1.2 million HCV+ people in the U.K. The results of this work were published in *The Journal of Hepatology,* 1994, Volume 20, p. 768, and were consistent with a simultaneous U.S. study. The numbers of patients now presenting at liver clinics are apparently statistically consistent with this estimate. The U.K. government has shown a marked reluctance to perform a more widely based prevalence study; further research proposals for prevalence studies have so far been rejected. In the U.S. a prevalence of 1.7% would equate to over six million people exposed to hepatitis C.

Dr. J. M. Guffens, a French specialist in liver disease working for the EC commission, reported the following findings of a report on HCV prevalence in France and Europe as a whole. Speaking at the first International Conference on Hepatitis C held at Regents Park College, London, in 1995, he stated:

> In Europe seroprevalence of HCV has been evaluated from blood donors with a North to South gradient. In Norway seroprevalence of HCV is 0.3%. Around the Mediterranean sea seroprevalence is between 1 and 2.5%. In Spain it is 1.2%.

In France seroprevalence of HCV among blood donors was 0.7% in 1991 and 0.28% in 1994 (D. Sicard, oral comment). Other epidemiological data is available. According to a study on more than 6000 pregnant women and more than 3000 outpatients of both sexes, the Reseau National de Sante Publique has estimated the number of patients with HCV infection to be around 500,000. A more recent French survey based on over 45,000 people chosen at random found that 1.18% had antibodies to HCV, indicating an overall infected population of 660,000 in France.

The reduction in the seroprevalence of HCV in blood donors between 1991 and 1994 demonstrates that this population is likely to be a very conservative sample. This is because of the introduction of rigorous screening between these dates.

In some parts of Japan hepatitis C is far more common than the 1.5% reported by the Red Cross survey of blood donors. The July 1993 edition of the medical publication *Kansenshogaku-Zasshi* carried an article entitled "Seroepidemiological study on hepatitis C virus infection in an endemic area of hepatitis C virus." It reads as follows:

> To clarify the prevalence of hepatitis C virus infection in a rural area with high incidence of chronic liver disease in Japan, sera from 412 inhabitants, aged 20–89 years, collected in 1989–1990

and sera from 483 inhabitants in the same area, collected in 1982 were tested for anti-HCV.... Anti-HCV was positive in 175 out of 412 sera collected in 1989–1990 (42.5%); prevalence was higher in male (54.0%) than in female (34.9%).

The results of a survey into the prevalence of hepatitis C among volunteer blood donors at a Cairo hospital were published in the October 1993 edition of the *American Journal of Tropical Medicine;* 22% were found to have HCV antibodies. This was particularly alarming since volunteer blood donors are classified as a "low risk" group because they are screened.

The *Review of the Institute of Tropical Medicine* in Sao-Paulo [35(1):45–51, Jan-Feb 1993] published the results of a survey into 29,833 blood donors in the Campinas region that revealed a prevalence of 2.6%.

A report by a French medical team working in the Ukraine found an anti-HCV seropositivity of 12.06% among blood donors in the city of Lviv and suggested that HCV might be a major influence on levels of morbidity there.

According to John Tindall, a practitioner of Traditional Chinese Medicine who visits China regularly, experts there estimate that 10% of China's 1 billion population have hepatitis of one sort or another at any one time, and that at least 40% of these are chronically infected with HCV.

There are thousands of fragments of information such as this that provide overwhelming evidence of widespread global infection, with average rates of 1 to 3% in developed countries and 2 to 6% in most of the developing world. Allowing for various factors, the overall number of people infected worldwide is at least 240 million.

In most countries the number of people diagnosed is a small fraction of those reckoned to have been exposed. For instance in the U.K. only about 10,000 people had been notified as having antibodies to HCV by 1997, yet the actual number carrying the virus is of the order of 1 million people. Australia has a diagnosis rate of over 50%, with 110,000 of an estimated 200,000 carriers notified so far. This reflects the early action taken by the government there.

As a public health problem it dwarfs HIV. The good news for

patients is that they are certainly not alone and that part of the "success" of this virus is due to the fact that it is much less likely to prove fatal.

Transmission

Almost everyone in the modern world will have experienced multiple possible opportunities for exposure to HCV. As the possible routes of infection are so widespread and involve commonplace procedures such as the receipt of vaccinations, dental treatment, and blood products, only individuals who have no history whatsoever of these could be described as being entirely risk free. Having said this, it is also now very clear that historical exposure to some routes carries a much higher probability of infection than others.

HCV is a blood-borne virus. This means that it is transmitted via blood-to-blood contact. It is known to be able to survive in dried blood for longer periods than many other such viruses like HIV—a figure of up to three months has been mentioned. (HIV can survive for considerable periods in bottled plasma.) In reality the survival period is undetermined, and no safe limit can yet be defined. HCV is uncommonly small and often inhabits blood cells—the virus can survive as long as these cells remain intact.

Because it has been effectively invisible until 1991, no one was able to monitor its global proliferation. However, patient populations reflect transmission routes. These groups have been broken down into the following categories.

Note that the exact process of international proliferation is unknown. The process presented here is based on the author's inference along with additional information provided by Dr. Peter Simmonds of Edinburgh University, the world's leading expert on HCV genotypes.

1. Patients Infected via Blood Transfusions, Operations, and Infected Blood Products

In most Western countries this group represents at least 15% of the HCV+ population. In the U.S. it may account for 25% because of factors described below. This group often contains many older patients who seem to have been infected as long ago as the late 1940s onwards until blood screening and other antiviral countermeasures in the early 1990s. In Europe and the U.S. that represents the "first wave" of the hepatitis C epidemic. Infected blood transfusions are believed to be a major cause of the HCV epidemic in Japan and is certainly the cause of infection in many of the older patients in Europe, North America, and Australasia.

The origin of these blood supplies is a sensitive issue, and at least one researcher has been threatened with litigation for speculating about the reasons for blood bank and blood product contamination. The fact that the genotypes of the hepatitis strain infecting some of these patients allegedly do not tally with the stated country of origin of the blood supplies means that there may be grounds for patients to feel disquiet about the blood supply industry.

Nearly all hemophiliacs born prior to 1986 have hepatitis C because of the presence of the virus in blood supplies and products. Measures taken to remove HIV from the blood supply in the mid-1980s seem to have also been quite successful at eliminating HCV, although donor screening for HCV did not begin until after 1990. CDC estimates that 300,000 U.S. citizens were exposed to HCV via contaminated blood products. Congressional hearings are currently underway to establish whether or not the situation was well managed by the authorities in charge of the blood supply.

Perhaps the most notorious case of infection through blood products is that of 1,000 Irish women infected with HCV via contaminated anti-D immunoglobulin in the 1970s. Anti-D is routinely given to rhesus-negative mothers after giving birth to a rhesus-positive child to prevent a future blood compatibility disorder (blue babies). The infected anti-D was made by the Irish state blood bank. As a result of sustained pressure from the group Positive Action, the Irish government has now agreed to compensate the women.

The Hepatitis C Society of Canada has finally managed to obtain a similar settlement despite bitter resistance on the part of the government, which was nearly toppled over the issue.

Studies in France demonstrate that among transfused patients and hemophiliacs type 1b is most common, whereas intravenous drug users (IVDUs) rarely have this strain. This type is also common in

Japan, particularly in patients with significant progression. Studies of U.K. hemophiliacs show a prevalence of type 1 and also a significant amount of type 2 and 3. Type 2 is also common in the Far East.

Thus the first wave of HCV proliferation appears to have involved extensive global intermixing of blood supplies, particularly between Europe, the Far East, and North America. The precise time and geographical origin of HCV cannot be defined. However, Peter Simmonds's analysis of the mutation process indicates that the genotypes recognized today are all derived from a single original strain:

> The radiation of the major genotypes can be predicted to have occurred 100 to 120 years ago. This reasoning would suggest that HCV is a relatively recent infection of humans, with relatively short evolutionary history compared to other human viruses.[1]

Although HCV has been classified into types, the reality is that there are hundreds of different genetic identities, and that these types represent "stills" from a constant evolutionary process. Many doctors describe hepatitis C as consisting of a family of viruses.

Having said this, it does seem likely that if there is a single point of origin, it is somewhere in the Far East. This is because the genetic diversity and numbers of people infected in that part of the world are greater than elsewhere, indicating a longer history. Some strains, such as that found in Thailand quite recently, indicate that the virus has been mutating for a long period of time in that part of the world. Although parts of Africa also demonstrate very high rates of infection, the genetic diversity appears to be lower than in the East, indicating a relatively recent "arrival" date. However, less research has been carried out into the African genotypes, and it would be wrong to make this a firm conclusion. It is not yet clear whether the rate of genetic diversification is sufficient to explain the presence of these differing types in terms of evolution from a single point of origin in the human population.

The penetration of HCV into so much of the population in Japan so long ago—a lot of patients are now elderly—implies a contamination of the blood supply as long ago as the 1940s, probably during the Second World War or in its immediate aftermath. Many researchers have speculated that traditional medicinal practices also played a role in the proliferation of the virus in Japan, being particularly implicated in the concentrated pockets seen there. Because surrounding countries don't have such advanced health services, it is difficult to make exact comparisons with those populations. Since the use of Western medicine involving blood transfusions was relatively rare in Japan prior to World War II, it does seem likely that the postwar penetration of Western medicine accompanied by the colossal scale of injury may have played a significant role in releasing HCV into the wider population in Japan.

The Role of Conflict in East Asia

The extensive intermixing of Far Eastern with European and North American blood supplies may have occurred during the period covering the Second World War and the Korean and Vietnamese conflicts. There is correlation between the genotype of older Japanese patients and that found in older U.S. hemophiliacs, indicating a strong link between the pattern of infection observed in these two countries. European figures indicate that infection may have begun as long ago as the 1940s, but most researchers suspect that the 1950s and 1960s are more likely.

The presence of hundreds of thousands of American military personnel in the Far East under conflict conditions will certainly have influenced overall prevalence in the U.S. Anyone who has been in a military field hospital or even seen an episode of *MASH* will be aware that it is extremely unlikely that opportunities for cross-infection could be effectively curtailed under such circumstances. There are also plenty of anecdotal stories of "shared needle" inoculations and vaccinations taking place in the military (both of the U.S. and other allied countries) from the early 1940s onwards.

Rates among U.S. veterans as a whole are still unknown because there has as yet been no overall follow-up antibody testing program. Thus many who are ill but have so far not been diagnosed will have been missed. However, the number of veterans who have presented with advanced liver disease has been investigated. According to one report:

In 1991, 6,612 individual patients were reported as positive for HCV antibody in the Department of Veterans Affairs system. This increased yearly from 1992 to 1994 with 8,365, 14,097, and finally 18,854 persons, respectively. This represents an increase of more than 285% during the four-year period.... Overall, total patients seen nationally in the Veterans Health Administration increased by only 4.87% during the same period, 1991 to 1994. Thus, the increase in persons positive for HCV antibody is not based on workload alone. The impact of HCV disease on patient well-being and health care costs cannot be overestimated.[2]

There has also been speculation that increased rates of lymphoma found in veterans may have been related to exposure to agents of chemical warfare. Investigations have failed to establish a causal link. It is more likely that these increased rates are linked to hepatitis C, which is known to be associated with certain types of lymphoma.

Many will have received blood transfusions derived from local supplies, gone home, and subsequently become blood donors. The blood industry was beginning to become internationalized at about this time, and this would have contributed to cross-contamination. Because HCV is so infectious, only tiny samples of blood would have been capable of contaminating large parts of the blood supply. This sinister and invisible process began to manifest in increasing numbers of patients turning up in hepatology units with NANB hepatitis in the 1970s and '80s. Japanese medical authorities noticed unexplained increases in rates of cirrhosis and liver cancer quite early and were convinced that some unknown pathogen was at work. Western doctors noticed that many hemophiliacs were coming down with NANB, but were unable to locate the exact cause within the supply of blood and related products.

Some Western governments are now instigating "look back" programs, inviting anyone who underwent transfusions or received blood products prior to the introduction of blood screening (see below) to be tested. Thus a high proportion of patients infected in this way will become aware of their HCV status.

2. Current or Ex-Intravenous Drug Users (IVDUs)

In most Western countries this group usually represents a significant proportion of the more recently infected HCV+ population. HCV seems to lend itself to this mode of transmission, and it is thought that a significant proportion—CDC estimates 38% in the U.S.—of the "second wave" of HCV infection in developed countries has been via IV drug use (genotypes 1a and 3 are prevalent in Western countries). The relatively great presence of the former type in the U.S. indicates the importance of this historical link to the Far East. Type 3 is prevalent in India and may have been originally contracted by Westerners on the so-called "hippie trail."

Overall infection rates of IVDUs are very high. Representatives attending the NADA conference in Chicago in 1997 reported rates of 80% plus in their clients with a history of IV drug use. U.K. figures for 1995 record an average infection rate of at least 60%; they rose to 71% in London and 77% in Scotland.[3] These figures conceal the fact that there tend to be "pockets" of infection where the incidence is even higher, running at up to 95%. It is also thought that many IVDUs contract the virus within the first year of injecting, so many people who merely flirted with injecting drug use will have been exposed to the virus. A recent report from Seattle suggests that HCV infection runs at a rate of about 30% from once-only experimentation with IV drug use.

The IVDU population is thought to have been harboring HCV since the early 1950s, which means that a number of ex-users who have had nothing to do with narcotics for many years are now being diagnosed as having hepatitis C. Many more will have HCV but will be unaware of it. Because HCV is so resilient, it appears to be able to survive the equipment-cleaning techniques recommended to prevent the spread of HIV, which may well have started far too late to arrest mass proliferation within this community. It is also thought to have been spread via the sharing of spoons, filters, and other paraphernalia as well as hypodermic needles and syringes. According to Neal Flynn, MD, MPH, speaking at the second HCV Global Conference, there are as many as 100,000 HCV virions in a droplet of infected blood, compared to only 5 virions of HIV in an equivalent infected droplet. Many IVDUs who have successfully avoided HIV have HCV.

There is some evidence that the rate of IVDU transmission may be declining in the U.S. A recent study in Maryland concluded that infection rates have declined since 1990.[4] This may reflect greater awareness of the risks within the study population and suggests the potential benefits of educational programs in reducing transmission.

On the whole this group is younger than those infected by transfusion, and the disease is therefore likely to be less advanced. Because HCV often seems to progress slowly but steadily, a lot of people in this category will go on to experience liver disease in later life. Those who contracted HCV through occasional or "one off" IV drug use are likely to be among the patients with a better prognosis and a lower viral load. Long-term IVDUs are more likely to have multiple-strain infection, which may mean that they are more difficult to treat. They are also likely to be in a generally weaker state due to their unhealthy lifestyle, which contributes to disease progression, accelerated liver disease, and the appearance of secondary symptoms. (Some of the patient groups in the section on autoimmune diseases contain high numbers of drug users—this may influence the reported incidence of these diseases.) Those who are also alcoholic are more likely to be seriously ill. Ex-long-term IVDUs with hepatitis C often require expert nutritional advice and health care in order to help them recover their health, and many do so. HCV seems to be a contributory factor to the high mortality rate among current IVDUs, although the exact effect is difficult to ascertain, partly because it is often impossible to follow up patients.

This group has been described as the "Woodstock Generation." This is a dangerous and misleading journalistic cliché, implying as it does that HCV primarily affects a group of hippies who shot drugs in the 1960s and '70s; it tends to externalize and pigeonhole hepatitis C as a disease that only affects a particular stereotyped minority—the facts demonstrate that no social group is untouched by HCV. It is also becoming apparent that IV use has been far more prevalent in drug users during the 1980s and '90s. The hippies of the 1960s and '70s seem to have been more attracted to psychedelic drugs and pot and were often antagonistic to injecting and "hard" drugs in general.

In the U.S. the African-American population has been hit particularly hard by HCV, with figures from CDC suggesting both a higher prevalence and a longer average duration of infection. This is probably linked to the targeting of inner-city ghettos by heroin wholesalers in the 1940s and '50s. IV drug use is known to have been popular among many of the personalities of the "jazz age" long before it spread to the wider population. HCV may well have contributed to the early deaths of many of the addicted musicians of this era.

In both the U.K. and the U.S. there is some anecdotal evidence to suggest that the crack cocaine epidemic has generated a wave of IV heroin use among exsmokers trying to get over withdrawal. Sadly this is underresearched.

It seems that somewhere along the line the overall number of people who have used drugs intravenously, be that occasionally or persistently, has been seriously underestimated. Roger Holmes, a researcher for the Institute for the Study of Drug Dependence in the U.K., has estimated that the HCV+ population infected in this way is at least 370,000. Since this number represents the 60% infected with HCV, the true figure is likely to be even higher, raising serious doubts about previous estimates of the prevalence of IV drug use. The Hepatitis C Virus Projections Working Group in Australia reports that 80% of patients there contracted HCV via IV drug use.

Unless radical alternative theories on HCV prevalence are true (see below), the IVDU-related epidemic is more rooted in contemporary housing projects and inner cities than the rock festivals of the hippie era. Since rates of infection are broadly similar across the developed world, it is likely that this analysis is equally true internationally. If journalists need clichés, perhaps they might talk about the "Nirvana Generation" or the "Reagan Generation." HCV transmission via IVDU is an ongoing process; it is extremely misleading to encourage the perception that hepatitis C only affects this seemingly remote social minority.

Other practices that may be specifically implicated in high developing world incidence of HCV include the practice of circumcision and tattooing in unsterile conditions, and the presence of "injection shops" in some countries. (Some people appear to have developed the idea that injections in themselves are medicinal.)

3. Tattooing/Ear Piercing/Electrolysis/Barbers

A significant proportion of the "sporadic" cases of HCV have been infected by cosmetic contact, particularly tattooing. They probably represent 3% of the overall numbers at most. Patients infected in this way baffled researchers in the past. A recent survey of barbers in Sicily showed a significant prevalence of HCV; the practice of reusing razor blades is implicated in this. The fact that people have been infected in this way demonstrates the infectivity of HCV and the fact that no section of society can afford to be complacent. Most countries have now introduced public health measures and education to counter these methods of transmission (see "Prevention of Transmission" below).

4. Acupuncture and Vaccination Programs

Although these are now entirely safe so far as HCV transmission is concerned, these outpatient medical practices have been strongly implicated as vectors in the spread of HCV in past years. In the Far East acupuncture or other forms of traditional medicine such as practices involving blood suction probably help to explain some of the local endemics of HCV. Although the cleaning of acupuncture needles has always been important, traditional measures may not have been sufficient to kill HCV. These practices probably helped to propagate HCV in local communities, once it had arrived there by other means. Since some acupuncture needles are made of gold or silver, they would certainly have been reused. In Western countries acupuncture will have played a small role, since standards of hygiene have been very high. Because acupuncture has become popular in the post-AIDS era, sterilization procedures have been extremely strict. Nowadays most acupuncture practitioners employ single-use needles, which means that this transmission route is no longer open.

In case the above information makes practitioners of Western medicine feel complacent, it is now known that a number of people have contracted HCV as a result of "shared needle" vaccination programs. This method of transmission is implicated in many countries;

because children were the primary recipients of these vaccinations, many have developed significant HCV progression over the years. Again it appears that there were cleaning procedures in place—typically a sterile swab or syringe boiling—but that these were inadequate to prevent transmission. This route explains up to 5% of HCV incidence in parts of Southern Europe and may be responsible for much higher rates in the "developing" world. In Egypt HCV infection correlates with a history of treatment by injection for bilharzia, and in Japan it is associated with attendance at particular health clinics. It is highly likely that this is the principal route of transmission in terms of worldwide incidence of HCV.

There are several reports of such shared-needle vaccinations taking place in schools both in the U.K. and the U.S. The possibilities for infection via other technologies, such as the "vaccine guns" have not yet been thoroughly investigated. It is likely that such procedures account for a few cases, particularly unrepresentative pockets of high HCV prevalence in otherwise low-incidence communities. However, because the children involved are likely to have had a very low background infection rate in Western countries, most recipients of shots administered in this way will be clear.

5. Sex

The evidence so far suggests that although HCV can be transmitted sexually, it is not easily passed on via this route. It is definitely not a major sexually transmitted disease. Studies of long-term heterosexual partners of hepatitis C patients demonstrate that rates are low in this group,[5,6] and many researchers suspect that transmission is more likely to have occurred via household contact. There is some evidence to suggest that those who are coinfected with HIV are more likely to be able to pass on HCV via sexual intercourse; [7] this may be related to higher viral loads in body fluids such as semen observed in coinfected patients.

However, there is evidence that heterosexual transmission does occur, particularly in certain groups. Studies of non-drug-using female prostitutes show HCV seroprevalence of between 9 and 12%.[8,9] Infection correlated with increased numbers of paid partners, traumatic sexual activities, failure to use a condom, syphilis, and years working as a prostitute. It does seem likely that any sex involving blood would pose a definite risk.

Studies of long-term male homosexual partners who have no declared history of IV drug use demonstrate an infection rate of 1.5%.[10] There are no conclusive figures for the risks attached to anal sex as opposed to vaginal sex. More recent data from small uncontrolled surveys suggests that some groups of homosexual men have rates of over 10%; sexual transmission in this group needs to be investigated further.

Again it is important to stress the overwhelmingly blood-borne nature of HCV and apply common sense. If blood-to-blood opportunity exists during sex, then the likelihood of transmission will be much higher than if it does not. In other words "traumatic sex" is a risk factor, while what one doctor referred to as "gentle marital sex" is not.

If sexual transmission was a common route, then many millions more people would have become infected. Given the fact that this virus has been present since the 1940s, a routinely viable sexual route of transmission would have yielded population infection rates of at least 50% or higher in the general population by now. Overall a small percentage of patients are likely to have contracted HCV via a sexual route. News reports warning of "numbers of sexual partners" being a risk factor are misleading.

6. Household Contact/Shared Razors or Toothbrushes

Household contact may account for more cases of intrafamilial transmission than the sexual route. Because the virus is so difficult to kill and can be harbored in invisible quantities of blood and may lurk in other fluids, albeit at low levels, there are a number of opportunities for it to jump to a new host within the home. The combination of bleeding gums and toothbrush sharing may favor transmission, particularly if the practice is prolonged over many years. The use of the same razor by more than one family member is another possible risk for transmission.

The evidence so far suggests that the likelihood of transmission gradually increases over many years.[11] The opportunities for transmission will vary according to the practices of family members and may also be linked to cultural factors.

7. Occupational/Needlestick/Dentist

Dentists who practice oral surgery and health workers who have needlestick injuries have an increased likelihood of exposure to HCV. Rates of infection arising from such accidents are thought to run at about 5%. The overall numbers infected are quite low, and probably represent about 2% of the HCV+ population, but cases have been caused by only minor breaches of guidelines. The fact that public health workers have been infected has influenced the attitude of some personnel towards hepatitis C patients and may be a cause of some difficulty in obtaining treatment.

8. Mother to Child

It is now consistently estimated that a mother with HCV has about an 8% chance of passing the virus on to her child in Western countries. (Rates are higher in developing countries, probably due to less sterile conditions.) It is now thought that the birth process itself is the most likely point of transmission and that the virus is not passed on in the womb. Mothers with both HIV and HCV have a higher probability of passing the virus on, thought to be about 25%. Children who have contracted the virus from their mothers will form an increased percentage of the HCV+ population over the next few years. This may be the fastest growing section of the patient population and represents a "third wave" (see chapter 6).

9. Air Filters in Oxygen Masks

Reports from Australia indicate that some hospital patients may have contracted HCV via minute blood traces in the filters of anesthesia masks.

10. Intramucosally/Via Blood-Soaked Rolled-Up Notes Used to Ingest Cocaine and Other Drugs

According to one survey of HCV+ blood donors, "The risks for exposure to HCV that were significantly associated with positivity for HCV were a history of blood transfusion (27%), intranasal cocaine use (68%), IV drug use (42%) and sexual promiscuity (53%) ..."[12]

The results of this survey do not amount to proof of intranasal transmission. Strictly speaking, they demonstrate a correlation only. However, they do indicate that public health authorities in the U.S. are taking this vector as a potential transmission route seriously. If HCV can be transmitted on specks of blood and mucus, it is a theoretically feasible route, particularly given the sensitive nature of the membranes in the nose and the sharpness of the edge of paper currency. Some doctors have recently reported this to be a major suspect in patients with sporadic exposure. This route was suggested as being of significance in an article entitled "The Shadow Epidemic" by Jerome Groopman, which appeared in the *New Yorker* magazine on May 11, 1998.

11. Via Insects?

The possibility that HCV could be transmitted via mosquitoes caused alarm in Australia and among tropical disease specialists a couple of years ago. Following analysis, doctors claimed that this route was impractical, on the grounds that HCV would not survive within the mosquito. This route appears to be extremely unlikely.

12. Via Electroencephalogram (EEG), Needles, Dialysis Equipment, and Other Medical Instruments

There has been one recent report suggesting that hepatitis may have been passed on as a result of using inadequately sterilized EEG needles. The use of electrodes is a safer method of administering this test.

There have been many reports indicating that renal dialysis patients did in the past run a high risk of infection. Changes in dialysis unit routines have diminished the risk considerably. Another report has shown that HCV has been transmitted by coloscopy; routine cleaning procedures were clearly not adequate. There are a few other reports of infected medical equipment being implicated in occasional instances of transmission. These cases are very rare indeed, but it does confirm that routine sterilization procedures are not necessarily adequate to kill HCV.

13. Unknown or Sporadic

Most surveys of the HCV+ population in Western countries come up with a number of patients with no identifiable risk factor. Typically this is about 10%, but it represents the most worrying section of the patient population because it suggests that transmission routes are still not fully understood and therefore that countermeasures may be inadequate to completely halt the spread of HCV.

Prevention of Transmission

No one can be blamed for passing on this virus prior to its discovery; to all intents and purposes it was invisible. However, now that the salient facts are known and high-quality tests are available, it is vital that information to safeguard against further transmission gets through to the individuals, institutions, and government bodies that need to know. Sadly the measures that have been taken so far are inadequate. Even when the information is getting through, the appropriate action and changes in behavior are not taking place; this applies to government bodies as much as to individuals. The following is a summary of what should be happening, not necessarily what is happening.

Action Required from Government and Public Health Bodies

1. Blood Supply and Blood Products

Most developed countries now screen blood donors for HCV. Lifestyle questionnaires and the medical history are checked, and the first batch of donated blood is tested. Belatedly some governments have introduced backup testing of the blood supply. However, even the most sophisticated PCR and RIBA tests are not 100% accurate.

Since 1986 donated blood products, such as clotting factors, have been subject to various treatments designed to kill viruses and bacteria. However, hemophiliacs are not convinced that these measures necessarily work and are campaigning for the availability of recombinant (genetically engineered) blood products. They are also suspicious that some blood products are derived from sources that are not properly screened and tested. There is also the fact that HCV antibodies may not appear in blood for up to five months after infection. Thus blood supplies that are tested with PCR occasionally demonstrate the presence of HCV, even though donors have been screened. In addition PCR tests do not pick up the presence of extremely low levels of virus that are probably infectious.

Hepatitis G (GBV) is another blood-borne virus that is present in the blood donor pool. There is little evidence so far that it is harmful, but research is still at an early stage. It is government's responsibility to see to it that tests for GBV are developed rapidly and that research into the existence of other undetected blood-borne viruses is properly funded. It is also government's responsibility to ensure that all blood products are produced according to strictly enforced rules, particularly those from countries known to have produced infected products in the past. If these cannot be enforced, then recombinant products must be made available to those who need them. (Taxation of these products must be removed.) The case for the use of recombinant products is well put in a hemophiliac commentary on the subject:

> The whole history of plasma products over the past twenty-five years indicates that it is inevitably the case that every few years we discover a new virus and it then becomes apparent that this virus has been present in the blood supply for several years.... How many more viruses have to be detected, and how many more patients have to be infected, before we all come to be convinced that the continued usage of these plasma-derived products makes people vulnerable to further viral infections?

International health bodies also need to ensure that all vaccination programs are carried out by personnel who are well aware of the risks of HCV transmission.

2. Public Health Education

The general public must be informed about HCV. They need to be told that they are many times more likely to contract this virus than HIV. The dangers inherent in any kind of blood-to-blood contact need to be reinforced. The public needs to know that HIV is not the only virus that they need to be taking steps to avoid, and that HCV has a wider range of transmission routes.

Hospital staff are already alert to the risk of blood-borne virus transmission via needlestick injury, but are less aware of the hazard presented by filters in face masks or EEG needles, for instance. More research and education is needed.

Dentists, barbers, practitioners of cosmetic surgery, acupuncturists, and tattooists need to receive reinforced hygiene instructions and details about just how infectious HCV is. Although most of these are already subject to strict rules, some groups, like barbers, may be less aware of the potential for contracting or passing on HCV.

Public Health and Personal Responsibility of HCV+ Individuals

Those known to have HCV need to be systematically provided with information that will enable them to avoid transmitting the virus to anybody else. Patients need to take action based upon this information. This includes the following:

1. Do not donate blood, eggs, bone marrow, or semen.

2. Do not register as an organ donor; if you are registered, then remove your name from the list.

3. Avoid sexual practices that involve blood-to-blood contact. If in doubt, practice safe sex. Sex during menstruation may be a remote risk. Oral-genital contact might pose a remote risk, if one or both partners have bleeding gums. Sadomasochism that involves bleeding is a risk.

4. Do not share razors, nail files, nail scissors, or toothbrushes. Avoid sharing any personal hygiene equipment.

5. Blood-stained tissues, swabs, tampons, and so on need to be disposed of carefully.

6. Blood spills must be cleaned up with bleach. Remember that blood is sticky, so washing of hands after any possibility of contact is vital.

7. Dress cuts and wounds with disinfectants and bandages.

8. Advise public health workers, dentists, doctors, tattooists, acupuncturists, and so on that you have HCV.

It is important to stress that HCV is actually very difficult to pass on. Anxieties in the normal work place are unfounded. Risks in the home can be countered.

Further advice, unrelated to transmission, may also include considering having hepatitis A and B vaccinations, or strictly avoiding risks for these viruses. See chapters 4 and 5 for more information.

HCV+ pregnant women need to discuss with the delivery team means of minimizing the possibility of transmission to the baby.

IVDUs: Policy Options—Harm Reduction and Narcotics Regulatory Reform

Professionals working in the fields of harm reduction, public health, and related research have assessed the seriousness of the situation and articulated the urgent need for coherent policy reform based upon their findings. Australia is at the forefront of hepatitis C management, having recognized the problem far earlier than other developed countries. The experience of leading Australian experts may therefore be of value to policy makers in other countries. Dr. Alex Wodak, director of the Alcohol and Drug Service at St. Vincent's Hospital in Sydney, Australia, has quantified the problem:

> Hepatitis C is undoubtedly a serious public health problem.... Complications arising out of chronic hepatitis C infection will result in many patients needing frequent hospitalization. Perhaps 50% of people with CHC develop a lingering illness with debilitating fatigue precluding employment and often home duties. Fatigue may be one of the most expensive aspects of the hepatitis C epidemic.... The overall health and economic burden of hepatitis C may be at least comparable with HIV because of the far larger pool of hepatitis C infection and the greater duration of the illness.[13]

In the same paper Dr. Wodak went on to discuss the kind of options that professionals working in the field commonly recommend:

> Needle exchange, at an annual cost of $10 million, was estimated to have prevented 2,900 HIV infections in Australia in 1991 and saved $267 million at a cost per life year saved of

$350. Needle exchange is an excellent example of the effectiveness, cost-effectiveness and minimal side effects of harm reduction ... there is still no good evidence that needle exchange increases drug use ...

If illicit drug use cannot be eradicated, it might be possible to virtually eradicate IDU by persuading would-be and current drug users to adopt non-injecting routes of administration (NIROA).... Adoption of NIROA has the probable additional benefit of reducing the number of deaths from overdose.

In a broader sense consideration of hepatitis C control forces us to consider difficult questions about the relationship between harm reduction and drug law reform. Australia will need to change the current debate from one about symbols and ideology to a real concern for outcomes and rationality.

Thus in needle exchanges, NIROA promotion, and legal reform there are three prongs to the health- and economics-based strategy suggested by experienced professionals.

Stuart Loveday, of the Hepatitis C Council of New South Wales, reports that needle exchanges coupled with education have proved to be highly effective in reducing prevalence in IVDUs: from HCV prevalence of 67% in 1988/89 in people who have injected for less than two years, to 15–20% in the same group in 1997. However, he has stressed that education is also a vital component in this package, particularly stressing that HCV can be passed on via paraphernalia. As well as providing clean equipment, such facilities are ideal opportunities for passing on educational material to users, particularly with regard to NIROA. Funding is essential. Money spent on the prevention of transmission via this route is likely to be a tiny fraction of that required for treatment. The establishment of funds for this specific purpose is a public health priority.

Education and resources must be concentrated in areas identified as being of particular importance. For example prison populations often demonstrate high rates of HCV prevalence. Drug education programs should include HCV, not just HIV. Users need to be aware that steps taken to prevent HIV transmission are inadequate to prevent the spread of HCV. It is thought that the sharing of spoons, filters, and even tourniquets can be responsible for HCV transmission.

Appropriate authorities need to ensure that the following information reaches this group in particular:

1. It is unsafe to share any injecting equipment. This includes spoons, water ampules, filters, syringes, needles, tourniquets, and swabs. Front loading and back loading, the practice of cooking up one "hit" and then sharing it by each participant drawing up an equal dose from a single spoon via a hypodermic syringe, is unsafe.

2. All equipment should be used once only. No sharing or reuse is safe.

3. Immersion in bleach for thirty seconds and boiling of equipment for twenty minutes may not always be sufficient to kill HCV, according to information used by the Mainliners Agency in London. If it is necessary to reuse equipment, then all components must be fully immersed in full-strength bleach for at least twenty minutes, rinsed, and then subject to the same process twice more. Note that ecologically friendly brands of bleach are not powerful enough to kill HCV. Glass syringes can be sterilized by boiling in water for at least twenty minutes. Spoons need to be thoroughly washed with pure alcohol and should also be boiled for at least twenty minutes.

4. Continuing to use drugs in general and hard drugs in particular may worsen the prognosis. If you do use drugs, then try not to drink alcohol as well because the combination is thought to be doubly harmful for HCV progression (see pages 398–400).

5. Information on where to seek help to stop using drugs.

Joey Tranchina, director of Harm Reduction Projects for the HCV Global Foundation, has pointed out that many addicts are unwilling to use bleach because of the possibility of accidentally injecting themselves with it, and that strength grades are often obscure. He echoes the point that no injecting behavior is safe and suggests the following additional measures and possible courses of action:

- Addicts should be encouraged to be creative about developing alternative means of consuming drugs.

- Addicts must be strongly discouraged from initiating other users into IV drug use. They must be warned that HCV is a serious condition, with a very high one-off transmission rate, and advised to counsel other users to abstain from IV drug use.

- Addicts should be encouraged to improve standards of personal hygiene. This is problematic for the homeless, but is also often a problem with affluent addicts.

- Professionals should explore the possibility of making blood-less or sterile injection technology available to addicts (this is along the same lines as "Powderject" products being tried for interferon administration).

Perhaps the most intractable challenge to reformers is the legal status quo with regard to narcotics regulation. It is the observation of many professionals in this field that the illegal status of narcotics is intimately linked to the switch from noninjecting use of narcotics and IV usage. They have noted that the switch often occurs due to factors that are logically linked to the illegal status of narcotics. For instance, heroin smokers frequently switch to IV use as a result of the need to maintain their dependence, which they cannot otherwise afford. Certain forms of narcotics are unsuitable for smoking, and if that form is the only one available, addicts may switch to IV use. These are not the only factors.

In general, professionals concerned with harm reduction and HCV control advocate policies based upon health and economic parameters. Political and ideological factors also play a powerful role in determining policy in this very important category. It could be that the issue of HCV prevalence and control will bring this debate to a head.

Professionals Working with Risks

Public health care workers are at additional risk of exposure to HCV, though prevalence figures in this group are hard to interpret. A study performed at the Royal Free Hospital in 1995 examined the seroprevalence of HCV antibodies in health care workers (HCWs), compared to the general population, and found that there was no significant difference. However, the results of a comprehensive long-term Italian study titled "Incidence of non-A, non-B and HCV positive hepatitis in health care workers in Italy" by T. Stroffolini et al. demonstrated that HCWs were at greater risk of contracting the virus compared to the general population, with needlestick injury being the major factor. The report concluded: "These findings strongly suggest that in Italy health care workers are at greater risk than the general population of acquiring NANB hepatitis, as well as HCV."

Medical professionals need to ensure that universal precautions are followed. These are as follows:

- Always use latex gloves (hypoallergenic or low protein) and plastic aprons (and visors if there is any risk of splashing, or aerosol of body fluids) when dealing with body fluids, especially blood or body fluids containing visible blood. Ensure the monitoring of skin integrity and that any abrasions are covered with waterproof dressings, and any dermatological complaints such as eczema are reported.

- In the event of an exposure, make the area bleed if there is a needlestick injury, do not suck the wound, clean with soap and water, and cover with a waterproof dressing. Report and document immediately and ensure occupational health follow-up, with a baseline serum sample to be saved and a three- and six-month test for HIV, HBV, and HCV. The serum samples are crucial to document the time of infection. Compensation payments will depend on such incontrovertible data.

- The duty to dispose of needles, blades, and other sharp instruments is always the responsibility of the user, via a recommended container adhering to British and U.S. standards no more than two-thirds full. Never resheath needles or similar objects and always ensure the risk to others during use is minimized. If equipment is to be reused, ensure that cleaning, disinfection, and sterilization are adhered to rigidly. Never multidose from the same vial for multiple patients, especially in anesthetics due to the risk of cross-infection.

Adhesion to these principles would ensure that infection of health care workers was reduced, and the possibility of long-term infection, infectivity, and disease were minimized. Infection may lead to effects on quality of life, longevity, life insurance, loans and mortgages, employment, and possible stigmatization, all of which could be prevented. There could also be a risk of transmission from HCW to patient, so the consistent practice of these measures may be expected to ensure a safer environment for everyone.

There is no HCV vaccine, or immunoglobulin as for HIV, and no guidance as yet on postexposure prophylaxis. Complacency is the single most common mistake alongside lack of knowledge.

It is also worth noting that it is now clear that there is new strain of blood-borne viral hepatitis, referred to as hepatitis G or GBV. It is possible that this virus is responsible for a small number of cases of fulminant hepatitis, although it is more commonly not an immediate threat to health. This reinforces the need for vigilance.

It is also obvious that infected HCWs have a far greater potential capacity for multiple transmission than lay people. A recent report from Spain suggests that one infected doctor managed to pass HCV on to a large number of his patients:

> This alarming article recounts the tale of an opioid addicted anaesthetist, Dr. Juan Maeso, who has infected 217 patients with HCV (with 3,000 being screened) at two hospitals in Valencia (La Fe and the Casa de Salud). Apparently he helped himself to opioid analgesia post-op and then administered the remainder to the patient with the same syringe! It is also alleged seven of his colleagues remained silent despite knowledge of this. The full report is expected in three months time. [Hepatitis C outbreak astounds Spain. Bosch X. *The Lancet,* 351:1415, 1998]

Thus there is a particular need for vigilance among HCWs. Nurses and other health professionals who do contract hepatitis C may face difficulties pursuing their careers, particularly if specializing in certain areas such as theater support. If you are working in health care, it is advisable to check that your employers carry insurance coverage in the event of becoming infected in the course of your professional duties.

Denise's Story

Denise has worked as a dental nurse for many years. She discovered that she had been exposed to hepatitis C two years ago. This is how she believes her work put her at risk:

> During the course of treating patients I was regularly required to change the long needles used for the administration of local oral anesthetic. This required me to screw and unscrew these units onto the syringe. New units needed to have the plastic casing snapped off after they had been attached. Old units needed to be unscrewed and disposed of.
>
> I would occasionally scratch myself with the needle during this procedure. It wouldn't matter that I had put on two latex gloves; the sharp would just slice through the latex like a knife through butter. I am pretty sure that I was exposed to HCV during one of these scratching episodes.

Other Theories about the Epidemiology of HCV

There is another school of thought about the current prevalence of HCV, which is included here to provide a comprehensive picture.

Some practitioners, particularly naturopaths, feel that there is a link between the appearance and proliferation of "modern" viruses such as HIV and HCV and certain developments in "global lifestyle" that have emerged during the twentieth century.

The book *A World without AIDS* by Leon Chaitow and Simon Martin (Thorsons, 1988) epitomizes this interpretation of these pandemics. The appearance of AIDS is used as a powerful metaphor. The book suggests that the whole world has a form of immune deficiency and that we are all implicated in the processes that are identified as causes of these outbreaks of viral illness. These diseases are seen as arising out of increased susceptibility. Certain developments are cited as being particularly damaging to global immunity and individual health. Among the factors identified as damaging immunity and increasing susceptibility are:

... the effects of air pollution, drinking water that fails to meet commonly agreed health standards, denatured food, the stress of overcrowding and noise, geopathic stress and electromagnetic pollution, radiation, pesticides and toxic heavy metals, food additives and contaminants, lack of exercise, psychological stress ...

... Although outwardly healthy, the truth is that we are getting weaker. And we are breeding future generations whose immune systems have been systematically weakened by vaccinations; random overuse of medical and socially acceptable drugs, poisonous air, toxic water and deficient food; and by their toxic parents—a fair proportion of whom were themselves sickly offspring of genetically damaged parents who only achieved some semblance of adulthood and reproductive capability by consistent medical intervention form conception onwards. (pp. 71–72)

My early research for this book suggested that Chaitow might have a basis for explaining patterns of HCV spread and progression. The observation that some patients cleared HCV spontaneously and others did not—the figure was initially put at 50%—suggested that varied susceptibility might well explain HCV disappearance in some and progression in others, and that an immunological deficiency might explain this, that some combination of exposure and inadequate immune responses was at work. Research into the immunology of opiate users had already demonstrated weakened responses (see chapter 22, page 402).

It seems that Chaitow and Martin were not so wide of the mark. It is now thought that the small proportion of people exposed to HCV who have undetectable virus often have a slightly different genetic makeup to those who don't. It is not known why this ability is present in some people and not in others, whether this is governed by distant genetic history or more recent environmental influences. Thus the case for acquired susceptibility to progression through lifestyle and environmental cofactors is still open to debate.

Chaitow has since done a lot of work on the interaction between vaccination programs and susceptibility to viral infection. It appears that live vaccines may transfer the immunity developed by the micro-organisms they contain to other unknown viruses or bacteria into the bodies of vaccinated patients. It is suggested that this might have adverse, unforeseen consequences,[14] perhaps resulting in the sub-version of the vaccinated subjects' own immune response. From the naturopathic viewpoint the nature of modern technological medi-cine and its emphasis on drugs is a prime cause of the increased pro-liferation of viral pathogens.

It is also known that alcoholics demonstrate a higher prevalence of HCV than the general population. It has been suggested that HCV might be a latent virus from the prehistory of human existence, whose reappearance has been triggered by a combination of unhealthy lifestyle factors, which represent deteriorations in immunological health. Research in Germany has tried to establish whether or not HCV is a latent virus. One study found that HCV-specific RNA sequences were present in HCV-antibody-negative people, indicat-ing the possibility of a "trigger" existing for the development of dis-ease. Thus the infectious agent may not be HCV itself but some other related entity, and the rises in HCV RNA in antibody-positive patients may be partly manufactured by the body. In turn these raised levels of HCV RNA may play a key direct role in extrahepatic disease pro-gression. The coauthor of the report, Reinhard Dennin, has also questioned whether or not HCV is a true virus.[15]

Although these views are persuasive and even attractive, they do not detract from the fact that HCV"s manifestation can nearly always be traced back to an event involving "blood-to-blood" con-tact. The most likely scenario is that HCV requires a combination of blood-to-blood contact and susceptibility to spread. Whether this susceptibility can be linked to episodes of vaccination or lifestyle pattern either in patients or their parents is a very interesting ques-tion which cannot be satisfactorily answered at present.

Looked at from still another perspective, the discovery of HCV, and possibly hepatitis G as well, could be regarded as a confirma-tion of the "viral cause" school of thought as opposed to the "whole world has AIDS" theory. Many of the illnesses cited by naturopaths as symptoms of global deterioration in immunological integrity, such as chronic fatigue syndrome and lupus, may also be explained as previously undiagnosed HCV or hepatitis G! On the other hand, recent genetic findings swing the argument back towards the susceptibility school of thought. As more facts emerge, the more difficult it is to fit them into any particular theory.

Contacts

For information on harm reduction in the U.S. and on a range of other related subjects, call the **Lindesmith Center** in New York City at (212) 548-0695 or in San Francisco at (415) 921-4987. Or visit their Website: http://www.lindesmith.org.

Or contact **Harm Reduction Coalition** (who also produce a newsletter): New York City: (212) 213-6376. Oakland, CA: (510) 444-6969. Email: hrc@harmreduction.org.

Website: http://www.harmreduction.org.

In the U.K. the **Mainliners Agency** may be able to help with information about harm reduction and hepatitis C. Telephone 0171 582 3338.

Or call the **John Morduant Trust:** 0181 846 6611.

Positive Action is based in Dublin, Ireland, and can be contacted at 353 1 676 2853.

References

1. Variability of hepatitis C virus. Simmonds P. *Hepatology,* 21(2):570–583, 1995.

2. A four-year review of patients with hepatitis C antibody in Department of Veterans Affairs facilities. Roselle GA, Danko LH, Mendenhall CL. *Military Medicine,* 162(11):711–4, Nov 1997.

3. The sleeping giant awakes. Waller T and Holmes R. *Druglink,* pp 8–11, Institute for the Study of Drug Dependence (U.K.), Sept/Oct 1995.

4. Incidence and risk factors for hepatitis C among injection drug users in Baltimore, Maryland. Villano SA et al. *Journal of Clinical Microbiology,* 35(12):3274–7, Dec 1997.

5. Transmission of HCV between spouses. Akahane T et al. *Lancet,* 339, 1059, 1992.

6. Risk factors for HCV seropositivity in heterosexual couples. Osmond DH et al. *JAMA,* 269:361, 1993.

7. Heterosexual co-transmission of HCV and HIV. Eyster ME et al. *Ann Internal Medicine*, 115:764, 1991.

8. Prevalence of anti-HCV in non drug-abusing-female prostitutes in Spain. Gutierrez P et al. *Sex Trans Dis*, 19:39, 1992.

9. Prevalence, infectivity and risk factor analysis in prostitutes. Wu JC et al. *Journal of Medical Virology*, 39:312, 1993.

10. Comparison of risk factors for hepatitis C and hepatitis B infection in homosexual men. Osmond DH et al. *Journal of Infectious Disease*, 167:66, 1993.

11. Intrafamilial transmission of the hepatitis C virus. Kao JH et al. *J Infect Disease*, 166:900, 1992.

12. Routes of infection, viremia and liver disease in blood donors found to have hepatitis C virus infection. Conry-Cantilena C et al. *New England Journal of Medicine*, 334(26):1691–1735, June 1996.

13. Injecting Nation: achieving control of hepatitis C in Australia. Wodak A. *Drug and Alcohol Review*, 16, 275–284, 1997, Australian Professional Society on Alcohol and Other Drugs.

14. *Vaccination and Immunization*. Chaitow L. pp. 101–102, CW Daniel, 1994.

15. Hepatitis C virus (HCV) specific sequences are demonstrable in the DNA fraction of peripheral blood mononuclear cells from healthy anti-HCV antibody negative individuals and cell lines of human origin. Dennin RH and Chen Z. *Eur J Clin Biochem*, 35(12):899–905, 1997.

3

Tests for Hepatitis C

Diagnosis

To Test or Not to Test?

THERE IS NO DOUBT that being diagnosed as having hepatitis C carries certain disadvantages. There is considerable stigma attached to the condition. The appearance of the diagnosis on your medical records will often influence the attitude of employers. Some patients feel that they have been dismissed or not employed in the first case due to their hepatitis C status. Life insurance policies, and therefore mortgages, are more expensive. Other financial packages can also be dearer. Schools can react badly if they discover that either children or parents have hepatitis C. Friends and relatives can respond unpredictably. Doctors often regard the presence of HCV as a "surrogate" for evidence of present or previous IV drug use, which can be infuriating. One can get the feeling that one is "marked down" as a second-class citizen.

Consent

Some patients have been tested and given diagnoses without their explicit permission. This seems to reflect the widespread, outdated view of the medical authorities that hepatitis C is not a serious condition. None of the procedures that have been adopted for HIV tests apply to hepatitis C at most medical centers. If blood is taken with the intention of testing for HCV, it is good practice to inform you and gain your consent.

Anonymous Testing

Anonymous testing facilities are available in some private clinics and genito-urinary medicine (GUM) centers; getting a result in this way would at least enable you to obtain a clear picture of your health status without being obliged to tell your doctor.

If you want the complete battery of associated tests and to try antiviral drug therapy, it will be very difficult without being officially classified as a hepatitis C patient. You will need to be tested and have the positive result in your medical records.

A Cautionary Note about Test Results

It is common for patients to experience levels of well-being or debilitation that are not reflected in the results of clinical tests, particularly liver function tests. It may be worth bearing in mind that some doctors now suspect that HCV is best understood as a systemic condition that would theoretically require regular scans, biopsies, and function tests for several major organs and body systems to establish a complete clinical profile. Even then the way in which HCV causes debilitation is not yet clearly understood. Therefore it is still advisable for patients to take into account their own assessment of well-being and not place absolute trust in the results of these tests.

Commonly Used Tests for Hepatitis C

Blood Tests for the Presence of HCV and Previous Exposure to It

1. Antibody Detection Tests

These tests check for the presence of antibodies to hepatitis C, not the current presence of the virus in the blood. The production of these antibodies may have begun at any time in the past upon exposure to HCV.

After the hepatitis C virus was discovered in 1989, it took a while to develop practical tests that could used to assess whether or not individuals had been exposed to the virus or currently had it in their blood. The first priority was a simple cheap test to assess the presence or absence of antibodies to hepatitis C. Two types of test were used.

ELISA stands for Enzyme Linked Immunosorbent Assay. The ELISA I test for hepatitis C was the first to be developed and was introduced in 1991. ELISA effectively searches the blood sample for certain biochemical sequences whose existence corresponds with the presence of antibodies to HCV.

The ELISA I test only searched for the presence of one particular genetically specific antibody to HCV and was soon shown to be unreliable, giving both false positive and false negative results. It was displaced by ELISA II in 1993, although this more comprehensive test was not introduced until 1994 in many countries. This test proved more reliable, but still fell short of being 100% accurate. ELISA III is now available; because it is relatively cheap and easy to perform, it is often used as the initial test today.

RIBA stands for Recombinant Immunoblot Assay. The RIBA I test was developed for use in hepatitis C partly because of the unreliability of ELISA I. This test incorporated a search for two different sets of antibody patterns and a test for the presence of a control substance. Pathologists have to visually assess the positivity of the result by comparison to controls.

A third generation RIBA test called RIBA III is now available. This is highly accurate, but still cannot be reliably described as 100%. Because the RIBA tests are more expensive than ELISA, they tend to be used as confirmatory tools.

Matrix Test is another variation on the antibody test using procedure that uses a technique known as "in vitro enzyme dot blot immunoassay." It is also thought to be highly accurate.

Important Note: It takes up to six months for antibodies to HCV to form in the blood. (This process is known as seroconversion.) Therefore it is important that people seeking a diagnosis after a recent suspected risk should get retested six months after the initial antibody test.

There are a number of people who had negative antibody tests in the past yet have subsequently turned out to have hepatitis C. This seldom happens now because the new tests, such as ELISA III, are much more specific and sensitive. There are also documented cases of people with HCV who cease to produce HCV antibodies (see chapter 6 for examples.) There are also some who have been told they are positive who later turned out to be negative. If you want confirmation of your status, then go back and get retested, particularly if your first test was prior to 1995.

2. Virus Detection and Analysis Tests

These tests try to assess the presence or absence of the hepatitis C virus itself in the blood and other body tissue. They are more definitive than the tests above. Because the virus is so small and elusive these procedures are sophisticated and expensive.

PCR stands for polymerase chain reaction. It is the most sensitive test available. Developed by a young American scientist with a taste for hallucinogenic drugs, it is a testing method that lends itself to detecting minute traces of any organic substance in any given medium; that medium is usually blood. In the case of HCV it works by taking a sample of the blood of the patient being tested and amplifying the nucleic acid associated with the virus many millions of times. This is the chain reaction—effectively a copying process. It brings the nucleic acid up to detectable levels. The amplification effect is consistent, enabling experienced technicians to assess how much of the original material is present in the sample.

The test is expensive and its use is sometimes rationed. Patients using hospitals with research facilities are likely to be offered this test more freely than others. This test does not rely on seroconversion and may be able to detect the virus after only three days of infection. There are a couple of problems with this test.

First, it tends to be more sensitive to some strains of HCV than others. This is because the nucleic acid it searches for is a closer fit in some genotypes than others. Thus viral load comparisons between patients with differing genotypes are not reliable. There is also the possibility that some quasi species variations of HCV may not be picked up at all, which raises the possibility of a need for a range of different HCV PCR tests geared to these variants.

Second, there is also a problem related to the fact that HCV levels in the blood tend to fluctuate. Therefore the result may have an element of "hit or miss" about it. The results of some patients undergoing antiviral therapy indicate that it comes and goes, often in quite an unpredictable way. Having said this, viral load does not fluctuate as wildly as ALT/AST (see the "Blood Tests" section on page 85), so a significant reduction in HCV PCR is highly likely to represent a "real" reduction in viral load.

Results are given on a logarithmic scale that is often expressed in different ways according to the protocols of the hospital concerned. Thus it is difficult to compare the results of these tests. However, there are general opinions; results of 1 million copies of HCV per ml or below would generally be regarded as low or very low. Results in the order of 5 million copies per ml might be regarded as "average." Results of 10 million per ml or above might be regarded as "high." Because infectivity is thought to correlate to viral load, quantitative test results could be used as a basis for counselling.

Being PCR negative does not necessarily mean that HCV has disappeared completely; it may still be present at undetectable levels in the blood, or it may be present in liver cells and in certain white blood cells. These can also be tested, although such extensive screening is rarely carried out. When it is, however, it seems that some patients judged to be clear of HCV by blood test alone actually still have traces of the virus in white blood cells.

Although PCR has these limitations, it is probably the most useful single blood test and can be used to assess the antiviral efficacy of any particular therapy.

b-DNA for HCV (branched DNA test) also tests for the presence of the virus in the blood, but is less sensitive than the PCR test. It generates an estimate of viral loads above a certain level—PCR can detect as few as 1,000 genomes per ml, while b-DNA only picks up levels over 350,000. It is often used, a quick test to assess infectivity and viral load. Sensitivity is improving, so check with your doctor if you want to know the significance.

A negative b-DNA test does not mean that you don't have HCV in your blood. Results of these tests may have caused confusion in some patients. You can be b-DNA negative and PCR positive. b-DNA has also been found to give false negative results in post-liver-transplant patients.

Some clinicians use the test to assess suitability for interferon-based treatment—they reckon that patients who are b-DNA negative stand a good chance of responding.

There is now a second-generation b-DNA test available, which claims greater sensitivity. b-DNA tests are also sometimes referred to as Quantiplex tests.

Note that the results of such tests require intelligent interpretation; having a high viral load dose not necessarily correlate with liver damage. This would depend upon a range of other factors, particularly the length of time since infection. A negative result may indicate either occult infection or the presence of a different pathogen causing symptoms of chronic hepatitis, such as hepatitis B.

Genotype tests assess which strain or strains of the virus are present. They are more difficult to execute than PCR, at least as expensive and are rarely performed. The usefulness of the test is related to the bearing of genotype on prognosis and responsiveness to treatment. This is debatable, with some doctors suggesting that viral load is a more important factor. However, the results of this test can be useful in making a decision regarding treatment selection.

Genotyping is usually performed through a technique called line probe assay. This test has recently been refined, which raises the possibility of wider access and reduced price. Some clinicians are using a "serotype" analysis technique to establish genotype; this examines antibodies for characteristics that reveal the genotype of the virus to which it is responding.

Liver Health Tests

There is a broad distinction between tests to assess the physical state of the liver as seen through the microscope (histology) and the efficiency with which it performs various functions. Because liver biopsy is expensive, time-consuming, uncomfortable, and potentially dangerous, a number of clinicians have been trying to find "noninvasive" methods of assessing liver histology.

Blood Tests

Liver function tests (LFTs) are the most commonly used diagnostic tools. As the words suggest, they attempt to assess the effectiveness with which the liver performs various jobs by measuring certain biochemical indicators known to be associated with these functions. These biochemical profiles reflect recent activity only.

LFTs are not always a good indicator of the health of the liver and they require skilled interpretation on the part of clinicians. Some patients plot their results over time. They test for the levels of the following substances in the blood, which are thought to reflect the efficiency of the liver as well as damage.

Alanine aminotransferase (ALT) and **aspartate aminotransferase** (AST) are the two most common indicators used. These are enzymes that are normally present in liver cells. When cells become damaged, they leak into the bloodstream, causing levels of these enzymes to be raised. Thus results can be interpreted as an indication of ongoing liver damage. ALT is thought to be a more accurate reflection of liver inflammation because AST can also be produced by other organs such as the heart.

ALT and AST can be poor indicators of the absolute level of damage to the liver. A patient whose enzyme levels have only been raised for a few months is likely to be in better shape than one whose levels have been high for years, even if the former has higher counts than the latter. A patient with HCV-related cirrhosis may have normal ALT and AST counts.

HCV patients often have a classic sine curve pattern of ALT/AST results, which mean that these tests would need to be performed frequently to gain an accurate assessment. The normal range of results is 5–40 international units (iu) per liter; some clinicians regard anything below 50 iu/l as normal.

While the absolute levels may be poor indicators of the health of the liver, some doctors believe that the ratio of AST to ALT may be a good indicator of the extent to which fibrosis has progressed. For instance, one recent report found a correlation between a higher AST:ALT ratio and cirrhosis. If the AST was greater than the ALT, patients were found to be likely to have cirrhosis.[1]

Alkaline phosphatase is the test most often used to detect obstruction of the biliary system, a problem associated with progressive disease. Levels are also raised in cases of gallstone disease, excessive alcohol intake, and drug-induced hepatitis. The normal range varies and should be checked.

If the result is inconclusive, tests for the levels of **gamma-glutamyl transpeptidase (GGTP)** may be carried out. This substance is more closely related to biliary problems. Results of GGTP have been cross-correlated with genotypes; preliminary findings suggest that genotype 3 may be more likely to cause biliary disease, suggesting that this subspecies is prone to causing a slightly different pattern of injury. Elevated levels of GGTP are traditionally associated with high alcohol consumption. This association has caused some doctors to jump to incorrect conclusions about their patients' drinking habits.

Bilirubin levels correspond to the health of the bile duct and the overall efficiency of the liver. It is a bile pigment that is usually extracted from the blood by the liver. In healthy individuals there should be little bilirubin in the blood. Increased levels are associated with the destruction of red blood cells or decreased efficiency of liver function. High levels are the cause of jaundice. The level should be lower than 1.2 mg/dl or 17 ml/L in healthy individuals.

Albumin is the major protein that is found in the blood. Levels correspond to the livers effectiveness in forming protein. The normal range is 35–50 g/l. Lower levels indicate problems with protein synthesis that correspond to chronic liver damage.

Prothrombin time is a test that assesses the efficiency of blood clotting. When the liver is damaged, it may fail to produce blood clotting factors. This test is a good indicator of liver damage.

Caffeine clearance testing is regarded as an accurate and inexpensive measure of general liver function by some practitioners. Because caffeine processing is particularly affected by reduced liver function, slow reductions in levels can be correlated to impairment.

Immunoglobulin G (IgG), procollagen III, propeptide (PIIINP), and **type-IV collagen (CL-IV)** have all been investigated for their value in predicting the advance of fibrosis or the presence of cirrhosis. Results so far indicate that although there are often general correlations, the relationship is not consistent enough to predict histological health. Of these PIIINP has been reported to be the most useful indicator of fibrogenesis.[2]

Japanese researchers have found that levels of **serum hyaluronan,** an enzyme linked to connective tissue health, are closely correlated to the degree of fibrosis.

Another approach to diagnosing cirrhosis via blood tests is to assess the levels of certain fats in the blood. Cirrhosis is normally associated with *lower* levels of these fats in the blood. The following substances are measured: **low-density lipoprotein (LDL), high-density lipoprotein (HDL), very low-density lipoprotein (VLDL),** and **total cholesterol serum levels.**

It is possible that clinicians will be able to devise a reliable set of blood test indicators and ratios that accurately predict liver histology for hepatitis C patients. Once the data is satisfactorily correlated with histological findings, a computer-based model could be introduced. Researchers based at the Royal Infirmary in Edinburgh reckon that they have managed to develop an intelligent computer system that enables them to predict the presence or absence of cirrhosis with 90% accuracy, using results from noninvasive tests.

Other Tests and Procedures

Liver biopsy is the process of extracting a tiny sample of the liver via a needle for the purpose of laboratory examination. It is a minor procedure. It is rightly regarded as the best way of accurately assessing the health of the liver. The results are often described as the "gold standard" for assessing liver status.

Consultants are often very reluctant to treat people who do not agree to a biopsy before drug therapy; only patients with obvious risk factors associated with biopsy, such as hemophiliacs, are excused, although some doctors are reluctant to exclude even this group.

Liver biopsy does carry a risk for patients. The procedure has been assessed as having a 1/10,000 death rate; some doctors reckon it is higher than this. It is sometimes carried out as an inpatient procedure, with patients lying down on their right-hand sides as still as possible for six hours or so after the biopsy, and remaining under observation for a further eighteen hours. This is to prevent bleeding, a dangerous complication, and to allow patient monitoring.

Other hospitals do biopsies as an outpatient procedure, only detaining patients for six hours or so. In some cases the biopsy is done in the X-ray department guided by an ultrasound scan; this may result in greater precision and a reduced need to go back "for a second bite."

While some patients have no problems, others report suffering varying degrees of discomfort. There seems to be a common problem with referred pain in the right shoulder, which prevents patients from lying still. This might be alleviated by analgesic sprays such as Ibuleve. Only local anesthetic is used during the procedure, and this can be quite disconcerting. Hospitals offer tranquilizers such as valium and mild painkillers such as distalgesic or paracetamol, although these are inadequate to counter acute referred pain, which may require the use of opiates.

Patients undergoing biopsy sometimes feel that they are being experimented upon. The profession argues that biopsies are necessary for a number of reasons: first to ensure that no contraindications to therapy are present; second to accurately determine the health of patients' livers—blood tests are unreliable for hepatitis C patients; and third as a tool to decide whom to treat with interferon—those with cirrhosis are less likely to respond and those with little or no liver disease may not need therapy.

It is hoped that a new generation of more sophisticated liver function tests may remove the need for liver biopsy. In the meantime it is an ordeal that many patients will have to face. Patients can reduce the risk of discomfort by having an experienced doctor and backup painkillers.

Biopsy Results and Classification Systems

It is sometimes quite difficult for patients and nonspecialist medical practitioners to interpret the results of liver biopsies.

The categories of injury referred to in chapter 1—chronic persistent hepatitis, chronic active hepatitis, chronic lobular hepatitis, and cirrhosis—have been superseded by more systematic techniques for assessing both the absolute and the relative nature and extent of liver injury. Doctors have become increasingly aware that distinct patterns of disease progression often correlate with particular causes of liver injury. For instance, the histological course of liver disease in a chronic alcoholic may be very different than that of a chronic hepatitis B patient. It now appears that particular features may be especially significant in the progression of liver disease in hepatitis C patients. One of these is the presence of "bridging fibrosis" between the portal tracts and the terminal hepatic venules—and the association with the progression of cirrhosis. Traditional classifications often excluded this kind of detail.

Biopsy results are graded and staged. The grade corresponds to the extent of inflammation. The stage corresponds to the extent of scarring and reflects the degree of progression.

A modification of the Knodell index is the most widespread system of biopsy classification. The following is a typical staging index:

No fibrosis	0
Fibrous expansion of some portal areas	1
Fibrous expansion of most portal areas	2
Fibrous expansion of most portal areas with occasional portal-to-portal bridging	3
Fibrous expansion of most portal areas with marked portal-to-portal bridging	4
Marked bridging with occasional nodules	5
Cirrhosis	6

Grading indexes are more complex; typically they divide the liver into four categories of injury and assess grade of activity:

A	Periportal injury	absent (0) to severe (5)
B	Confluent necrosis	absent (0) to severe (5)
C	Focal necrosis, inflammation, and apoptosis	absent (0) to severe (5)
D	Portal inflammation	none (0) to marked (4)

Ultrasound Scans and CAT Scans

This is a nonintrusive method of assessing liver health. The procedure is simple; some gel is smeared over the liver area and a device shaped like an ice cream cone is moved over the surface. An operator is than able to "see" your liver and other internal organs on a screen. (Disconcertingly, so are you!)

Unfortunately this procedure will not detect the detailed progress of liver injury, although cirrhosis often can be diagnosed because of the distinctive nodular and irregular surface associated with the condition. Much depends upon the skill of the operator. Ultrasound scans can reveal lymph node abnormalities in the abdomen, a useful contribution.

CAT scans, which involve the three-dimensional modeling of X-rays, can yield useful results, but are expensive.

References

1. AST/ALT ratio predicts cirrhosis in patients with chronic hepatitis C virus infection. Sheth SG, Flamm SL, Gordon FD, Chopra S. *Am J Gastroenterol,* 93(1):44–48, Jan 1998.

2. Serum assays for liver fibrosis, Schuppan D et al. *Journal of Hepatology,* 22 (Suppl. 2):82–88, 1995.

4

Other Types of Viral Hepatitis

FOR THE PURPOSE OF CLARITY a brief summary of the characteristics of the other types of viral hepatitis is included. Many people, including some health professionals, are confused about the
distinctions, and it may be helpful to be able to communicate the
differences. The word "hepatitis" simply means inflammation of the
liver. The different types of viral infection that are responsible differ
greatly from each other.

Hepatitis A (HAV)

Identified in 1973, this is a cytopathic virus. It is transmitted via food
or liquids exposed to feces. Shellfish are particularly prone to hepatitis A contamination and may also carry other bacteria or viruses.
Transmission can be prevented by the adoption of rigorous standards of hygiene, particularly where food is prepared. There is now
an effective vaccine available. Called "Havrix," it provides protection for up to ten years.

Symptoms include diarrhea and vomiting. It causes acute illness—
in other words, effects are felt quickly but are short lived. The virus
is cleared from the body shortly after infection ('self-limiting" in
medical jargon) and can be fatal to elderly patients in the acute illness. Hepatitis A is common in developing counties and poses a
threat to travellers. It is reported to be on the increase in the U.K.
and not uncommon in the U.S. and Canada.

An episode of hepatitis A on top of chronic hepatitis C infection can be life threatening (see chapter 5 for details and notes about vaccines).

Hepatitis B (HBV)

Identified in 1965, this is an immunopathic virus. It is transmitted from mother to child, via infected blood and blood products, using needles contaminated with blood, and sexually. Transmission is prevented by blood screening, the use of sterile injecting equipment, and safe sex. There is now a highly effective vaccine available that is actively contributing to significantly lower global prevalence of this virus, which infected several hundred million people at its peak. (The development of a vaccine was made simpler by the fact that HBV is a relatively stable virus compared to HCV.)

Acute HBV infection tends to cause more severe symptoms, but is rarely fatal. About 7% of adults infected fail to clear the virus and become chronic carriers; the rate is higher in young children. Chronic means that the virus persists after the acute phase. Chronicity can lead to long-term liver problems, such as cirrhosis and cancer.

Hepatitis D (HDV)

This virus requires the presence of HBV for its own replication and is therefore found exclusively in HBV patients. The two viruses may be contracted at the same time (coinfection), or an existing HBV carrier may become infected with HDV (superinfection).

Both coinfection and superinfection tend to lead to more severe acute and chronic liver disease.

Hepatitis E (HEV)

Identified in 1990, this is transmitted via the fecal-oral route, most commonly causing disease in humans via contaminated drinking water; it causes high levels of mortality during pregnancy. It is largely confined to developing countries, though cases do occasionally occur in the West.

Explicitly mapped in the early 1990s, it is a single-stranded RNA virus without an envelope. A vaccine will hopefully be available soon.

Hepatitis F (HFV)

It is inferred that this virus exists.

Hepatitis G (GBV)

Three new flavivirus-like strains were identified in 1995. Collectively referred to as HGV (hepatitis G virus), the disparate strains are termed GBV (standing for GB virus) types A, B, and C. They are most closely related to each other but are also similar to HCV, and may even be a mutation of the same basic virus. A PCR test is now available. No antibody test has been developed yet, but specialists suspect that the numbers infected may compare to HCV. One survey of London blood donors, a heavily screened group, revealed a prevalence of 1.5%. This is potentially worrying.

Some doctors have been quick to conclude that the virus is harmless, or at least not a major cause of liver disease. It is worth noting that this is what they said about HCV when it was first discovered. The jury is still out.

Around 20% of HCV patients may be coinfected with hepatitis G. It may play a role in the pathogenesis of secondary conditions such as lymphoma. GBV is thought to be more easily transmitted via sexual intercourse.

TTV

This is another "new" virus recently discovered in Japan and found to be present in 10% of "healthy" blood donors in the U.K. according to one small study. The relationship between TTV and other forms of viral hepatitis and its role in the development of liver disease either as a single agent or as a cofactor is unclear. Research into TTV is still in its infancy.

Note

The discovery of GBV and TTV and the detection of significant numbers of people across the globe who have been exposed to these agents raises serious questions with regard to international public health. It is now clear that so far as viruses are concerned the world really has become a much smaller place.

5

Coinfected Patients

Hepatitis A and Hepatitis C

PEOPLE WITH CHRONIC hepatitis C may be at particular risk of life-threatening episodes of fulminant hepatitis if they are exposed to hepatitis A. One recent study followed 432 patients with chronic hepatitis C for seven years. Seventeen chronic hepatitis C patients contracted hepatitis A during this period.

> Fulminant hepatic failure (severe liver failure with hepatic encephalopathy) developed in seven of the patients with chronic hepatitis C but none with chronic hepatitis B. None of these seven individuals with chronic hepatitis C had cirrhosis. All but one of the patients with chronic hepatitis C and HAV infection with fulminant hepatic failure died. None of 191 control individuals with acute HAV infection alone had fulminant hepatic failure. These results suggest that individuals with chronic hepatitis C may be at an increased risk of developing fulminant hepatic failure and death if infected with HAV.

Other studies paint a less gloomy picture. Nonetheless doctors recommend that people with hepatitis C obtain hepatitis A vaccination, particularly if travelling abroad (see page 91 for more details).

Hepatitis B and Hepatitis C

Acute hepatitis B is dangerous and can kill patients on its own or in synergy with hepatitis D, which is linked to B, although this is rare. Some doctors feel that the likelihood of this happening is increased in patients who already have hepatitis C; they therefore recommend that HCV patients at risk from hepatitis B (homosexual men and IVDUs in the main) get vaccinated against HBV. However, the vaccination is regarded as posing a health risk in its own right by some commentators, who claim that it may be linked to M.E. Several patients have reported an upsurge in HCV symptoms following an HBV vaccination. This experience is difficult to quantify but seems to be unusual. Patients need to make up their own minds. Obviously minimizing or eliminating the prospect of infection is also a good option (see "Transmission" section in chapter 2).

Less than 10% of those exposed to hepatitis B as adults go on to become chronic carriers. In theory these two viruses, dangerous enough on their own, let alone combined, should cause more serious damage at a faster rate. The immunopathic elements of HBV might be expected to be synergistic with the cytopathic and immunopathic characteristics of HCV. The carcinogenic qualities of both viruses might be expected to result in earlier instances and higher rates of liver cancer.

In practice this is not proven. Some reports into coinfection conclude that HCV may actually suppress the replication of HBV.[1] It seems that other factors such as alcohol consumption have a greater influence over the chances of developing liver cancer. Therefore the prognosis for patients with both viruses is probably worse, but not dramatically so. More research needs to be done here.

So far as drug treatments are concerned, interferon alpha has been used in both conditions and would be the obvious choice to try to "kill two birds with one stone." However, some reports suggest limited effectiveness. Traditional Chinese Medicine is also a viable option—it simply treats patients as they present, although patients should tell practitioners that they have both viruses. The anticarcinogenic measures outlined in various parts of this book are particularly relevant. Hypericin (derived from St. John's wort—see chapter 16) may be active against both viruses.

Human Immunodeficiency Virus (HIV) and Hepatitis C

Being both HIV+ and HCV+ is regarded as extremely serious by most doctors. It seems that hepatitis C does not cause a more aggressive course of HIV-related disease. However, HIV-related immunosuppression may be associated with a more malign course of HCV-related disease. Because immunosuppression causes lower liver enzymes, this indicator of damage is unreliable in these circumstances.

CD4 cells are thought to play a key role in immune response to viral infections. (See the notes on the immune system in Part 5). While patients with reasonable CD4 counts may not have worse than average HCV symptoms, it seems that more advanced cases of HIV and the AIDS status may be associated with more severe liver damage and faster progression than would otherwise be the case.[2] The levels of fibrosis were more advanced than expected from the overall severity of liver inflammation, suggesting that HIV may directly augment liver damage caused by HCV.

Patients with lowered CD4 counts have been found to have higher levels of HCV viremia in their blood. This indicates the important role of the immune system in countering HCV; if the immune system itself is under attack, as is the case with HIV, then damage may proceed more rapidly.

Some HCV antibody markers may disappear when HIV is also present, a factor that may have caused some positive patients to have tested negative for HCV with the early tests. Some researchers interpreted this as a sign that HIV inhibits the replication of HCV; unfortunately this is not the case.

There is also the theory that autoimmune diseases associated with HCV are less likely to occur in immunocompromised HIV patients. The picture seems to indicate the prospect of more severe liver damage and less severe autoimmune disease. Again more research needs to be carried out. It has been shown that patients who are coinfected with HIV and HCV are more likely to be infectious than others. The exact reason for this is not known, but it probably has something to do with higher viral loads in body fluids. Thus coinfected patients need to be particularly careful when it comes to preventing transmission.

So far as treatments are concerned, these two conditions can make life very awkward for patients and doctors alike. Many HIV drug treatments carry a risk of liver inflammation (e.g., AZT and ddI), although this does not necessarily amount to a clear-cut contraindication. Doctors are quite likely to adopt a "suck it and see" approach if patients are keen to try. It seems that if HCV treatment is carried out before AIDS has developed or CD4 count has declined too far, then the prospects for success are the same as for individuals with HCV alone. Interferon alpha is sometimes used to treat Kaposi's sarcoma, although its results as an HIV treatment have been disappointing. Generally, interferon-based therapy is contraindicated for HIV patients with dropping CD4 counts as it may lower counts further.

Analysis of the results of coinfected patients treated with the newer HIV antiviral drugs provides mixed conclusions. In one individual case, treatment with protease inhibitors had no impact on HCV but helped to resolve serious secondary cryoglobulinemia. Improved CD4 counts are thought to have helped.[3]

A second study of nineteen coinfected patients treated with protease inhibitors found that both HCV titres and liver enzymes rose during the therapy, indicating an adverse impact.[4]

A more positive aspect of HIV and HCV is that the technology used to develop treatments developed for the former may enable the design of more effective treatments for the latter. Much depends upon the ability to develop HCV cell lines for laboratory analysis, a task that is proving challenging to the technologists concerned.

Some of the herbal medicines developed to treat HIV might be tested for activity against HCV. Todoxin or some of the Chinese herbal formulations tested in China and East Africa spring to mind as possibilities. Metanalysis of the antiviral or "heat clearing" herbs in the Chinese materia medica has demonstrated the presence of naturally occurring nucleoside analogues, protease inhibitors, and noncompetitive reverse transcriptase inhibitors. The organic messaging model of cellular antiviral activity developed by John Babish looks like a promising basis for identifying the plants that may contain specific anti-HCV and anti-HIV ingredients.

Alternatively, hypericin, an extract derived from the plant St. John's wort, has been suggested by researchers as a suitable therapy for HIV and HCV coinfected patients. This is because it is thought to exercise a broad effect on both of these types of virus (see chapter 16 for more details).

The compound Todoxin is an option worth exploring (see pages 304–305 for details). N-acetyl cysteine would also seem to be a useful therapeutic resource for HIV-HCV patients (see pages 339–343).

A further observation is that HCV-HIV coinfected patients are more infectious with regard to HCV than other patients. Coinfected mothers are more likely to pass HCV on to their children at birth. Coinfected men may have higher viral loads in semen, which may reach sexually infectious concentrations, thought to be very unusual in men with HCV only.

Hepatitis C and Hepatitis G (GBV)

Research into hepatitis G is still at an early stage, but it seems to indicate that it is not an important cause of liver disease or other detectable illnesses on its own. However, some recent studies suggest that coinfection with hepatitis G may be a factor in accelerated progression. One report concluded:

> GBV-C RNA was detected more frequently in patients with liver cirrhosis or hepatocellular carcinoma than in those with chronic hepatitis in the present study. This could reflect a possible role of GBV-C in aggravating liver disease in co-operation with the other hepatitis viruses. The studied patients with chronic hepatitis were younger than those with liver cirrhosis or hepatocellular carcinoma, however, leaving the duration of disease as another contributing factor for the progression of liver disease.[5]

However, it may be the case that some of the other conditions associated with hep C, such as lymphatic disorders, may be linked to coinfection with hep G. HGV levels can be reduced or rendered undetectable by interferon-based therapy, although rates of response are low, say, 20–30%.

A Note about HIV and HCV

A lot of the work that has been carried out in HIV research has proved to be vital in the development of an understanding of HCV. Without the technological advances made by HIV researchers, it is arguable that HCV might never have even been discovered, let alone understood.

Breakthroughs in the understanding of HIV seem to be mirrored a short time later in HCV. For instance, Dr. Ho's theories of the relationship between the immune system and viral progression are applicable to HCV, particularly the notion of "reservoirs." The discovery that some people are effectively immune to HIV because of certain human leucocyte antigen combinations was quickly followed by an analysis of HCV patients that suggested a similar mechanism. Hopefully the story will be concluded by a similar discovery of clear-cut cures for both viruses. The prospects do not seem as remote as they once did.

References

1. HBV replication in patients with HCV + HBV dual infection. Mathurin P et al. Sce d'Hepatogastroenterologie, Hopital Pitie-Salpetiere, URA CNRS 1484.

2. Influence of HIV infection on hepatic lesions related to HCV infection. Benhamou JP et al. Service d'Hepato-Gastroenterologie, GH Pitie-Salpetiere, 75651 Paris Cedex 13, France.

3. Arthralgias and cryoglobulinemia during protease inhibitor therapy in a patient infected with human immunodeficiency virus and hepatitis C virus. Monsuez JJ et al. *Arthritis Rheum*, 41(4):740–743, Apr 1998.

4. Impact of treatment with human immunodeficiency virus (HIV) protease inhibitors on hepatitis C viremia in patients coinfected with HIV. Rutschmann OT et al. *J Infect Dis*, 177(3):783–785, Mar 1998.

5. Infection with GB virus C in patients with chronic liver disease. *Journal of Medical Virology*, 51:175–181, March 1997.

6

Children and Parents

Thanks are due to the Children's Liver Disease Foundation and Professor Giorgina Mieli-Vergani, director of the Pediatric Liver Service, Kings College London, for helping to compile and edit this chapter.

THIS IS A VERY IMPORTANT, difficult, and sensitive area. Relatively speaking, children with hepatitis C are probably the fastest-growing section of the HCV+ population in Canada, the U.K., and the U.S. The following is an attempt to answer typical questions and relate both the expert advice of doctors and the experiences of parents and children coping with hepatitis C.

Prognosis, Progression, and Spontaneous Clearance

The prognosis for HCV+ children as a whole is unknown because positive diagnosis has only been possible since 1991. With average normal life expectancy now in the seventies in many Western countries, the full picture will only become clear with the benefit of hindsight in many decades' time. It seems highly likely that effective and well-understood therapies will be widely available before then, which may normalize life expectancy.

Babies who are infected with HCV at birth (6–7% according to Dr. Mieli-Vergani) are the most theoretically likely group to experience diminished life expectancy. This is simply because the virus has a longer period to evolve and is therefore more likely to cause serious problems. Data is not yet available to assess how many become chronic virus carriers or the rate and degree of progression of this group. It is not yet known how the immature immune system responds to the virus, although it is known that HCV antibody formation may not occur until a year or two later. Thus the PCR or b-DNA tests need to be used in this group. The situation is further complicated by the fact that some mothers pass on HCV antibodies to their babies but not the virus itself. Thus a HCV-antibody-positive baby may not have HCV. Doctors are currently trying to recruit HCV+ babies for further study.

According to Dr. Graham Alexander, consultant hepatologist at Addenbrooke's Hospital in Cambridge, HCV may not "like" young liver cells. Infection may be present, but replication does not take place until later, when certain substances known as "transcription factors" appear in liver cells. This theory is subject to further investigation and verification. In addition he believes that the overall mother-to-child transmission rate is 8%, lower figures being based upon the inadequacy of detection methods. The good news is that he believes that a youthful immune system is more capable of identifying and engaging the virus, resulting in a more "educated" response by the immune system. Thus prognosis may be better for children than for people infected in later years.

The situation for infants and children infected after birth is clearer. There has been some work done on children infected by blood transfusion in Japan. The study looked at HCV progression over a period of three years in forty-eight children with an average age of twelve years. Remarkably the clinicians found that four of these children (8.3%) cleared the virus from their blood spontaneously during this period. However, it was later found that one of these still had HCV in their liver tissue. (This is an important qualification to the claims of "clearance" in all patient groups.) This finding would tend to confirm Alexander's theory of the relative efficiency of youthful immune response. Likelihood of spontaneous remission was positively associated with low viral load:

A low serum titre of HCV RNA and a significant decrease in the serum titre of anti-HCV core were associated with spontaneous remission in children with chronic hepatitis C. Intrahepatic HCV RNA assessment is necessary to confirm complete remission.[1]

Another significant group with HCV are those who have been exposed during treatment for childhood leukemia. Because such patients are very likely to have contracted HCV through this route only and the dates of treatment are known, it is possible to draw inferences about progression over a longer period, stretching back to before the introduction of tests. An Italian study found that ninety-four out of 114 patients who had been treated for leukemia prior to blood screening and treatment became HCV antibody positive; thirty-three of this ninety-four ceased to react to the HCV antibody test over the follow-up period ranging from eleven to twenty-seven years after presumed infection. Only four patients demonstrated persistently abnormal liver enzymes, and none showed signs of advanced liver disease over this period.[2]

Thus it appears that a significant proportion of patients infected during childhood effectively neutralize the virus, while most of the others tend to have normal liver enzymes. However, biopsy does reveal a degree of progression in children with normal liver enzymes. Professor Mieli-Vergani reports:

> I have performed follow-up biopsies in some of these children and have observed worsening of liver disease, albeit not dramatic.... It is likely that in children, as in adults, the viral genotype, the viral load and presence or not of iron in the liver, may be important facts in determining the severity of liver disease.

Thus the overall situation appears to be far from dire. The observation that a much higher proportion of children appear to deal with the virus naturally compared to adults is good news. This accords with the view of some practitioners that children's constitutions are usually more "balanced" than those of adults. Rapid progression appears to be rare, but cannot be discounted; as is the case in adults, children with depressed immune response may be more likely to progress.

Symptoms

It seems that most children do not present with significant symptoms, although, as with adults, some manifestations of HCV can be subtle and very difficult to quantify. One factor relates to the response of parents, who may unconsciously transmit anxiety to their children. Professor Mieli-Vergani reports:

> Generally speaking children with chronic hepatitis C virus infection have no symptoms. This experience is not only mine, but also in larger series like the ones from Professor Vegnente and Professor Bortolotti in Italy. What I have observed is that once the parents know that the child is HCV positive, they become tremendously anxious and their anxieties certainly filter to the child. I have therefore seen psychological problems related to hepatitis C infection, but to me they seem to be mainly related to the fact that there is knowledge of having a chronic infection.

Response to a Child's Diagnosis and Related Family Issues

This issue is often more problematic for the parents of those children diagnosed than for adults receiving the bad news (this is covered in part 2). Having to take responsibility for making decisions about another person's health is more difficult than making decisions on one's own behalf.

Sue has a son, Christopher, who contracted hepatitis C during treatment for lymphoblastic leukemia.

> Thankfully after many infections and stays in hospital, Christopher appears to have beaten the leukemia. However, about two years ago, the hospital contacted us and said that Christopher needed to be tested for hepatitis C, as there was a chance that he could have been infected by a blood transfusion given to him during treatment in 1991–2. This test proved that Christopher was in fact hep C positive.
>
> We were devastated and angry at first. To think that he had

beaten leukemia (as far as is possible), but now had another disease through no fault of his own, but that it was certainly someone's fault!

We were referred to the liver unit, again at the Birmingham Children's hospital, and we took some comfort in knowing that the unit had a very good reputation and that Dr. Deirdre Kelly was one of the best hepatologists in the country.

Christopher underwent a biopsy, and the results confirmed that there was "significant" damage to his liver. We were told that when treatment became available we would be contacted. Christopher knows about the hep C in as much as it is another cross for him to bear. It is over a year now, and we have heard nothing. I think I might ring the hospital now and ask if anything is in the pipeline.

James, the father of an HCV+ seven-year-old daughter, Amie, relates his experience:

The diagnosis came as a shock, although I was assured by the doctor that there was no immediate cause for concern. The implications only began to sink in when I started to hear stories about hep C sometimes causing cancer, at which point I decided to research it myself. My wife and I, who are now separated, became wary of the drug therapy and have been exploring other available avenues of approach in detail. We have not told Amie yet. I would like to be able to tell her after she has been cured. That would be nice. But I don't know what will work. Because she has an unfavorable genotype and also because of some excellent personal recommendations, we are going to try a highly regarded and appropriately specialized TCM practitioner. I have also looked at hypericin in depth.

The question of whether, when, or how to tell a child that they have hepatitis C is very difficult. There is no correct solution. It is advisable to seek expert advice if you have any doubts, particularly as this is now readily available. Specialist counselors will often tell clients that there are no such things as secrets in families. Children "know" that something is wrong long before they are explicitly told;

subtle changes in family dynamics and the "messages" given out by parents will be "picked up" by all family members, whether they are privy to facts or not. Such therapists will often conclude that it is healthier to share such information openly as early as is reasonable.

Teenage Issues

Andrew has had hep C since birth but was only diagnosed at age twelve. The doctor explained the situation in a very reassuring way, stressing the usually benign course. However, the restrictions imposed by hep C soon began to affect his life. The crunch came when he was fourteen and started to drink beer after school with his buddies—peer pressure I believe. He was also beginning to smoke cigarettes and pot. Having learnt enough about hep C to know that this was particularly dangerous, I decided I had to lecture him.

Andrew found it difficult to take on board. I think the worst thing for him was feeling that he couldn't behave like his friends, that there was something setting him apart. I now realize that I had become very protective towards him and that he needs to face his situation. I cannot alter his reality or make things different; I'd be doing more harm than good.

Sex is another important area, where briefing kids with hepatitis C on the need for "safe sex" is likely to be particularly difficult for both parents and teenagers. Again professional counselors may be able to help.

Treatment

Professor Mieli-Vergani reports on drug therapy in children:

Results of treatment in children are very similar to those in adults, although there are currently only two small studies. In both of them results appear to be more promising than in adults because there was a 50% viral clearance. I am in contact with both researchers, and both of them tell me that quite a number of their patients have relapsed now, having stopped the treatment. I think that probably 22–25% of the children treated with interferon have a sustained response, a fraction better than the results in adults. We are currently discussing a pilot study using interferon and ribavirin with Schering-Plough.

What I have noticed is that children with hepatitis C infection tolerate interferon much less well than children with chronic hepatitis B infection. They appear to have many more side effects, particularly behavioral side effects, and they become very tired, very withdrawn, and upset. I often have to modify the dose because of the side effects.

Chapter 8 includes results from young patients taking drug therapy.

Children are thought to respond better than adults to other therapeutic approaches such as homeopathy and Traditional Chinese Medicine.

Overview of the Situation for Children and Parents

Professor Mieli-Vergani comments:

It is difficult to give clear messages to parents. My message is usually that we still do not know enough about chronic hepatitis C infection in children, that vaccination is not likely to be available very soon, that current treatment is not particularly satisfactory and therefore new forms of treatment need to be investigated. I feel very strongly, however, that they should only be investigated in specialized centers where a significant number of children can be recruited so that meaningful results are produced. The major risk is that everybody starts treating these children, for example with interferon, so there will not be any children in whom to try new modes of treatment, starting from zero. This is happening in America where, although interferon is well recognized as being not so effective, it is now prescribed to practically all children with chronic HCV infection.

Experiences of Treatment

Kari D. is the mother of eleven-year-old daughter A., who has hepatitis C.

I had A. tested only after talking to my ex-partner, who was aware of the potential for mother-to-child HCV transmission. She was diagnosed when she was eight. At that time she was lethargic, skinny and underweight, looked run down, had black bags under her eyes, and didn't want to get up in the morning. There was a general air of lethargic despondency about her. I was aware that this was unusual for kids of that age, who were usually full of energy.

When we went to the specialist, I soon felt that I was being pressured into letting her have a biopsy with a view to taking interferon. The implication was that by refusing to give my permission for this course of action I was being irresponsible. This was never said outright, but I nevertheless got this impression. I felt that my role as parent and mother was being challenged. It was also very clear that they were looking for children to study, and I felt that they were passing this need for "guinea pigs" onto me. This was incredibly insensitive—I think this is an astonishing way to behave toward a caring mother. I felt that they would rather mislead me than admit that they did not know. Partly because of this pressure, I changed specialists. The new doctor, an Australian, was far more open minded.

At about this time I was given the name of John Tindall as another approach. I believe in self-healing, and so the herbal approach seemed more appropriate. I felt that the biopsy process was tantamount to tampering with my daughter. The thought of her having injections in her stomach was just awful. So I insisted upon trying the Chinese herbal approach first. By this time the Australian doctor was also applying pressure to have her on drug therapy, informing me that they knew of one child infected at birth who had needed a liver transplant at the age of eighteen.

The new doctor agreed to support the herbal approach, but

stated that if there were no clear clinical improvements within six months he would recommend the biopsy and interferon route.

Things started to improve straightaway after starting the herbs. She started to put on weight, to the extent that she is now quite plump, she got up early, and generally became a bright, happy, and healthy child. Tindall stressed the importance of learning to relax, and we now take time out together, doing nothing in particular, going for a walk. At first she hated the taste of the herbs, so I tried mixing them with honey or fruit juice. John Tindall talked to her, suggesting that she imagine the medicine as her friend, helping her to be well. Now she takes them religiously; her whole attitude is to make herself better.

The Australian doctor was very surprised and impressed, to the extent that he now recommends that we continue this approach. He asked me, "Who is this John Tindall?" He seemed to be quite literally stunned. Her blood tests have shown continuing improvement over the past eighteen months. The change in her general health is unmistakable.

I feel vindicated in making this choice. I think there is a lot to be said for this approach.

Parents thinking of following up this approach should refer to the sections "Finding a TCM Practitioner" and "Safety, Toxicity, Quality Control, and Other Considerations" in chapter 15.

I interviewed the doctor managing Kari and A.'s case, Vas Novelli, consultant pediatrician in infective diseases at Great Ormond Street Children's Hospital in London. He reported that A.'s HCV PCR tests had recorded a steady decline since starting treatment with John Tindall. The results were

- 2 million copies per ml of blood prior to treatment in February 1996

- 1.14 million copies per ml of blood in September 1996

- 194,000 copies per ml of blood in February 1997

- 79,000 copies per ml of blood in December 1997

Thus a steady decline in HCV viral load occurred during treatment by John Tindall using Chinese herbs; the level at the time of the last test represents 4% of the initial level, indicating a very significant improvement.

Novelli stressed that not enough is known about the natural history of the virus in children to draw any firm conclusions from this one case, but did describe the results as very encouraging, commenting, "It would seem very unlikely that this would happen on its own."

He also defended the right of parents to select complementary therapy, pointing out that he was getting good experience as a result. He went on to stress the importance of lookback programs to identify any other children who might have been exposed to HCV. He dismissed the principal objection by the governing authorities, who resist lookback on the grounds of there not being effective treatment. His experience of both conventional and TCM treatment confirmed that therapy is available and that parents of HCV+ children should be told. Asked about specific areas where more research was required, he commented that more needed to be known about the immune response of children both pre- and postnatal. Novelli is looking forward to the results of a current study into natural history of HCV being funded by the U.K. government at the Institute for Child Health.

Christine is the mother of James, who is thirteen, hemophiliac and HCV+:

> James was diagnosed as having NANB hepatitis when he was very young, three or four years old. He was positively diagnosed with HCV in 1991. This was later confirmed as being type 1b at the level of 5 million copies per ml. His hepatitis was also described as being "aggressive" on biopsy.
>
> By nature James is a very strong character, lives life like there is no tomorrow, and has a very positive attitude. He is very fit, keen on games, and excels both in the classroom, where he often gets As, and on the sports field. Although he knows about the hep C, he has never restricted himself in any way; he only gets grumpy when he is cooped up indoors.
>
> In 1995 we were referred to a specialist center for the treat-

ment of liver disease in children and told about a new treatment called interferon. We were warned that it had side effects
and that the chances of success were 50:50 or so. We decided
to go for it, and treatment commenced in September 1996.

James was very brave but was also obviously frightened. He
knew he had a chance and wanted to try. I think they put him
on 6 million units of interferon three times per week. He spent
the first three days in hospital, and they showed him how to
cope with the drug and syringe packaging and do the injections.
Later in the treatment we attended a regional center for blood
tests and general monitoring. A few weeks later they changed
the packaging, and this caused a lot of problems to James. I
told them he was having these difficulties and asked them if
they could change back to the original.

The local doctor was quite snotty about it, saying that the
packaging could not be changed back. When I asked him about
how James was doing, he refused to share the results or explain
how James was doing. When I questioned him he threatened
to discontinue the treatment if I continued to make a fuss. He
also scared James, who said that the doctor was making him
feel uncomfortable. I feel very strongly that only doctors with
specific experience of dealing with children should be seeing
kids in this position. What he did eventually tell us was that
James's blood counts were dangerously low and that they were
considering taking him off the drug. James started to lose confidence at around this point. This crisis was eventually overcome, and his blood counts returned to normal; his viral load
went undetectable. I refused to see the same doctor; the rest of
our consultations were with somebody with a lot more sym-
pathy and empathy, so that side of things improved.

Throughout the treatment James had severe side effects. His
personality changed, toward being introspective and quiet. The
school, who knew he was on interferon, became very concerned.
He was very, very tired, falling asleep in the classroom; he was
losing his hair, he turned very pale, developed dark bags under
his eyes, and his appetite was terrible. He lost his twinkle, his
luster, and he was just not the same boy. He stopped growing

for the whole year he was on interferon. Yet he wouldn't admit to being in pain and kept positive. At night, after his injections, he would try to imagine the good that the drug was doing him. This was the worst thing that James has ever had to go through.

The treatment finished in September 1997, and soon afterwards he began to recover quickly, although he is still a bit "off-color." Otherwise he is nearly back to his old self and has started to grow again. The hospital tells me that it takes three years for the interferon to leave the system. Unfortunately the hepatitis came back. We found out in April. It is at the same level it was before treatment, so we are back to square one. I would never, ever put him back on it.

For detailed information on both the disease and treatments, please refer to the specific chapters elsewhere in the book.

Contacts

U.S.

American Liver Foundation—Children's Liver Council
See the Resources for ALF details.

Children's Blood Foundation
424 East 62nd Street
New York, NY 10021

U.K.

The **Children's Liver Disease Foundation** provides emotional support to children and families affected by liver disease. Specifically, it can provide counseling to address the feelings of isolation and despair that sometimes arise after a diagnosis. It also carries out a number of other important activities such as funding research and providing education for parents and health care professionals.

The **Family Support Officer** and the Children and **Adolescents Support Officer** can be contacted at 0121 212 3839. Or write to the Children's Liver Disease Foundation, AXA Equity and Law House, 35–37 Great Charles Street Queensway, Birmingham B3 3JY.

References

1. Spontaneous remission of chronic hepatitis C in children. Fujisawa T et al. *European Journal of Pediatrics,* 156(10):773–776, 1997.

2. Prevalence and natural history of hepatitis C infection in patients cured of childhood leukemia. Locasciulli A et al. *Blood,* 90(11):4628–4633, Dec 1, 1997.

7

Hepatitis C and Hemophilia
or Related Bleeding Disorders

This chapter was largely written by Lucy McGrath, hepatitis worker, the Hemophilia Society (U.K.).

What Is Hemophilia?

THE GENERAL TERM "HEMOPHILIA" describes a group of inherited bleeding disorders in which one of the proteins responsible for the clotting of the blood is missing or present at a very low level.

This means that the blood does not clot normally, and so if a bleed takes place, someone with hemophilia bleeds far longer than normal. In people with severe hemophilia, bleeds can take place spontaneously. Many of these bleeds can occur in joints and, unless treated quickly, can result in joint damage.

Hemophilia mainly affects men, but both men and women can suffer from similar bleeding disorders, such as von Willebrand disease. Women who are "carriers"—that is, they carry the genetic defect that may lead to hemophilia in their sons—may also suffer from bleeding problems, although these are not usually so severe.

What Relevance Has Hepatitis C
to People with Hemophilia?

In the late 1960s there was a big step forward in the treatment for hemophilia with the introduction of clotting factor concentrates obtained by pooling plasma from thousands of blood donors and then fractionating out the required clotting factor.

Some hemophiliacs treated with clotting factor concentrates from the 1960s, 1970s, and early 1980s developed an acute, then unknown, form of hepatitis, known as "non-A, non-B." It is now known that most of these cases of "unknown" hepatitis were caused by the acute stage of hepatitis C.

In 1985, after the discovery of the HIV virus and the realization that it could be transmitted through blood and blood products, heat treatment to destroy the virus was introduced into the production of clotting factor concentrates. At this time the hepatitis C virus had still not been identified. After it was identified and a reliable test became available (1991), many hemophiliacs were tested, and subsequent studies showed that nearly 100% of hemophiliacs treated with clotting factor concentrates between 1967 and 1985 in the U.K. were infected with the hepatitis C virus. Rates of HCV among the people with hemophilia who received clotting factor before the mid-1980s in the U.S. have been reported to be as high as 90%.

Records of the exact number of people infected in this way have not been kept, but, it is likely that about 5,000 people with hemophilia or a related bleeding disorder were infected in the U.K. In the U.S. it is theorized that at least 70% of people within the hemophilia community have been infected with HCV. This includes not just people with severe hemophilia who require regular treatments, but also those with mild or moderate hemophilia who may have been treated once or twice in their life. It includes both men and women with von Willebrand disease and some women carriers. About 1,200 of these people were also coinfected with HIV.

Many hemophiliacs were tested for hepatitis C without their knowledge, and then not informed for several years. This has caused a great deal of anger.

People living with hepatitis C and hemophilia are affected by and respond to their infection in a variety of ways. Many of the issues will be similar to issues faced by others living with hepatitis C acquired by a different transmission route, but there are some differences, as follows.

Health Issues

Treatments

Some studies suggest that people with hemophilia have significantly lower long-term sustained response rates to interferon-alpha than other hepatitis C sufferers. This may be for various reasons: hemophiliacs are often found to have genotype 1, which is thought to respond less well to treatment with interferon; people with hemophilia were repeatedly infected with hepatitis C and may carry many different strains of the virus; and length of time since infection—most hemophiliacs have been infected for about twenty years or more.

Liver Biopsy

There is much debate in the hemophilia community about the use of liver biopsy, due to the possibility of bleeding complications. If a liver biopsy is performed in someone with hemophilia, care is taken to ensure that the levels of clotting factor proteins in the blood are raised to normal levels. While biopsies are increasingly being performed, usually with very close collaboration between a hematologist and a hepatologist, many hematologists still regard it as a risky procedure and choose instead to monitor their patients through a combination of blood tests, ultrasound, and so on. Liver-biopsy-related deaths have occurred.

Liver Transplantation

Liver transplants may well become more common in the management and treatment of hemophilia. Twenty-six transplants performed on people with hemophilia have been reported in the literature, and survival rates are comparable to other patients with hepatitis C who have a transplant, although with the added bonus for people with hemophilia that their hemophilia is cured.

Coinfection

About 1,200 people with hemophilia in the U.K. were coinfected with HIV. Of these about 600 people are still alive. There is still much work to be done to understand how HIV and hepatitis C interact, but it appears that hepatitis C can progress more quickly in people coinfected with HIV.

Psychological and Social Impact

Many of the issues facing people with hemophilia and hepatitis C are those faced by other hepatitis C sufferers, including the major problem that it is not yet possible to predict which individuals are likely to develop cirrhosis, liver cancer, or other more serious non-hepatic complications. While some will remain well, they all have to live with uncertainty over their future health and the stress and anxiety this creates.

Other issues may include problems getting life insurance and mortgages, living with fatigue, disrupted schooling or employment, and dealing with stigma and discrimination.

Anger at what has happened is a feature for some people with hemophilia, often those with mild hemophilia whose lives have been far more affected by hepatitis C than they ever were with hemophilia. Partly as a result of this anger, a fairly high-profile political campaign to try to obtain financial assistance for people with hemophilia infected with hepatitis C was launched in 1995.

Guilt is another feature found among people affected by hemophilia and hepatitis C. Many parents of children who have been infected carry feelings of guilt and responsibility for having administered the treatment that gave their child the infection.

The impact on individuals varies according to personal circumstances, but because hemophilia is an inherited condition, families are often affected through several generations. In some families, uncles, brothers, and nephews have all been infected by hepatitis C.

Conclusion

People with hemophilia, once a life-threatening condition itself, have seen treatments improve radically in the past fifty years. While these advances have brought many benefits, they have also brought many problems through the introduction of viral infections, particularly hepatitis C and HIV.

HIV affected about one-fifth of people with hemophilia and has devastated some families. Hepatitis C has affected far more people, as nearly everyone with hemophilia who received treatment before 1986 was infected. Given the nature of hepatitis C, and the fact that some people may live without symptoms for very many years, it is not really possible to quantify the full impact of this virus on the hemophilia community. For those infected the main hope for the future lies in the development of new and more effective treatments.

For those in the U.K. with hemophilia who have not been infected with hepatitis C, most of whom are children, hope for the future now rests in making genetically engineered clotting factors as widely available as possible. There is no guarantee that these products are "risk-free," but the hope is that they will reduce or prevent the possibility of further viral infections in the future.

Contacts

U.S.

The National Hemophilia Foundation
Soho Building, Room 303
110 Greene Street
New York, NY 10012
Tel: (212) 219-8180
Fax: (212) 966-9247

U.K.

The Hemophilia Society
Chesterfield House
385 Euston Road,
London NW1 3AU
Tel: 0171 380 0600
Fax: 0171 387 8220
E-mail: info@hemophilia-soc.demon.co.uk
Website: www.hemophilia-soc.demon.co.uk

The Hemophilia Society offers support, advice, and information to people with hemophilia or a related bleeding disorder.

Ireland

The Irish Hemophilia Society, Dublin
01872 4466

8

Thalassaemia/Cooley's Anemia
and Hepatitis C

I am indebted to Dr. Beatrix Wonke, MD, FRCPATH, MRCP, consultant hematologist at the Whittington Hospital, London, for providing much of the following information.

This aspect of hepatitis C is included both as a service to thalassaemiac HCV patients and because certain findings from studies of this group of patients may cast light on questions for the general HCV+ population. Two areas of interest are the treatment of younger patients and factors that may influence the overall response to drug therapy. (Thalassaemia is known as "Cooley's anemia" in the U.S.)

What is Thalassaemia and Cooley's Anemia?

Thalassaemia is an inherited blood disorder characterized by the inability to make sufficient hemoglobin—the oxygen-carrying liquid in red blood cells; because life is unsustainable without this substance, patients need to receive blood transfusions on a regular basis—typically every month—throughout their lives. Prior to the availability of blood transfusions, many with this condition died, usually before reaching the age of five. In the words of Dr. Wonke, "This is the first generation of survivors."

Because of this dependency on transfused blood, many thalassaemiacs have hepatitis C. Overall HCV infection rates in thalassaemiacs vary; in Italy it is nearly 75%, but only 35% in the U.K.

The introduction of blood donor screening and treatment in industrialized regions such as North America and Western Europe has effectively cut off this route of infection in these areas. Thus patients born in these countries now have virtually nil rates of infection. However, immigrants from Asia, the Middle East, and the Mediterranean region—thalassaemia is mainly confined to these particular areas of ethnic origin—still harbor high rates of exposure to HCV. (Note that a related hereditary disorder, sickle cell anemia, is found in people of Afro-Caribbean origin.)

Hepatitis C in Patients
with Thalassaemia and Cooley's Anemia

Because thalassaemia presents very early in life and requires life-long monitoring, HCV progression can be followed closely. Although there is no direct synergy between thalassaemia and hepatitis C, some secondary factors may make the situation more serious.

As with all groups dependent upon blood and blood products, there is a higher prevalence of other blood-borne viruses such as hepatitis B and HIV, which will mean that overall prognosis will theoretically be poorer than average.

A second factor is the presence of abnormally high levels of iron in liver cells and in the blood, recognized as being a common feature of thalassaemia; this is thought to be caused by regular blood transfusions, which introduce high levels of iron. As demonstrated in chapter 1, higher concentrations of iron in liver cells are associated with accelerated liver disease progression and reduced response to interferon. Although high iron or ferritin levels in the blood do not necessarily indicate cellular overload,[1] they are worrying. It has also been shown that thalassaemia patients with HCV have higher levels of serum ferritin compared to those who are HCV negative. This implies that HCV infection exacerbates this problem. The authors of the report commented:

> Our results show that the serum ferritin concentration is roughly doubled by ongoing chronic necrosis and inflammatory changes in patients with iron overload and chronic hepatitis C.[2]

Thalassaemia patients with elevated levels of serum ferritin may be prescribed a medicine called Desferal (desferrioxamine), which reduces levels of cellular iron and prevents associated damage.[3] It appears that those with HCV may require higher doses.

Patients may be advised to avoid food with high iron content such as prunes. Vitamin C should be generally avoided because it causes increases in levels of iron absorption from the gut except when taking Desferal, when it enhances the effect of the drug.

A further adverse factor is the increased risk of spleen enlargement as a result of frequent blood transfusion. Sometimes the organ has to be removed. Because the spleen acts as a blood filter and plays a role in overall immune function, patients who have had a splenectomy have more frequent episodes of bacterial infection.

Response to Drug Therapy— A "Well-Behaved Population"

Despite these adverse factors, thalassaemia patients appear to have an excellent response rate to interferon and interferon/ribavirin drug therapy. Dr. Wonke reckons that her patients' results are the best found anywhere; patients are started on interferon alone; if there is no response after three months, ribavirin is added to the therapy. She reckons that 30% have a sustained response to the interferon alone and a further 40% to the combination therapy, leading to an overall sustained response at six months post-therapy of 70%.[4,5] (Treatment regime of 3 MU IFN three times per week plus 1 g of ribavirin daily.) Sustained responders also demonstrated reduced blood ferritin levels.

Dr. Wonke reckons that the relative youth of her patients is the key factor determining this high rate of response and concludes that all thalassaemic children should be tested for hep C every year and quickly referred for treatment if found to be positive. The median age of her patients undergoing combination therapy was twenty-five years old. Wonke also thinks that relative youth also contributed to the ability of her patients to tolerate treatment with few problems. Findings from these studies would also seem to provide strong evidence supporting the need for early detection of HCV infection in the wider population.

A second factor unique to this group of patients is the frequent receipt of blood transfusions while undergoing therapy; the side effects of ribavirin necessitated increased frequency of blood transfusion. Frequent blood replacement might be a factor worth investigating for its bearing on viral clearance.

Contacts

U.S.

Cooley's Anemia Foundation Inc.
Gina Cioffi
National Executive Director
129/09 26th Avenue, Suite 203
Flushing, NY 11354
Tel: (800) 522-7222 or (718) 321-CURE
Fax: (718) 321-3340

Children's Blood Foundation
424 East 62nd Street
New York, NY 10021

U.K.

U.K. Thalassaemia Society
107 Nightingale Lane
London N8 7QY
Tel: (0181) 348 0437

References

1. Serum ferritin in patients with iron overload and with acute and chronic liver diseases. Prieto J, Barry M, Sherlock S. *Gastroenterol,* 68, 525–33, 1975.

2. Antibody to hepatitis C virus in multiply transfused patients with thalassaemia major. Wonke B, Hoffbrand AV, Brown D, Dusheiko G. *J Clin Pathol,* 43, 638–40, 1990.

3. *What is Thalassaemia?* Vullon R, Modell B, and Georganda E. pp 47–52. Published by The Thalassaemia International Federation, 1995.

4. Alpha interferon in the treatment of chronic hepatitis C in thalassaemia major, Donohue SM, Wonke B et al. *British Journal of Hematology,* 83, 491–497, 1993.

5. Combination therapy with interferon alpha and ribavirin for chronic hepatitis C virus infection in thalassaemic patients. Telfer PT et al. *British Journal of Hematology,* 98, 850–855, 1997.

9

The Liver

ALTHOUGH THE LIVER is not the only organ affected by hepatitis C and a number of symptoms are unrelated to liver disease, it is usually the site of the most potentially life-threatening HCV-related injury.

It is the largest organ in the abdomen. Situated on the right-hand side of the torso beneath the ribs, it is classified as part of the digestive system. The hepatic portal vein, which is the major source of blood supply, also drains the stomach and the bowel; it conducts the products of digestion such as amino acids and vitamins to the liver, where they are screened for toxins and then metabolized for availability by the rest of the body.

The cytochrome P450 enzyme system (described in detail in chapter 22, pages 372–378) plays a major role in the screening process. Nontoxic substances are converted into chemical products needed by other parts of the body. The liver can be seen as the body's central chemical regulator, converting raw materials into essential products and regulating a number of metabolic processes. The liver has to deal with everything that enters the body and a large proportion of the chemicals that are produced by other organs, which is why diet, alcohol, drug intake, and other lifestyle factors are thought by many doctors to have a strong bearing on the rate of disease progression.

The liver also produces bile, which is stored in the gallbladder. Bile is an important component in the digestive system, and low concentrations of bile in the intestine may be associated with some symptoms due to difficulty in digesting fats. This is why cholagogues are often prescribed to patients.

The biochemical functions of the liver include

- Energy storage and production
- Regulation of cholesterol levels and other fat levels
- Maintenance of hormonal balance
- Site for the storage of vitamins, minerals, iron, and sugars
- Production of blood clotting agents
- Site of production of proteins
- Bile production, essential for digestion
- Neutralization and destruction of toxins
- Removal of bacteria from the blood
- Metabolism of alcohol
- Regulation of levels of chemicals and drugs in the blood
- Cleansing the blood and discharging waste products into bile
- Forming blood before birth
- Production of certain immune factors
- Regeneration of its own damaged tissue

Because the liver plays such a central role in so many vital life processes, liver disease is highly likely to have a "knock on" effect on other parts of the body.

The liver also has certain important classical functions. For instance, in Chinese medicine it is seen as having certain personality- and character-related functions:

- It is the "Minister of Decision."
- It governs the ability to accept reality.
- It is the seat of kindness and courage.
- It regulates "Qi," ideally delivering a "free flow" of energy.

Thus signs of poor liver function may manifest in personality traits such as indecision, denial, anger, negativity, and malaise. Likewise a person with good liver function might display the characteristics of clear decision making, charisma, leadership, acceptance, kindness, generosity, positivity, spontaneity, and a high capacity for work and play.

Thus when it comes to assessing one's progress in terms of both treatment and lifestyle change, we can take into account a wide range of markers. The personality and subjective factors are not necessarily less important than the biochemical indicators, which are often inconclusive.

Some practitioners of "natural" medicine, particularly those from ancient systems, see the manifestation of disease as "tests" or "challenges." Thus a hepatitis C diagnosis might be seen as a particular challenge to an individual to develop the positive qualities and eliminate the negative qualities associated with the liver. They might even suggest that this is a transcendent challenge, offering the opportunity to improve karma for future lifetimes. This is fiercely contested by other doctors, who point out that such notions can induce feelings of guilt and blame. The view taken will relate to belief systems, which can always change.

Part
2

A Positive Diagnosis

10

Responding to a Diagnosis

Christine Beveridge, professional HCV educator and cofounder of the first support group in the U.K., contributed to this chapter.

IN THE FIRST INSTANCE, you will be given a test for the antibodies to HCV (anti-HCV) to establish whether you have ever been exposed to this virus. If you have been exposed, then your immune system will most probably have produced antibodies. As a minority of people clear the virus, it is necessary to perform a second test to establish whether the virus is still present. This will be a polymerase chain reaction (PCR) test or HCV-RNA test, which establishes the presence of the virus itself in your blood. It is only after receiving a positive PCR test that an individual can deem themselves HCV positive.

How much information you are given at the time of your diagnosis depends on the type of center (GUM, DDU, GP, etc.) as well as the information available in that geographical area. The quality of the information available is sometimes poor and is almost always inadequate to make much sense of hep C or what to do about it.

Quite often the HCV test is given at the same time as an HIV test under "HIV and related viruses." This is misleading as HCV and HIV are not related. Often when testing for HCV along with HIV, the emphasis is on the HIV virus. Pre- or posttest counselling for HCV may not exist at all. It is not uncommon for the HIV result to be given in person on the same day, but the HCV result to be given up to three weeks later over the telephone, in writing, or in one case left as a message on an answering machine.

However you found out that you have hepatitis C, or even if you are not sure but suspect that you might be positive, it is worth bearing in mind that a diagnosis is just a piece of information.

It is quite normal to go through a range of emotions that may include anxiety, fear, guilt, remorse, anger, indifference, futility, feeling doomed, denial, disorientation, shock, and grief. Much depends upon how much you know about the virus or what you are told at the time of diagnosis. Because there is an almost complete lack of pre- and posttest counselling procedures in place and also because there is so much ignorance surrounding hepatitis C, patients have had a wildly varied experience of receiving a positive diagnosis. A classic pattern has emerged, with the following identifiable phases:

Minimization

Where information has accompanied a diagnosis, it has tended to be dismissive of the implications. The phrases "extremely mild" and "nothing to worry about" featured in the blood transfusion service's standard letter to those who have been found to have HCV antibodies in their blood samples. GPs often adopted the same kind of line, leading to patients shrugging off the implications and carrying on as normal. For patients with a lifestyle that is healthy with a view to hepatitis C, this may not have caused too much damage. For those with lifestyles likely to accelerate progression, it has been an act of serious mismanagement and a lost opportunity to intervene for positive change. Given the fact that most evidence suggests that early treatment is more likely to be successful, all patients given a misleading "no need to worry" type of diagnosis have been badly let down.

Maximization

What tends to have happened in the past is that some of the more alarming "facts" about hepatitis C have reached patients via a different route, such as through a friend or the tabloid press. Often these bits of information have been given out of context or are downright inaccurate. The result is that patients feel scared and misled by the medical authorities, which can lead to distrust of doctors. Some of these patients react badly. If there is a history of destructive behavior, there is a distinct risk of relapse in some patients; others react in the opposite way, responding to the bad news by determining to make positive changes.

Finding a Balance

Making decisions about treatment and lifestyle based upon good information is a great way of coming to terms with a diagnosis. The central purpose of this book is to show you that there are many ways forward. Even if these choices are only provisional, they can help to ground you, generating the feeling that you are doing something to address your situation, that certain actions can lead to a material improvement in how you feel.

By reading through this book and talking to others it will be possible to make these choices. If as a result of making these choices you start to feel better, you will probably begin to feel a little more confident in your ability to successfully live with hepatitis C or even obtain an effective cure. Thus you can begin the process of empowering yourself and disempowering HCV.

One other consideration that is not covered in detail in this book is how to adjust to the idea of being ill. Many patients find this quite difficult. The following story covers this important issue quite well.

Patient's Experience: Helen

My experience of having symptomatic hepatitis C is fairly typical, I think. I am lucky enough to be in good health now and would like to share how I got from A to B.

Firstly, I need to say that by "symptomatic," I do not mean that I have progressed to significant liver disease but that I have suffered various other symptoms. At one time I was diagnosed as having M.E., as the way I felt—extreme fatigue, fever, aches and pains, and depression—were, at that time, not considered to be related to hepatitis C infection.

My story begins with me getting flu in 1992 while working as a temp in—of all places—the liver unit of a big teaching hospital. I went back to work after a week off sick—temping means no work, no pay, so I couldn't take longer even though I still felt really rough. On my first day back I collapsed and had to go home. At about this time I was hearing a lot of people in my support network talking about this new hepatitis virus and saying that it made you feel tired a lot. As an ex-injector I knew that I had been at risk, and it seemed like this could be what my problem was.

I went to my GP and asked for a hepatitis C test. She had never heard of it and assumed that I had started injecting drugs again. Eventually I got her to realize that I was worried about something that had happened years ago and that the virus was common among my ex-drug-using peers. She agreed to test me, took blood, and sent me home. One week later she rang me to say that it was positive, but that it was nothing to worry about. She did, however, refer me to a hepatologist in a liver unit. There I was given further test and assured that although, yes, I did have HCV-RNA, which means I still have the virus, my flulike symptoms were unrelated. Also because my liver enzymes were not sufficiently raised, I was not a candidate for their interferon trial.

I returned regularly for a year, being monitored for liver function, which was always just above normal. The last time I went there I was so poorly that I arrived in tears. On seeing this, the consultant said that he considered that what I needed was a psychiatric referral and that he could not help me. Everybody wanted to tell me that it was all in my head; my GP was trying to get me on antidepressants, and even the hospital receptionist had an opinion on my mental state!

I was convinced that there was more than just emotions going on here! Eventually through a friend I heard about a natural health clinic that was available at the National Health Service if you could persuade your GP to write the referral. I decided that I would try anything, and I went along. On the first visit

I saw the acupuncturist, who asked me more questions than I have ever been asked by any medic in my life. I told him what the doctor had said and he asked me what I thought was wrong with me. I said, "I think it's physical and to do with hepatitis C." He said, "I agree," and I burst into tears. I was so relieved to be heard at last.

Since then I have gone regularly for acupuncture and also a course in Chinese herbs. When you start this type of treatment, you need to make a real commitment because for a while I was going three times a week to the other side of London. It took up most of my time. A lot of people don't last the course because of how time-consuming it is. I had to keep it up; illness does not sit easy with me. I'm a doer and can't stand to be sitting still for too long. It was like a slow torture for me having to spend so much time resting. Now I only go back once a fortnight, and I have been back in paid work since February 1994.

I am convinced that the acupuncture and herbs played a major part in my return to health. Many people are cynical and say that it only works because I want it to. Well if that is the case, I don't care. I don't need to understand it, or know why it works, only that it does, and I am grateful.

I put everything I had into getting well during those long months, and this included listening to Louise Hay tapes every night as I was going to sleep. This form of mild self-hypnosis slowly convinced me that I had the right to expect full health and that I deserved it. These tapes build on the belief that we in some way have a hand in creating our own illnesses, and although part of me hates that idea, I found that listening to the tape was soothing and did calm me. I also started on a low-fat, almost dairy-free diet and cut down on coffee and tea. I drank a lot of mineral water too. And most importantly when I was tired, I rested. Many of us who have this virus are naturally busy people, and my instinct was to keep pushing through the tiredness, but I found that with that kind of fatigue, I just couldn't. I would lie down—even half an hour would have me feeling better again.

I also got some counselling from somebody who had good experience of people with chronic illnesses, and I think this helped enormously. I found that for me, that a lot of what I was feeling wasn't so much to do with being ill, but about how I viewed myself as an "ill person." I discovered that I hated myself for being sickly! Self-hatred is never likely to be a good basis for recovery from any type of illness so I had to deal with that in order to get past it—if you know what I mean.

In retrospect, I can see that in the worst stages I was actually depressed and that the doctor had a good basis for making that diagnosis, but I believe that the depression was secondary to the physical symptoms. Anybody who had flu for a year would be depressed. Add that to being disbelieved by every doctor I consulted and you can see a real basis for the anger that I was internalizing.

The turning point may have come for me when I became involved in the hepatitis C support group at Mainliners, which has empowered me, informed me, and given me a focus. I would recommend that everybody gets involved in some kind of self-help group. If twenty people have the same symptoms, we can't all be imagining them, we can't all be wrong. And twenty times the symptoms means twenty ways of dealing with them!

I am happy to say that many doctors are now a bit more enlightened, and few people are likely to have to run the gauntlet of disbelief and skepticism that I faced. Remember that when you are feeling low that you know best what you are feeling and that you have a right to be listened to.

I don't know what the future holds for me. I don't discount the possibility of interferon treatment, but I do fear the side effects. I hope a cure is found soon but I'm not holding my breath. I do know that whatever happens, I will never feel that bad again because I will know that my opinions are valid and that the help is there.

Contacts

Christine Beveridge is an experienced hepatitis C educator who runs a number of courses on the subject; she can be contacted at 44 (0)171 209 0993. Or write to:

Christine Beveridge
P.O. Box 13036
London, NW1 3WG, U.K.

Or visit the hepchandbook.com Website for updates on training courses.

11

Talking with Doctors

T HE MAIN AIM OF THIS BOOK is to empower you, the reader, with the ability to decide for yourself how to proceed with your life following an HCV+ diagnosis. While changes in lifestyle can be made independently of others, obtaining treatment necessarily involves talking with medical practitioners. Having made a decision about your preferred treatment, the next step is to negotiate the meeting of your needs with doctors. This process can sometimes be trying.

You may need to learn how to apply pressure and assert yourself. Many patients benefit from being able to draw upon the strength of other people who have been through a similar process; attending a support group may help.

One of the reasons why so much detailed, referenced information is included in this book is because it will provide you with the "ammunition" that is sometimes necessary to convince doctors that HCV is a serious medical condition requiring the expert attention of specialized practitioners. Confronted with the substantiated facts cited in the first chapter of this book, no doctor will be able to dismiss you as having "imagined" symptoms without running the risk of being charged with incompetence. Many patients are particularly bitter about their treatment by doctors in this respect.

Unfortunately it is also sometimes necessary for patients to have a basic understanding of the medical aspects of hepatitis C in order to weed out incompetent or poorly informed practitioners. This charge can sometimes be levelled at doctors and medical advisors of all types including complementary and alternative practitioners, who sometimes lack the requisite knowledge of HCV to be able to correctly diagnose symptoms, let alone treat them.

The following is a list of the broad categories of practitioners that patients may need to talk to, together with likely scenarios and how to cope with each one.

General Practitioners/Primary Care Physicians and Getting Referred to a Specialist

Though the situation is not as dire as in the mid-1990s when very few GPs or PCPs had the ability to recognize and treat hepatitis C, encounters with this class of doctor can still be trying. Because they are often your first point of contact with the medical profession, it is important to have a good one. Ideally he or she will discuss options with you, refer you for detailed tests, and support you in gaining access to your treatment of choice. However, there are very few binding protocols for hepatitis C management in place, which means that patients are still likely to experience inconsistent treatment.

Patients may find that the response they receive also depends upon the attitudes of the doctors that happen to be in the area or personality factors such as individual ability to negotiate with them. The attitude and approach of doctors to hepatitis C patients are erratic. Some are excellent, being open-minded, supportive, and sympathetic. Others are high-handed and dismissive. If your doctor is supportive and gives you the referrals you ask for, then there is no need to adopt an assertive attitude. If, however, your doctor is obstructive, then there are some steps you can take.

The Problem of Ignorance

GPs and PCPs, even sympathetic ones, can be poorly informed about hepatitis C. If you have read the first part of this book, you will almost certainly know far more than your GP or PCP—unless, that is, they have also read it. If you suspect that straightforward ignorance is the problem, then invite the doctor to read some of the facts stated there, and check the authority of the references. You can also invite them to contact the American Liver Foundation or the British Liver Trust, which produce medical information packs for doctors.

There are consistent reports from patients in both Europe and America of their doctors misdiagnosing hepatitis C. An example is of the doctor who misinterpreted HCV-related skin disease as acne:

> I told my GP that I had no energy and felt exhausted after a day's work. My skin was unbearably itchy; if I scratched, it became worse. In the past I had always had a good complexion, but now I started to get spots, particularly before my periods. Premenstrual acne was accompanied by mental confusion and lack of coordination—I had a three-second memory, would spill and drop stuff all over the place, and misjudge distances so as to walk into door frames.
>
> He told me that I had acne, commenting that it was common for women in their thirties to have a resurgence of acne, and prescribed the antibiotic tetracycline. Despite the fact that this had no effect, he prescribed a second course of the same drug three months later. I was surprised and worried by the doctor's decision as I had always been under the impression that antibiotics were potentially harmful. The doctor, however, reassured me that this was quite normal. I took the pill for a further two months, then threw away the remainder.
>
> Next I consulted a TCM doctor who also diagnosed acne and hormonal imbalance. Even though I told him about an attack of jaundice and acute hepatitis in my youth, he did not link my symptoms to chronic liver disease. I mention this because I now think that the best approach is a combination of Western diagnosis and TCM treatment. Hepatitis C was finally diagnosed by a blood test two years later.

Another approach is to check your symptoms against those listed in chapter 1. Some of these symptoms can be tested. For instance, if you are experiencing joint pains, then request a blood test to see if rheumatoid factor is present in your blood. Remember that liver function tests are not necessarily a good indicator of the severity of hepatitis C symptoms.

If your doctor is still unsupportive, you have two options. You can complain or change to a new one; some hepatitis C support groups keep lists of sympathetic doctors.

Claiming Benefits or Medical Insurance

Hepatitis C can often render patients unable to work or need home help. Some patients undergoing drug therapy may also need to make claims even if they were capable of work before treatment. Again it is necessary to carefully go through all of your symptoms and have these clinically assessed if possible. Seek the advice of claims consultants and benefits advisors—they will help you to complete the necessary forms to your best advantage. They will usually advise you to describe your symptoms on a "bad day." Some patients' claims have been rejected at first, but accepted on appeal. Medical insurance policies often contain unwelcome "small print" qualifications that severely limit payable benefits and liabilities for medical costs. Policies need to be checked carefully. It may be necessary to obtain extensive legal and professional medical backup to substantiate claims. Do make use of the information in this book, particularly in chapter 1. Support groups can be very helpful if you are struggling to obtain an insurance settlement. Also refer to the Resources, page 456.

Complaining about Doctors

If you continue to have problems, inform the doctor concerned that you are not satisfied with their performance. At this point it is sometimes useful to point out that you do appreciate that they may be under a lot of pressure, especially if you suspect that your doctor is under stress from overwork or restricted resources; this gives the doctor the opportunity to take on board the seriousness of your concern and to react in a more sympathetic manner. If the doctor does not change their attitude, inform him or her that you will be writing a letter of complaint.

Letters of complaint should be addressed to the appropriate governing authority or the managers of the medical institution concerned. Use your common sense to decide who to write to, and do not be afraid to copy the letter to political representatives; this often secures a prompt response. Be clear about the nature of your complaint. For example, state that you feel that the practitioner has failed to accurately record or test for your symptoms, has acted rudely, or failed to provide treatment.

You will almost certainly find that there are formal complaint procedures open to you. Because these are lengthy and sometimes frustrating, it is often best to wait until you receive a reply to your letter.

It is helpful to be in communication with other HCV sufferers so that you can gauge what the problems may be with doctors. You may be able to get an idea of what levels of support and responsiveness other patients are receiving, and therefore be better able to know what to expect.

Obtaining a Referral for Your Selected Treatment

Complementary Practitioners

If you have decided to use complementary medicine, it is important to have a broad-minded doctor. Many doctors are extremely wary of the whole sector, so it is important to stress that this is your personal decision and to insist on your right to exercise this option.

Use the information supplied in the book to back up your case. Professionally administered Traditional Chinese Medicine is highly efficacious in the treatment of HCV. (A number of the leading hepatologists in London and Australia acknowledge this fact. Some hepatologists will refer you to complementary medicine practices with good records of HCV treatment, even if your doctor will not.)

Reassure them that you will be using a qualified practitioner; in the U.K. there are registers of qualified complementary therapists. Some doctors will be antagonistic to these approaches no matter how reasonable you are. In this instance it is probably best to change your doctor—talk to other HCV patients to find a sympathetic one.

Conventional treatment

Contrary to the general impression a considerable number of doctors are resistant to referring their patients on for currently available drug therapy. Some object on grounds of dubious efficacy; one doctor responded to his patient's request for guidance on whether or not to take interferon with the following comment: "What? You're not sick enough already?"

It is therefore apparent that that there is little consensus on appropriate treatment and wildly inconsistent responses on the part of doctors.

Funding Problems

Another problem becoming increasingly frequent is that of a shortage of financial resources limiting the availability of treatment. In state-financed health care systems doctors, are increasingly concerned with the cost of therapy and are subject to strict cost control. Insurance companies often have small print exclusion clauses for chronic diseases such as hepatitis C. Since the drugs used to treat HCV and the associated tests are expensive, this is often an issue.

A number of patients have been told that the treatment is too expensive by their doctors. In some cases doctors appear to be acting in accordance with policy decisions taken further up the management chain. This raises serious ethical and economic questions. Patients wishing to be referred for less expensive complementary therapy are also frequently turned down, raising questions of inconsistency, medical bias, and failure to offer real choice despite the fact that premiums have been paid. While some insurance companies and medical practices have behaved honorably and flexibly, these are too often the exception to the rule.

In the U.S., patients may be asked to pick up part of the bill for therapy. Pharmaceutical manufacturers offer assistance schemes for hard-up patients; call these numbers for prices and other details:

Schering-Plough: (800) 222-7579 or (800) 521–7157

Roche: (800) 526-0625 or (800) 443-6676

Amgen: (800) 282-6436 or (888) 508-8088

A Note for People with Drug or Alcohol Problems

Some doctors are apparently reluctant to offer treatment to patients with drug and alcohol problems. In some instances this extends to people who no longer use drugs or alcohol and merely have a history of such difficulties.

Any doctor who withholds treatment on this basis is breaching their ethical code. The U.K. Department of Health produced a document "Drug Misuse and Dependence—Guidelines on Clinical Management," published to report the findings of a medical working group in 1991. Section 3 of this document, "Principles of Clinical Management—Applicable to All Doctors," states the following:

> It is unethical for a doctor to withhold treatment from any patient on the basis of a moral judgement that the patient's activities or lifestyle might have contributed to the condition for which treatment was being sought. Unethical behavior of this kind may raise the question of serious professional misconduct.... Drug misusers have the same entitlement as other patients to the services provided by the NHS. It is the responsibility of all doctors to provide care for both general health needs and drug related problems.... Patients need to feel confident of a sympathetic hearing and the availability of effective health care.

Complementary and Alternative Practitioners

Ignorance about hepatitis C is not confined to the conventional medical profession. Homeopaths, naturopaths, aromatherapists, and other specialists will often jump to conclusions when they hear the word "hepatitis" and prescribe treatments more suited to type A or B. Many will encounter secondary symptoms, such as fatigue or arthritis, and try to treat them without knowing that these are symptoms linked to the presence of HCV, which actually affects many different parts of the body.

It is important to ask complementary practitioners whether they have experience of treating hepatitis C and what benefits may be expected from their therapy. If you have doubts, you can quiz them about the condition and find out if they know what they are talking about—some don't.

Some TCM practitioners are reluctant to treat patients with liver disease because of adverse media coverage that has suggested that

Chinese herbs cause liver damage. For instance, a recent article in a national newspaper suggested that a female patient had died and a number of others had been injured as a result of taking Chinese herbs to assist in a radical weight reduction program in Belgium.

The article failed to mention that the subjects were also taking amphetamines, undergoing rigorous exercise, on crash diets, were being prescribed herbs by an unqualified person, and had not informed any of their medical practitioners about this treatment. (Readers should note that it is important to inform doctors and therapists about their whole treatment program.) The subject of the safety of Chinese herbal medicine is discussed in chapter 15. (It is safe if registered practitioners are consulted and the herbs are from reputable suppliers.)

The upshot of this is that some practitioners of TCM do not use the herbs that affect liver function, the very ones that can most benefit patients. They may prefer to prescribe formulae rich in ginseng, for instance, which can benefit patients, but are not as efficacious as the long-term use of personally prescribed herbs with known action on liver disease.

As always it is a good idea to ask the practitioner what benefits are likely and roughly how long these will take to materialize. Despite strong skepticism to begin with, some hospitals are now building bridges with TCM clinics, which is very encouraging for patients seeking to "mix and match" their treatment.

Consultants—Hepatologists and Gastroenterologists

The best consultants seem to be those who concede that they do not yet have all of the answers so far as hepatitis C is concerned. They tend to be frank in their assessment of the chances of getting cured and are often blunt about the need for certain lifestyle changes such as reducing alcohol intake or giving it up altogether. Some are a little overenthusiastic about the benefits of interferon therapy—remember that you have a choice.

On the whole they are excellent, particularly given the immense stress of their workload—they are bearing the brunt of the explosion in the numbers of patients being diagnosed with HCV. However, patients will still sometimes encounter problems along the following lines.

Minimizing or Misinterpreting Symptoms

Because HCV has a large number of symptoms that are not fully understood and have been poorly researched, there can be a problem when it comes to asserting their existence and seriousness. Some doctors still use the word "anecdotal" to describe HCV symptoms; what they seem to mean by this is unproven, possibly imagined, and not serious. The word is often used in a patronizing manner with the intention of minimizing the experience of the patient.

Where there is doubt regarding the prognosis for those infected, doctors sometimes insist on taking an optimistic line despite the fact that they do not have any data regarding the long-term impact of HCV. Some hepatologists collude in this view; one stated the following in a talk in the autumn of 1994: "In most people the infection is 'benign,' indolent (inactive), with a long natural history and low mortality." The truth is that this speaker could not possibly know the long-term impact of HCV. The use of the word "benign" is totally misleading—an offense against the English language, in fact, since the literal meaning is "favorable, gracious, kindly" *(Collins Dictionary)*. This doctor's use of words reflects the attitude that patients may come up against.

Some informed doctors have now started to take this problem seriously. This is reflected by serious investigation of hepatitis C symptoms in some hospitals. A good example of a report covering this aspect is "Chronic hepatitis C infection causes a significant reduction in quality of life in the absence of cirrhosis," Foster G et al. *Hepatology,* 27(1):209–212, 1998. If you have a doctor who is unable to come to terms with the symptomatic profile of hepatitis C, it may be worth referring them to this report.

It is a good idea to write down a list of all of your symptoms before your consultation. This will give the doctor a clearer idea of the need for additional tests and a basis to assess the degree of progression. Here are two examples of common symptoms and the experience of patients when trying to assert the reality of these symptoms to doctors.

The Fatigue Problem

Fatigue is a good example. Many patients report that doctors tend to categorize this as "normal" and "just part of life," effectively dismissing the symptom. One patient I have met described the common experience of finding himself subject to sudden frequent attacks of complete exhaustion. This patient is a male in his early thirties, takes regular exercise, eats a healthy diet, and abstains from alcohol, cigarettes, and drugs. When describing these attacks to a specialist hepatologist, he was told that this was nothing to be unduly concerned about, that tiredness was just a part of life.

It is well known that the liver plays a central role in the generation of the body's energy. For instance, the liver produces and retains glycogen. It would seem to be quite obvious that people suffering from hepatitis would be most likely to suffer from energy-related problems, yet some doctors will still try to deny the reality of the impact of the illness in this respect. It seems that they want to promote a "stiff upper lip" attitude to patients—an attitude that they themselves are obliged to adopt during their education and conditioning. The rigors of medical training are well known, particularly in the U.K., where the scandal of the hours worked by junior doctors, often 140 per week, have been highlighted in the media. Doctors will often project this conditioning onto their patients and may well censor themselves when it comes to acknowledging the reality of pain and suffering undergone by patients.

Another important aspect of fatigue is that it is difficult to measure. Doctors are often conditioned only to accept quantitative evidence of disease. Such scientific conditioning renders them unable to cope with highly complex phenomena such as HCV-related fatigue, which cannot be reduced to single blood test with a numbered "result." Those doctors who have started to investigate the subject have confirmed the difficulty of measurement and the complexity of fatigue; one report concluded:

Chronic fatigue results from an altered (probably centrally mediated) homeostatic mechanism which is deranged independent of the severity and etiology of liver disease. This mechanism is poorly understood and requires further study.[1]

As with other symptoms it is vital that you refuse to accept this projection on their part. You need to be aware of exactly when the doctor starts to minimize or dismiss your symptoms and to firmly reassert the reality of your fatigue. Remember that the doctor cannot possibly know what you are experiencing; remind the doctor of this and insist that your symptoms are written down in your file exactly as you report them. Suggest to the doctor that they listen, that you do not require their interpretation for the time being. Be as clear and as honest as you can.

Mental and Emotional Symptoms—Malaise and Depression

These and similar symptoms have traditionally been described as "liverishness," indicating the common sensical linking of these characteristics with liver problems. Unfortunately many doctors do not share this common sense view, which is fully acknowledged in traditional medicine.

Of all the symptoms these are the most difficult to get accepted by the medical profession. Again it is common medical knowledge that the liver performs the vital chemical producing and balancing functions in the body. Yet it can be extremely difficult to persuade doctors that such symptoms are linked to HCV and not some neurotic disorder. These extremely debilitating conditions are frequently dismissed, often in a very offhand, patronizing way.

It appears that female HCV patients in particular have a hard time in getting doctors to take these symptoms on board. This may reflect the lingering tendency of the medical profession to be male dominated and to dismiss feelings, especially when they are articulated by women, as signs of "hysteria." The problem is not confined to male doctors or female patients, but this combination is more common in the most prominent examples of bad practice.

A female HCV patient had the following experience during a consultation with a senior hepatologist at a major hospital in London. On describing the above symptoms the specialist interrupted her and suggested that she was in need of antidepressant drug therapy. In other words the specialist dismissed her experience as being a mental problem, nothing at all to do with HCV. The patient was taken aback and immediately confronted the doctor, suggesting that the cause of her problems was indeed the hepatitis. The consultant dismissed this notion, insisting that there was no evidence to support such a link.

This experience played a large part in persuading her to seek treatment elsewhere, in her case from Traditional Chinese Medicine. She found them to be far more receptive to her condition and received a course of herbal medicine that treated the cause of these symptoms without having to recourse to antidepressants. The consultant concerned became hostile when he discovered that she was using herbal medicine.

Another female patient found that her doctor insisted that she was suffering from psychiatric problems when she described her mental and emotional symptoms. (This patient rightly felt that the only course of action open to her was to change her doctor; see section below for more information.)

Again it is vital that the patient persistently insists on the reality of his or her experience. It is important to stress the fact that so far as you are concerned these symptoms are a reality of HCV, that they are common, and that the lack of research on "proven" links between HCV and "liverishness" should not be used to discount a link that is entirely logical. Emphasize the fact that medical research is still at a very early stage and that the lack of it should not be used to dismiss your experience, and that liver function test results such as ALT and AST are only very crude indicators of severity of both disease and symptoms. Point out that M.E. and a range of autoimmune disorders are linked to HCV (see chapter 1). Insist that on the contrary for this very reason it is vital that these symptoms be put on the record, so that more information is available to collate. Above all insist that you are not "asymptomatic" if you feel that you are definitely suffering. If the doctor writes "asymptomatic" on your medical records, you will not be considered as suffering any adverse consequences from HCV.

Patient's Experience: Beth

I was told in February 1995 that the various symptoms I was experiencing were due to the hepatitis C virus. My GP knew little about the disease at the time (but has since diagnosed many more patients), and referred me to a gastroenterologist at the local hospital.

While waiting for that first appointment I collected information about the disease and treatment from the local health authority, the British Liver Trust, the Internet, and relatives in Australia. This was a very stressful and crucial period for me. The information I received was gloomy, inconclusive, and inadequate, and it became apparent that while procedures varied throughout the world, success rates after treatment with interferon were collectively low.

During this period I also consulted a Traditional Chinese Medical gastroenterologist who, I was very encouraged to hear, was confident that my condition could be stabilized by Chinese herbs. I saw the hospital specialist well armed with information and a plan of action. He was also very positive that due to my histology I would benefit from a twelve- to eighteen-month course of interferon. However, I explained to him that before possibly embarking on interferon, I would firstly undertake a few months treatment with Chinese herbs. I did just that.

When it came to picking up my first prescription, the pharmacy was unable to supply the interferon. There was a funding problem. I was irate. I explained to them that I had sent my children away to be looked after and had specially arranged for friends to come and nurse me through the first few weeks. I had prepared myself for the drug therapy mentally and practically and was devastated when it looked like the local authority would refuse to pay. My gastroenterologist seemed embarrassed and said that he would call the next day. I think that in the end I went through as a "test case."

By the time I started the interferon I had been taking TCM herbs for over three months. Blood tests taken after one week of interferon revealed that my ALT levels had dropped from nearly 300 to "normal" and that a quantiplex assay couldn't detect the virus. Fifteen months into an eighteen-month course reveals all monthly PCR tests have been negative and ALT levels consistently normal. I continue to take Chinese herbs and interferon.

I am really pleased with the results gained from both forms of treatment. I still have symptoms, some from ongoing but reduced sites of inflammation in the liver and others from the interferon. My symptoms started to decrease immediately I embarked on the Chinese herbs, and because they are individually prescribed each week or two, I am actively keeping abreast of symptoms and changes in my condition.

I can't say that the consultations and decisions have been easy, but I am confident that my research and assertive approach has enabled me to take the bull by the horns and ensured that during consultations I didn't waste either my time or the doctors by having to go over the basics. During a period of anxiety I sought counselling through my GP surgery, which was extremely beneficial as it helped me sort out emotional issues and child care and helped me, through their library, to develop a positive attitude. I thoroughly recommend that patients do as much as they possibly can themselves to keep pressure off their liver, including decreasing alcohol intake and stress.

Reference

1. Chronic fatigue in patients with liver disease; a preliminary study. Plevris JN. University of Edinburgh Dept of Medicine, American Association for the Study of Liver Diseases, 1996.

12

Change, Recovery, and Hepatitis C

We would rather be ruined than changed;
We would rather die in our dread
Than climb the cross of the moment
And let our illusions die.

W. H. Auden

A number of people contributed to this chapter.

CHANGING BEHAVIOR CAN BE a hard, slow process. Yet the need for change and the adoption of a different lifestyle is often pressing for hepatitis C patients. Learning to adapt, to cut out certain patterns of behavior and replace them with new ones, to alter attitudes and assumptions, can be challenging to say the least. Human beings don't seem to like change, particularly if it is forced on them by circumstances.

Yet the process of altering behavior, of adjusting or transforming outlook and actions, can be terrifically rewarding, giving a sense of having a new lease of life, a feeling of fluidity and self-respect that can become a compelling reason in itself for perpetuating the process. It does seem that a high proportion of people with hepatitis C are prone to addictive, repetitive patterns of behavior. Some of these patterns are life-threatening, and help is usually required to obtain lasting results.

There are a number of institutions and organizations claiming to be able to offer this kind of help; there are plenty of options in the change market. The techniques available vary widely—therapeutic, religious, psychoanalytical, artistic—the list is endless. Some want your money, others your immortal soul, a few want both. There are too many to detail here, although there is one that stands out because it is so commonly used by patients, particularly to address the very dangerous problem of craving for, and addiction to, alcohol and drugs.

Twelve-Step Programs

The "Twelve-Step Program" was developed by a couple of alcoholics who desperately wanted to stop their destructive drinking and had tried numerous methods in the past, none of which had worked for them. The method they eventually developed enabled them to stop drinking alcohol and has worked for many thousands of people throughout the world. Although it is not the only way of arresting destructive behavior, it is widely accessible and free of charge. While the language of these programs is clearly influenced by the social and religious environment of 1930s America, and can therefore seem quite alien in the cosmopolitan 1990s, most people find that they can adapt these ideas to suit themselves, although this process is not always easy.

If you use drugs addictively or drink alcoholically, then changing this behavior will be at the top of the list of beneficial lifestyle changes to be made. Many patients with a history of these problems attend meetings of Alcoholics Anonymous (AA) or Narcotics Anonymous (NA) in order to arrest this destructive pattern of behavior; although they are by no means the only effective way of addressing chemical dependency, they are widely regarded as being effective for some people. For patients in twelve-step programs, practicing the first part of the first step of NA or AA will be a prerequisite for living with hepatitis C.

The facts about alcohol and drug use in conjunction with hepatitis C make it clear that health is incompatible with compulsive drug or alcohol consumption. Continued abuse of alcohol and drugs is quite likely to be life-threatening, or at least to accelerate the progression of HCV. Secondary symptoms also seem to be more common in active alcoholics and addicts.

Likewise, active eating disorders will also be extremely hazardous for patients. Codependency and other emotional or mental disorders are also likely to stand in the way of developing a comfortable lifestyle with a minimum level of stress, so important for patients.

Thus patients "in recovery" can be confident that they are on the right track so far as dealing with both hepatitis C and addictive/compulsive behavior. The techniques for change outlined in these recovery programs can also be utilized to change other aspects of lifestyle, such as diet and exercise. The notion of powerlessness, the concept of acceptance, and the seeking out of a source of energy to power change are highly relevant to learning to live with HCV and adapt in order to attain the best possible level of well-being. Accepting the fact that you have hepatitis C and all that entails is the basis on which change can be founded. The support networks that these programs provide are extremely useful in the process of ongoing change and of taking the knocks that life inevitably entails.

Added Complications in Getting Clean and/or Sober for People with Hepatitis C

Addicts and alcoholics often decide to get clean and sober because they are "sick and tired of being sick and tired." The implication here is that getting clean will lead to not being "sick" or "tired" any more. However, for some people with hepatitis C, putting down the drugs and alcohol may not alleviate all of the physical symptoms. Many symptoms associated with withdrawal from chemicals, such as fatigue, nausea, flulike symptoms, and so on, are also symptoms suffered by some people with hepatitis C. This can be confusing and very painful for people trying to get clean. It can sometimes be difficult to tell where the disease of addiction stops and HCV starts.

Patient's Experience: Anonymous

I found myself in an expensively decorated and beautifully located treatment center in a converted country house. At first

I thought it would be easier to go through withdrawal here than in my dingy flat in London, but despite the nursing care, I still had a very bad time. My withdrawals seemed to go on for much longer than the other people in the group. The professional opinion was that I was malingering, and it was an opinion that I shared. This hardly contributed to my already minuscule self-worth; was I really just a coward? I remember being half dragged, half carried into group therapy and doing my "therapeutic duties" of cleaning the staircase, on hands and knees. I did not think I was going to make it, and I probably wouldn't have if I hadn't been in the middle of nowhere with no financial means.

Thank God, I made it and am still clean today, but it took a long time before I began to feel physically better, and I now accept that it is unlikely that I will ever return the level of robust good health that I enjoyed prior to hepatitis C, but I am a whole lot better than I was.

Some people fail to complete detoxification programs because they just feel too ill—it seems that a high proportion of these patients may be HCV+. There is therefore a need for doctors and other practitioners to take note of the fact that an individual has hepatitis C when they are guiding that person through the process of detoxification and treatment. The main thing is for clinicians to be aware of the possibility that a patient with hepatitis C is likely to be slower to regain their strength and that expectations of the speed of recovery may need to be modified.

How Fast to Change?

Talking to other HCV+ people trying to change can be particularly beneficial. One problem that often comes up is "How far, how fast?" On the one hand, there are so many beneficial changes that can be made, and on the other, there is the fear of destabilizing the whole process by taking on too much. Many hepatitis C patients have a particularly pressing need to alter many aspects of their lifestyle and will derive great benefits from such changes. However, it can sometimes be difficult to adopt the more challenging lifestyle alterations that are suggested when most other people in twelve-step recovery programs seem to be stuffing themselves with burgers, coffee, chocolate, sugar, and cigarettes—not that they necessarily are, but sometimes it just seems like that. For people with hepatitis C, stopping drinking or using drugs addictively is a vital start, but is often not enough. It can be difficult when others seem to be getting healthier by the day and you are still in a precarious situation. Support for more comprehensive lifestyle changes is not always forthcoming; some people in recovery seem to resent such ambition.

In the end only you can decide when you want to change. It is useful to remember that giving up smoking, changing diet, taking up exercise, and so on can be seen as ongoing processes. It often takes several attempts to stop smoking, and years to transform an unhealthy diet into a healthy one. These are things that you can afford to fail at and try again at a later date. Talking to others with HCV can really help in this process. Learning to take what you need and leave the rest is important; sitting in a meeting you can sometimes get the impression that other people know what is best for you. They often don't.

Other Methods

There are plenty of other methods of achieving change. For those who don't have chemical dependency problems, patterns of destructive behavior, or who simply find twelve-step programs unhelpful, the following have proved useful to some patients.

Will power and self-discipline—these much maligned techniques of cutting out unhealthy behavior work for some people.

Meditation is a powerful tool for change, if not transformation. There are many different forms available. Because practice is usually associated with particular religious sects, it is sometimes difficult to obtain instruction without making some kind of commitment. One organization that offers safe, basic meditation tuition is the Friends of the Western Buddhist Order (FWBO). They have a number of centers throughout the U.K., Europe, North America, India, and Australasia. The largest center in the U.K. is based in London;

the telephone number is 0181 981 1225. In San Francisco: (415) 282-2018. Seattle: (206) 726-0051. Boston: (617) 576-7345.

Mental and Emotional Complications Arising Out of Hepatitis C

Undiagnosed patients will often have had a sense that something was wrong long before they found out that they had hepatitis C. This feeling of unease and a sense of "not rightness" is dangerous and also easily mistaken for classic alcoholic or addict personality traits. In the case of undiagnosed hep C the instinct is subsequently shown to have had a valid basis, although it doesn't detract from the general sense of "dis-ease" or "unease" often associated with an addictive personality.

There is no doubt that the additional problems caused by hep C can make recovery more difficult than usual. It seems possible that some relapses can partly be ascribed to symptoms, particularly tiredness, depression, and, in some cases, drug therapy. A "jaundiced" view of the world is quite common in patients; it can be quite difficult to replace this with the faith and positivity that is often advocated by the recovery movement. Many traditions of medicine associate liver diseases with depression, negativity, denial, fear, anger, and so on.

If you are diagnosed as depressive or as having some kind of mental disorder, then it may be helpful to try to identify how much of this is due to the hepatitis C and how much may be intrinsic. If you and your doctor conclude that it is intrinsic, then the question of treatment will arise. This will usually consist of antidepressant drugs and perhaps group therapy as well. In practice, group therapy is frequently less accessible than the drugs. The decision whether or not to take antidepressants isn't easy for anyone in recovery; it may help to talk the decision through with other patients. Some antidepressants are less stressful to the liver than others. It often takes experimentation to find one that is suitable for you.

Appreciating that hep C is associated with mental and emotional symptoms that are often difficult to pin down, it can become hard to locate the source of negative emotions; the usual recovery and therapeutic techniques may not be appropriate.

Knowing that one is susceptible to HCV-related symptoms, it can be hard to know whether or not a particular emotional state is "valid." For instance, some patients become angry when they deal with doctors. It is sometimes hard to assess whether or not this is due to bad practice by the doctor (e.g., dismissing a symptom or refusing to refer), or an emotional symptom simply caused by the hep C while the doctor is acting reasonably (no resources, all you need is some antidepressants, etc.). This uncertainty can lead to an erosion of patients' self-confidence and ability to know themselves, to feel integrated. Sometimes it can feel as though one's emotional compass is subject to severe electromagnetic interference. It can seem hard to know which way is up and which way is down.

Patient's Experience: Anonymous

Having chronic hepatitis C is a major issue for me in life and in recovery. It is very real in my life and affects how I live to a large extent. I have had to be willing to change many things: how I work; how I play; how I rest; what I eat; who I have in my life; and most importantly, my expectations of myself. In changing these things, I have had to be willing to go through the whole grief process in letting go of my old ways. Elisabeth Kubler-Ross lists this process as denial, anger, bargaining, sadness, and finally acceptance, and I have denied the need for change, got very angry when I realized I had to change, attempted to strike a deal with hepatitis C, and sobbed my heart out at the realization that my life would never be the same. I get to a point of acceptance over one issue, like for instance, the decision not to have children, only to find that I have to go through the whole process again around my career. However, if I work through my twelve-step program, I do have the tools to get through these feelings, be it kicking and screaming!

At the end of most NA and AA meetings in the U.K., we say the "Serenity Prayer," which goes, "God grant me the serenity to accept the things I cannot change, the courage to change the things I can, and the wisdom to know the difference." I find that the concepts outlined in this simple verse very helpful. If I can change it, I will, even if it is hard. If I can't change it, I will have to learn to live with it, however difficult. The degree to which I am willing to do these two things greatly affect my level of comfort.

Drug Therapy and Recovery

Interferon therapy can be challenging, particularly in early recovery. The decision about whether or not to take this treatment is even more difficult for patients in the early stages of abstinence from alcohol or drugs. Those who have been on a course of interferon while in recovery stress the severity of mental side effects, particularly the depression. Interferon is contraindicated for people with depression; this qualification is no joke. People have described the mental effects of interferon as like a process of uncovering and exposing unconscious or semiconscious fears and insecurities. People who are prone to depression or anxiety can find that interferon turns these conditions into suicidal impulses and paranoia, respectively. Likewise, people with eating disorders should note the warnings about anorexic-like side effects. Sometimes these effects take some time to clear after the cessation of therapy.

It's a good idea to talk it through thoroughly before making a decision. The support available from fellowship members can make all the difference when undertaking a year or more of chemotherapy.

Practices That Can Be Used to Enhance
Physical, Mental, Emotional, and Spiritual Recovery

Many people use natural treatments, at least to begin with, looking for therapies that counter the debilitating symptoms and make them feel better. Some patients are drawn to "natural medicine" because they find its aims and methods more compatible with their approach to recovery. Some of the physical/mental disciplines associated with complementary medicines, such as Yoga and Qi Gong, can become an important ingredient in the overall process of change, providing a link between physical and spiritual health. Mental clarity seems to be a benefit of persistent practice for some patients. The ability to distinguish between emotional states and to have a sense of being grounded are frequently reported reasons for patients staying with these disciplines.

Three Anonymous Patients' Experiences

I've been following the Qi for seven years now. Of course I still go to meetings. I see this as a way of practicing steps three and eleven. I don't know if I'd have made it without Qi Gong, I really don't. It simultaneously addresses my physical, mental, and spiritual health needs. The hep hasn't been so much of a problem, and I put that down to the practice.

Qi Gong has given a sense of internal balance and calm which I've found invaluable. I am certain it has accelerated my recovery and got me through situations I might otherwise have relapsed over. It has given me a real sense of who I am and what I can become. The sense of complete and total relaxation is an incomparable benefit both to my recovery and the state of my liver. I am absolutely confident that this is the right way forward for me.

Recovery is a physical, emotional, mental, and spiritual process. It is necessary to look after all four areas. If you concentrate totally on the emotional side of things, you may neglect your physical well-being and complicate your disease.

If you become too tied up in the depression, it is possible to overlook the great benefits to be enjoyed from having a spiritual dimension to life, whatever that may be for you. Being stressed mentally or emotionally can lead to physical symptoms, so it is of great benefit to go to a meeting, share how things are for you, and leave feeling emotionally lighter, and therefore physically stronger.

For Those Working with Addiction and Recovery

Hepatitis C is highly prevalent within the recovering community. Because it precipitates a wide spectrum of physical, mental, and emotional disease, it may be helpful for counselors and other recovery workers to be able to identify and delineate the problems caused by hepatitis C as opposed to addiction; clients with such a dual diagnosis will have additional needs. There are avenues of approach that may help infected patients to turn a serious situation around to the advantage of both their recovery and their overall well-being.

The Scale of Hepatitis C Infection

Prevalence rates for exposure to the hepatitis C virus are around 1–2% in the general population in Western Europe, the U. S., and Canada.[1–6] However, the figures are dramatically higher in current and former intravenous drug users, typically ranging from 50 to 100%,[1,7] and are also significantly above average in other groups with a history of chemical dependency (see below).

While it is not the case that all people with hepatitis C have a history of chemical dependency, this group has been repeatedly shown to have been at a far greater risk of exposure to this blood-borne virus compared to the general population.[6,8] HCV is particularly easily transmitted via IV drug use, and epidemiologists strongly suspect that this is linked to the sharing of paraphernalia as well as the actual hypodermic syringe and needle.[7] This theory is substantiated by pointing to the much lower rates of HIV infection in IVDUs, apparently achieved as a result of education about the dangers of "sharing needles" and the provision of clean injecting kit. Researchers also point to the much greater resilience of HCV compared to HIV; it is suspected that HCV can survive outside the body for weeks or even months[9]—the time period has yet to be accurately determined—while HIV usually dies relatively rapidly outside the host.

Several reports have also established that prevalence is significantly higher than average in alcoholics[10–12] and cocaine snorters.[13] It is not so clear why. It may be the case that people in these categories choose to deny having a history of IV drug use when they are questioned. Despite assurances of confidentiality, many interviewees will be averse to having any mention of IV drug use appear on their medical records, perhaps being particularly aware of the possibility of employers gaining access to this information.

They may also be unwilling to admit to themselves that they have used drugs intravenously, which is still something of a taboo. They might well have had negative HIV and hepatitis B test results in the past and assumed that they had got away with IV drug use; many people in this category are likely to want to forget the whole episode. Naturally it is also quite possible that some of these respondents have genuinely forgotten episodes of IV drug use or that these occurred during a "blackout."

It is also important to appreciate that some people in these categories will be telling the truth. Almost everybody in the general population will have had several exposures to potential HCV transmission risk through routine practices such as dental work or having a vaccination, although these routes are associated with much lower rates of infection. The overall picture is of a very high percentage of people in recovery from chemical dependency infected with HCV.

Addiction Disease Progression and Hepatitis C

Unlike hepatitis B, where over 90% of those exposed to the virus as adults do not become chronically infected, HCV very rarely becomes "inactive" or disappears.[14] Many doctors, particularly older ones, are still unaware of this basic distinction and may also misinform patients about the seriousness of HCV, often having been taught that non-A non-B hepatitis is harmless. This has generated a great deal of confusion among patients. In fact almost everyone exposed to HCV in adulthood goes on to develop disease, although severity and symptoms do vary.[14–16] It has been observed that the use of alcohol, narcotics, and some prescription drugs is strongly associated with more aggressive disease and aggravated debilitating symptoms; [10–12,17–21] therefore it is reasonable to assume that all HCV+ clients will be experiencing symptoms, although these may be partially masked by drug use, which presents particular problems during detoxification and early recovery.

The onset of debilitating hepatitis C symptoms and the beginnings of deleterious impact on key body organs such as the liver and kidneys, frequently precipitate overt crises in the lives of using addicts earlier than would be the case if they were not infected. In particular the commonly reported symptoms of fatigue, depression, aches and pains in the upper torso and joints, outbursts of anger, alcohol intolerance, impaired thinking and memory loss, underlined and validated by the continuing emergence of a formidable array of clinical evidence of linked conditions,[22-29] are likely to lead to even committed substance and alcohol users realizing that something is obviously wrong. Such changes can make the difference in the perception of the costs and benefits of using, even to the most obsessive addict. HCV symptoms can easily contribute to events often associated with "rock bottoms"—losing employment through poor attendance or performance and the breakdown of relationships through a range of dysfunction.

Properly handled, together with a balance of information on both hepatitis C and addiction progression, this pattern can be used to show the client who has yet to commit to recovery a powerful and persuasive set of circumstances, which suggest the overwhelming logic for attempting to achieve abstinence. For infected clients the physical facts about hepatitis C can make a good substitute for the somewhat abstract concept of addiction disease, which may be assimilated at a later date. Thus a counselor can use the facts about hep C—significantly raised possibility of OD, for which there is consistent strong anecdotal evidence from both drug abuse professionals and users, cirrhosis, and various types of cancer—if using is not arrested; counselors may also stress that continuing to use addictively with hep C will cause diminished quality of life with a likelihood of chronic deep depression and the need for ongoing medical and/or institutional support. It is no exaggeration to state that the prospects for the HCV+ addict who continues to use are extremely poor. The positive side to this is that feeling terrible can provide a strong incentive to change direction in life. Gary, an HCV+ recovering addict, had the following to say:

There is no way that I would have stopped using if it hadn't been for the hep C symptoms. I was too committed to my drugs and quite prepared to pay the price for the problems they were causing. However, my condition deteriorated rapidly in my early thirties. I was completely incapable of getting out of bed in the morning after only a few pints of beer and a bit of puff the night before. Whenever I used speed or heroin it seemed to take up to four weeks to recover, and I felt absolutely devoid of life and deeply depressed for all of that time. Even smoking cigarettes seemed to make my skin go all puffy and precipitate depression. I began to find myself having to plan my "fun," trying to ensure that I had a recovery period, or having to admit that I would be incapable of doing any work if I used. It slowly became obvious that something was seriously wrong with my situation, even in my addled state.

In the end I had to accept that my only chance at any sort of life worth living was to stop drinking and taking drugs. I tried ignoring the self-evident impact of my using both on my work and my health. In the end I just couldn't face killing myself, knowing what I was doing. I now choose to think that getting hep C was part of God's will for me; I do not believe that I would have hit a rock bottom for many more years otherwise; so I feel that I would not have recovery or any of its benefits without hep C.

Another very important point is that chemical dependency in HCV+ addicts may be involved with the self-treatment of debilitating symptoms. In the case of those addicted to prescribed pain killers and antidepressants, by no means uncommon, chemical use may be exclusively linked to hep C treatment. Such a situation creates a strong logic for the treatment of symptoms using non-mood-altering methods during detoxification and recovery. All too often those with addictions to illicit drugs have also been prescribed medical drugs to treat HCV-related disease and symptoms, creating complex and deep dependencies that are hard to treat, difficult to unravel, and highly dangerous. Problems can also be exacerbated by certain non-mood-altering drugs; for instance, all anti-inflammatory drugs (prescribed to address frequently presenting arthritic symptoms) present a danger to HCV patients, largely on account of their immunosuppressant qualities, which are thought by some doctors to lead directly to increased viral load and a worsened prognosis.[30,31]

Intervention Counselling

The development of life-threatening disease in hep C patients has now been strongly linked to alcohol consumption and also associated with cigarette smoking.[17,32] The incidence of hepatocellular carcinoma (HCC or liver cancer) is much higher in heavy drinkers. Less hepatotoxic drugs, such as opiates, are also likely to lead to higher rates of disease through their link to impaired immune function, the stress caused by adulterants, and poor lifestyle factors closely linked to active or chaotic drug dependence. Rates of non-Hodgkin's lymphoma (NHL), a form of lymphatic cancer, appear to be much higher in people with HCV; unlike HCC this condition can occur in younger patients or in those with few signs of liver disease. (It is possible that HCV is the principal reason for the recent dramatic rises in rates of NHL worldwide).

Another point to make to HCV+ addicts is that the prospect of sudden drug-related death may also be much higher. It is now strongly suspected that HCV+ drug users are more likely to suffer from overdoses, although this has yet to be proved. It has been shown that HCV infected the African-American population in the 1940s and '50s, most probably through the proliferation of heroin use in inner-city ghettos (consult Harold Margolis of the Center for Disease Control, Atlanta, for details). HCV infection may well have played a symbiotic role in the early demise of a number of the great but chemically dependent jazz musicians of that era. Autopsy reports featuring heavy organ damage, often associated with much greater age, indicate that more than just chemical dependency may have been at work.

Therefore there is a pressing need for patients to take all of the steps they can, as early as possible, to minimize risk. Continuing to use alcohol and narcotics is the single most damaging activity someone with HCV could undertake.

In general, a knowledge of hepatitis C may lead to professionals in the fields of medicine, public health, and chemical dependency making new insights into previously unchallenged or ignored questions. For instance, an appreciation of the prevalence of hepatitis C and knowledge of the linked symptoms has caused some to draw links to chronic fatigue syndrome, M.E., and the dramatic rise in the incidence of lymphoma throughout the western world.[28] The subject has also reignited some old questions such as "If heroin is a relatively undamaging drug, why are so many opiate addicts so ill?" HCV may help to substantiate what many of those familiar with the heroin scene have long suspected, ergo, that something else was making addicts so ill. It is likely that following the emergence of more information about hepatitis C will allow professionals in the field of addiction to make increasingly incisive links with both the symptoms of some of their clients and the corresponding logic for treatment approach.

A Note about Methadone

Methadone is considered to be a very useful tool by some professionals working in public health, with advantages in terms of addiction management and prevention of further HCV transmission. However, counselors encountering clients on methadone maintenance should be aware that this form of medication may contribute toward accelerated progression. In particular, the linctus form of methadone, containing chloroform and ethanol, will place additional stress on the liver. It is unlikely that any doctor with a knowledge of liver disease would countenance the long-term prescription of any medicine containing such ingredients to patients with HCV under normal circumstances. Therefore, if stabilization and a reduction in dependency has not been achieved within a short period, alternatives, such as ear acupuncture, need to be considered and possibly suggested to clients. It is also important to note that immunosuppression has been observed to precipitate increases in viral load, another indicator for more serious disease progression.[31]

Hepatitis C Symptoms and the Importance
of their Recognition and Acknowledgment

Hepatitis C exerts a powerful influence on the dynamics of both addiction disease progression and the recovery process. Regardless of the causal mechanics, emerging research into HCV clearly demonstrates that a wide range of serious, sometimes fatal, and routinely debilitating medical conditions are either caused by hepatitis C or are strongly associated.

The ability to recognize typical hepatitis C symptoms will be very useful in the course of recovery counselling. While the subjective symptoms of HCV such as depression, extreme fatigue, indigestion, aching joints, emotional lability, night sweats, "floaters," dizziness, poor short-term memory, and impaired cognitive function may be easily confused with those of active chemical dependency (see references for symptoms at the end of chapter 1), they stand out quite clearly in those who are in recovery. Counselors who are able to identify these symptoms will be able to help their clients to select appropriate treatments for these symptoms. Although twelve-step work may help to address some of these, such as mood swings, it will not directly address problems caused by chronic liver disease.

Misinterpretation of symptoms and the suggestion that twelve-step or counselling work is the only appropriate tool for addressing these problems is very likely to result in powerful feelings of being "misunderstood" in clients. Such clients are sometimes too physically exhausted and mentally dispirited to undertake recovery activities with any degree of vigor or enthusiasm. This phenomenon will be familiar to counselors, although the possibility of an underlying physical reason may not. Addicts in early recovery are in particular need of sensitive and informed management. It is now quite common to encounter HCV+ addicts who have been poorly advised, particularly in primary and secondary treatment.

A common complaint is that the extreme fatigue that is typical in HCV patients has been solely interpreted as a lack of willingness, emotional blockage, or other such labels that are routinely applied in treatment, particularly where "tough love" is the guiding principle. It is extremely difficult to communicate the devastating and extreme nature of the fatigue that can be caused by hepatitis C.

Tim, a chronic hepatitis C patient, describes HCV-related fatigue as "feeling as though I have been laid out by a professional boxer. It often comes on suddenly and means that I have to stop everything that I am doing immediately and go and lie down. I think that people sometimes think that I am just tired, when in fact I am completely incapable of any activity whatsoever."

Some former clients of treatment centers, who have now made the link between hepatitis C and these symptoms, are resentful toward their treatment providers, particularly when they have been pressured into taking part in activities while suffering an attack of fatigue. Helen, a recovering addict who is now a professional hepatitis C and recovery educator, has the following recollection of treatment:

> I felt as though I had to be carried into groups, and when I got there I wasn't capable of any meaningful participation. Therapeutic duties were just a complete nightmare. Looking back I do not know how I got through treatment, and I wonder why the counselors did not appreciate that I had a physical problem—the implication was that it was all emotional and would therefore improve with recovery work. Unfortunately this has turned out to be untrue, although my recovery has allowed me to increase my awareness of hep C and related problems, allowing me to take appropriate action, which in my case means taking professionally prescribed Chinese herbs, getting acupuncture, or relaxing.
>
> I feel that this is a very important issue that needs to be appreciated by everyone working in recovery, particularly by staff in treatment centers. I conclude that addicts with hep C do not have their needs appreciated. I think that many of them will have given up on recovery, at least partly because of this misassessment. I certainly felt completely misunderstood by the therapeutic staff at my treatment center, and I am quite astonished that I managed to make it through. The mistaken application of "tough love" in circumstances of medical incapacity comes very close indeed to both abuse and professional mis-

conduct. I feel that the failure to recognize and acknowledge my fatigue as a physically rooted disability undermined my already shredded integrity; the lack of acknowledgment meant that I felt that I could no longer even trust my basic physical feedback. I no longer trusted my most basic senses, and my version of reality was challenged by people with power over me.

Hepatitis C also causes mental and emotional symptoms of varying severity;[22,25] research has now shown that these are significantly debilitating and will present challenges to recovering clients and their counselors. For many years patients have been complaining of short-term memory loss, cognitive dysfunction ("brain fog"), depression, and dramatic mood swings; the impact of hepatitis C on the brain is currently being researched at Charing Cross Hospital in London.

Mood swings, particularly the sudden outbursts of anger and impulsiveness commonly reported by HCV patients, are seen as classic signs of liver disease by John Tindall, a renowned practitioner of Traditional Chinese Medicine and manager of the Gateway Clinic, a well-known center in London. He notes that female HCV+ clients are particularly prone to exaggerated problems with premenstrual syndrome (PMS) and menopause, both seen as being linked to impaired liver function in TCM. In turn these instabilities can make relapse more likely; the combination of poor cognitive function, impulsive behavior, emotional lability, and generalized debilitation mount up to present a formidable array of problems for the HCV+ addict in recovery. He states:

> Wherever there is a pathogen disrupting liver function, there is an increased likelihood of problems relating to poor or wildly fluctuating energy flow, lack of acceptance, and denial. Clients with hepatitis C are often on a short fuse. Female clients have particular problems with PMS and menopause, and these are seen as being related to poor liver function in TCM. Such symptoms can often be improved through the use of Chinese herbs, ideally backed up by ear or whole body acupuncture. Long-term success in treating these symptoms is greatly improved if the client can learn to relax. If there are long-term unresolved issues contributing to tension or anxiety in clients, these need

to be urgently addressed through counselling, physical or spiritual work, whatever proves to be effective. My experience in treating HCV+ clients suggests that this work is very important in most cases.

Thus Tindall points toward the potential medical benefit of step and counselling work in the treatment of both addiction and hepatitis C—this is an important point to make to clients—recovery work can play a crucial role in forming a basis for the active treatment of hepatitis C, as well as enabling abstinence, a prerequisite for health in most HCV+ addicts. Coming to terms with oneself, developing acceptance, and standing a better chance of achieving a greater degree of ease and a relaxed approach to life is an extremely valuable therapeutic goal in itself for HCV+ clients.

Additional Risks of Relapse Related to HCV

1. HCV+ clients who achieve abstinence but still feel debilitated may be vulnerable to relapse. Seeing HCV-negative people in recovery reaping the benefits in terms of improved well-being, while they are still feeling jaded and ill, can be frustrating. This is particularly true where clients have hep C but are undiagnosed, or are diagnosed but do not appreciate the link between these problems and their status. Such people are quite likely to ask themselves the question "If this is failing to make me feel any better, why am I bothering?" or start thinking along the lines of "At least the drugs got rid of these aches and stopped me turning homicidal on account of the slightest problem." Counselors need to be aware of such "drifts" toward relapse and take appropriate action.

2. Drug therapy featuring interferon, either on its own or in combination with other agents such as ribavirin, is a possible relapse risk. Interferon can precipitate depression, increased cognitive dysfunction, and extreme anxiety, as well as a host of physical side effects. Not everybody experiences these effects, and some emerge from treatment with few problems. However, it is rare to come through interferon therapy without some degree

of mental and physical discomfort, and this is often significant, fairly frequently severe enough to cause the discontinuation of treatment (in about 15% of cases). Although a history of depression is a relative contraindication, this factor is sometimes skipped over by prescribers. The drug is also taken by injection, which presents obvious risks to patients with a history of IV drug use. Kevin, an HCV+ addict, had the following experience of interferon treatment:

> A few weeks after being diagnosed with HCV and having a battery of tests, I was advised by my hepatologist that I was suitable for interferon therapy and that he considered that this would be a good course of action. I agreed without really asking myself what I was letting myself in for. Just before my first injection the nurse asked me if I had a history of depression. I replied, "Yes, I have long history of depressive illness." She said, "Well we'd better keep an eye on that then," and proceeded to give me the shot. I fell into a severe depression and was also profoundly disorientated, which meant that I was not clear enough to realize what was happening or what action to take. Six weeks later I found myself shooting up heroin in the toilet. I had been clean for eight years, had a wife and kids, and a good job in a new career. About three weeks after that I attempted to kill myself. Needless to say I cannot overstate the anger I feel toward the treatment providers and would advise anybody with a history of depression or drug problems, which are usually associated anyway, to think very long and hard before taking this drug.

Experiences such as this suggest that patients need to be wary of "giving their power away" to doctors; it is also wise to assume that they will be unaware of addiction and recovery issues. They may need to inform themselves in detail of the pros and cons of drug therapy, and need help from counselors with this process. Active addiction will usually be more immediately life-threatening than chronic hepatitis C.

Those who do opt for interferon-based drug therapy should be advised to arrange maximum support from friends, family, doctors, fellowships, hepatitis C support groups, and counselling professionals. Although this treatment rarely amounts to a cure,[14] response rates are improving, particularly with combination therapy,[33] and so it will appeal to many patients. Serious side effects are not ubiquitous, but therapy can last for up to eighteen months. Note that some other drugs, such as amantadine and thymosin (common trade name Zadaxin), rarely precipitate such side effects, although they are also of limited benefit.

3. Mental and emotional problems, particularly disorientation, pronounced mood swings, and depression, comprise serious obstacles to recovery. While twelve-step programs and counselling can help to address the relapse risks posed by depression and mood swings, the threat posed by the cognitive problems collectively described as "brain fog" by patients is difficult to treat through these methods.

Methods of Addressing
These Risk Factors and Contacts

1. "Illness in recovery" meetings can be very helpful; typical issues can be raised, experiences reinforced, and practical solutions shared, all in the context of the fellowships. (Refer to twelve-step fellowship directories for details.)

2. Hepatitis C support group meetings can be extremely useful, particularly for having symptoms affirmed, and also for the sharing of experience and information. (See the "Resources" section at the end of the book.)

3. Chinese herbal medicine is a particularly effective approach to the relief of debilitating symptoms and can improve clinical indicators. Standard, quality-controlled formulations are now available. These can be taken from the first day of abstinence and may help to "level the playing field" between those

with and without hep C in recovery. Fatigue, depression, and digestive problems are often responsive to this approach. These are suitable for individual use and may also be useful to primary and secondary residential resources with hep C + clients. Refer to chapter 15 for details.

4. The NADA network can provide ear acupuncture and ear acupuncture training that will help HCV+ clients, particularly in synergy with herbal medicine. In the U.S., call (360) 260-8620 and in the U.K., call 0171 820 9892 for details. The U.K. branch offers a hepatitis C manual.

Conclusion

The attitude that symptoms associated with hepatitis C are insignificant or entirely secondary to the recovery process is no longer defensible. On the contrary, emerging findings about the pathogenesis of HCV and the wide range of related physical, mental, and emotional symptoms demonstrate that effective treatment for hepatitis C must be integrated into recovery provision in order to afford a reasonable likelihood of success. The status quo in the recovery professional community, where many of the symptoms of HCV infection are mistaken for symptoms of "addiction" and treated by twelve-step work and/or psychotherapy, needs to be changed. Although it is true that an HCV+ addict must be treated for addiction as a prerequisite, it is also true that failure to address symptomatic HCV will result in increased likelihood of relapse, unnecessarily poor quality of life, impaired functionality, increased likelihood of life-threatening disease, pronounced emotional problems, and associated reduced longevity.

Further Reading

Alcoholics Anonymous, Narcotics Anonymous, and other fellowship "Big Books."

For a perspective of recovery that includes acupuncture try *Transformation and Recovery*, Alex G. Brumbaugh, Stillpoint Press, 1995.

Or *Fighting Drug Abuse with Acupuncture,* Ellinor R. Mitchell, Pacific View Press, 1995.

References

1. Hepatitis C: The clinical spectrum of disease. Alter MJ. *Disease Weekly Plus*, p 36, June 9 and 16, 1997.

2. "This report indicates that hepatitis C has reached alarming numbers in the United States, yet public awareness of the disease is dangerously low," said W.G. Hardison, MD, president of the San Diego Chapter of the American Liver Foundation.

3. HealthWire. March 16, 1998. The American Liver Foundation (ALF), San Diego Chapter, calls on all public health officials and the state's lawmakers to follow the recommendations of a new report by the California Center for Health Improvement (CCHI).

4. The epidemiology of viral hepatitis in the United States. Alter MJ and Mast EE. *Gastroenterology Clinics of North America*, 23(3), September 1994.

5. See chapter 2 and references.

6. Chronic Hepatitis C, Roche Biocare Consultants Report. Thomas HC. pp 6–8, 1994.

7. The sleeping giant awakes. Waller T and Holmes R. *Druglink*, pp 8–11, Institute for the Study of Drug Dependence (U.K.), Sept/Oct 1995.

8. Histological activity in hepatitis C virus (HCV) infected English intravenous drug users (IVDU). Wali MH, Elias E, Mutimer DJ et al. Liver and Hepatobiliary Unit, Queen Elizabeth Hospital, Birmingham, England. Paper presented at the American Association for the Study of Liver Disease. Abstracts from conference, 1996.

> The vast majority of HCV infection in England is IVDU-acquired. We have reviewed 100 consecutively referred HCV-positive ex-IVDU [75 male: 25 female, median age 38 (21–55).

9. *Hepatitis C Virus.* Simmonds P. Topley and Wilsons Microbiology and Microbial Infections—Arnold, Sept 1996.

10. Hepatitis B and C virus infection, alcohol drinking and hepatocellular carcinoma: A case control study in Italy. Donato F et al. *Hepatology*, 26(3):579–584, Sept 1997.

11. Hepatitis C infection in patients with clinically diagnosed alcoholic liver diseases. Sata M et al. *Journal of Viral Hepatitis*, 3(3): 143–8, May 1996.

12. Interactions between alcohol and hepatitis viruses in the liver

[Review]. Brechot C et al. *Clinics in Laboratory Medicine,* 16(2): 273–87, June 1996.

13. Routes of infection, viremia, and liver disease in blood disease in blood donors found to have hepatitis C infection. Conry-Cantilena C et al. *New England Journal of Medicine,* 334(26), 1996.

14. Interferon treatment of chronic hepatitis C. Davis GL. *The American Journal of Medicine,* 96 (supplement 1A), 41–46, Jan 1994.

15. Natural history of liver fibrosis progression in patients with chronic hepatitis C. Poynard T et al. *Lancet,* 349(9055):825–832, Mar 22, 1997.

16. Natural history of hepatitis C. Seeff LB. *Hepatology,* 26 (3 Suppl 1):21S–28S, Sept 1997.

17. Prevalence of hepatocellular carcinoma in patients with alcoholic cirrhosis and prior exposure to hepatitis C. Yamauchi K et al. *American Journal of Gastroenterology,* 88: 39–43, 1993.

18. See chapter 22 and associated references.

19. Opiates and immune function consequences. Rouveux B. *Therapie,* 47(6):503–12, Nov 1992.

20. Study. Levier DG et al. *Fundamental and Applied Toxicology,* 24 (2):275–84, Feb 1995.

21. Macrophage functions in drugs of abuse treated mice. Pacifi R et al. *International Journal of Immunopharmacology,* 15, series 6, (7):6–11, Aug 1993.

22. Psychological stress, depression and quality of life in patients with liver disease due to hepatitis C virus. Singh N et al. Veterans Affairs Medical Center, Pittsburgh, PA. Paper presented at the 1996 American Association for the Study of Liver Diseases, November 8–12, 1996.

23. Increased risk for diabetes type II with chronic hepatitis C infection. Zein NN et al. Mayo Clinic, Rochester. Paper presented at the 1996 American Association for the Study of Liver Diseases, November 8–12, 1996.

24. Nonhepatic manifestations of and combined diseases in HCV infection. Hadziyannis S. *Digestive Diseases and Sciences,* 41(12):63s–74s, December 1996.

25. Cerebral ischemia in patients with hepatitis C infection and mixed cryoglobulinaemia. Petty GW et al. *Mayo Clinic Proceedings,* 71(7):671–8, July 1996.

26. Hepatitis C virus—associated membranoproliferative glomerulonephritis in renal allografts. Cruzado JM et al. *Journal of the American Society of Nephrology,* 7(11):2469–75, Nov 1996.

27. Viral hepatitis and autoimmunity: chicken or egg? Strassburg C, Mann M. *Viral Hepatitis Review,* June 1995.

28. Chronic hepatitis C and B-cell non-Hodgkin's lymphoma. Ferri C et al. University of Pisa, *Quarterly Journal of Medicine,* 89(2):117–122, Feb 1996.

29. Hepatitis C infection and clonal B-cell expansion. Sansonno D et al. *Clinical and Experimental Rheumatolgy,* 14 Supplement 45–50, Jan-Feb 1996.

30. Hepatitis infection in immunocompromised patients. Gitnick G. *Gastroenterology Clinics of North America,* 23(3):515–521, September 1994.

31. Influence of HIV infection on hepatic lesions related to HCV infection. Benhamou JP et al. Service d'Hepato-Gastroenterologie, GH Pitie Salpetiere, 75651 Paris, France.

32. Nicotine metabolism in liver microsomes from rats with acute hepatitis or cirrhosis. Nakajima M et al. *Drug Metab Dispos,* 26(1):36–41, Jan 1, 1998.

33. Combination therapy with interferon alpha and ribavirin in interferon alpha relapsers. Ricchiuti A et al. Clinical Gastroenterology Unit, University of Pisa, Italy. Paper presented at the 1996 American Association for the Study of Liver Diseases, November 8–12, 1996.

Part

3

Treatment Options

13

Treatments Overview

HEPATITIS C IS OFTEN responsive to treatment. No particular
approach offers the solution to every patient's needs. Most of
the medical paradigms included here offer partial solutions; they all
have pros and cons. It is also apparent that what works for one
patient may not help another. It is often necessary to experiment in
order to find out what approach suits you best—the same goes for
lifestyle. It seems that patients often need to assess their own situation as clearly as the treatment they are contemplating. Much will
depend upon individual disposition and character. An open-minded
and fluid approach will increase the chances of finding a satisfactory
set of solutions.

It is becoming clear that personal belief systems play an important role in influencing the response to hepatitis C diagnosis. One
recent study of newly diagnosed patients attending a large London
teaching hospital found the following:

> A large proportion of patients (39%) with newly diagnosed
> hepatitis C infection do not want to undergo further investi-
> gation. Of those patients who do attend for further treatment,
> a large proportion with severe hepatic fibrosis (42%) do not
> want to undergo currently available treatment.[1]

The report concluded:

> Current strategies aimed at investigating and treating chronic
> hepatitis C are not acceptable to a large proportion of patients.

Thus there is clearly a need for the introduction of new methods of addressing the needs of newly diagnosed patients and a requirement for the development of more broadly based treatment strategies. Failure to incorporate such options may result in further polarization between alternative and conventional modes of treatment and fragmentation of health care as a whole. It is apparent that many patients have very little faith in the ability of mainstream medicine to address their health needs. The relative youth of most hepatitis C patients may underlie this aspect, but the providers of health care and producers of medicines also need to review the acceptability and efficacy of their products; in many cases patients' concerns have basis in fact.

The treatments listed in this part of the book demonstrate that there is no shortage of options worthy of consideration; it is by no means an exhaustive list.

One of the main problems is the fact that there is a constant war of words between the various traditions and their philosophical underpinnings. The best source of information often proves to be other patients who can demonstrate the effects of treatment; they are a primary source of valid information. It is extremely hard to find a genuinely disinterested medical opinion. Therefore attending a support group may be an excellent way of helping to make a treatment choice.

The issue of treatment validation is central. The fact that treatment A has been through fifty double-blind placebo-controlled trials demonstrating a 50% drop in viral load in 75% of selected patients, for example, does not necessarily mean that it is superior to treatment B, which might have been used for a thousand years but doesn't warrant trial on account of its lack of potential for profit generation.

Drug treatments only receive official sanction after lengthy and expensive trials, which are funded by the providers of the medicines undergoing tests. Obtaining a license for any given medicine is also expensive, around £80,000 in the U.K. and $250,000 in the U.S. These sums are dwarfed by the budgets now required for global marketing of such products. Figures of $400 million and upwards have been quoted as a typical budget. Many critics of this system have pointed out that this means that inexpensive medicines or those advocated by suppliers without extensive resources do not stand a good chance of receiving official sanction. It is also the case that most medical research is funded by pharmaceutical companies, who clearly have a vested interest in developing and marketing profitable products. Conversely, expensive drugs like interferon would never have been developed by commercial organizations if there weren't a prospect of making a profit.

Because there is no significant detached and disinterested source of treatment research, it is very difficult for alternative products to obtain official sanction. Therefore they will always be open to the accusation that they are "unproven." The catch phrase "evidence-based medicine" sounds entirely reasonable, but upon close inspection what it actually means is that medicines that are not potentially capable of generating profits on a very large scale over a considerable period of time stand virtually no chance of being studied on equal terms. The words "alternative" or "complementary" could actually be substituted for the term "unprofitable" and the word "conventional" with regard to licensed drugs could be switched for "patentable/profitable." The same goes for conventional medical treatments that do not include the use of pharmaceutical drugs, such as immunotherapy. Thus it is clear that economic rather than medical factors are dominant in determining what is available from mainstream medicine.

Having said this, there are a growing number of factors coming into play that may radically change this general use of only a very narrowly based selection of medicines. The factors include changes in the laws governing patenting biotechnology and the development of certain biological "fingerprinting" techniques. These are discussed in the "Future Treatments for Hepatitis C" section in chapter 14. Another notable influence for change is the vast and possibly impractical cost implications of treating hepatitis C with such expensive medicines on the scale required. Both governments and institutions such as insurance companies may need to instigate alternative lines of research. Phytopharmaceutical medicines in particular look well placed to fill the gap that exists for affordable products.

Many patients feel uncomfortable around the word "cure." In

the past doctors have been careful to avoid using the word, but recently some have started to make extravagant claims. What constitutes a cure is another key question. Antiviral treatments often result in considerable debilitation, and it is difficult to assess whether or not HCV RNA has actually been removed. If it lingers, there is always the potential for HCV reemergence. The health "cost" of antiviral drug treatment should also be considered. Many think that chemotherapy permanently undermines immune function. The truth of this will only become apparent in the long term. Some other treatments can minimize or even halt liver inflammation but may not be able to reduce levels of HCV, necessitating long-term ongoing treatment, although quality of life may improve. Thus there are several different approaches to treatment with varied parameters of "success" that fall short of a proven cure.

What Constitutes Successful Treatment?

- The elimination of HCV from all body fluids and tissue? The restoration of full function and life expectancy?

- The suppression of the virus so that it remains undetectable in the blood for a reasonable period of time? The inhibition of viral replication, preventing associated damage?

- The arrest and reversal of HCV-related injury, resulting in improved or normal functionality and a reasonable expectation of an average life span?

The aims of treatment and the measurement of its success can also include other factors apart from the elimination of HCV. There are four basic parameters:

- Viral load

- Organ function

- Functionality/quality of life

- Modification of the course of hepatitis C-related disease

None of the currently available treatments have been systematically validated against all of these.

Because the dynamics of hepatitis C-related disease are not yet fully understood, an element of faith is sometimes required. For instance, finding a treatment that restores vitality may not necessarily mean that long-term prognosis is improved.

While it may be logical to infer that reduced symptoms and higher quality of life indicate improved prospects of survival, the necessary research has not yet been done to prove this. In a sense all treatments are quite literally experimental. The only way that one method can be conclusively shown to have worked is when large numbers of patients who have tried it die of causes completely unrelated to HCV.

It is quite likely that you will be able to find a combination of treatment and lifestyle change that will significantly improve your quality of life. It is possible that you will be able to get rid of the virus and all of its symptoms with the options presented here. It is probable that more effective treatments will appear in the near future and that the efficacy of the methods described here will become clearer.

Which Treatments Mix and Which Do Not?

If you are seeking to combine treatments always tell the practitioners concerned.

- TCM or herbs can be mixed with conventional medicine, but you must tell both sets of practitioners. The usual approach is to start with TCM and then use drug therapy after qualitative benefits have accrued.

- TCM or herbs can be used as adjunct therapy during drug treatment. Usually neither side is particularly happy about the other, but many patients have successfully combined these two approaches. Western doctors are usually quite happy to have patients using acupuncture, but they can become concerned when herbs are used.

- If you are taking a course of Western herbal medicine for instance, you should not simultaneously take courses of Chinese or Ayurvedic herbs. The same goes for any of these choices; stick to one approach if using off-the-shelf products.

- Some herbal practitioners use herbs from Western, Chinese, and Ayurvedic materia medicas, so you can gain access to a range of resources in one treatment. It is important to put yourself under the care of one herbalist only.

- Naturopathy and homeopathy usually don't mix well with taking medicines of any type, although practitioners will advise.

- Acupuncture is compatible with any other treatment.

In general, approaches can be classified as follows:

- Surgery and operational procedures aim to resolve a specific problem with a particular part of the body.

- Procedures such as phlebotomy or colonic irrigation address wider physical problems via mechanical means.

- Drug therapy usually represents a very specific therapy with narrow but clearly measurable aims. Drugs usually contain concentrates of "active ingredients."

- Vitamins, minerals, and amino acids will have wider ranges of less-pronounced action compared to drug therapy; measurement of benefit is often impractical.

- The use of single herbs will have specific aims, but these medicines will often have effects that overlap with those of drugs or vitamins. For instance silymarin may be used to protect the liver, but also has a general antioxidant effect and modest antiviral action as well.

- The use of complex herbal formulations can have powerful multi-faceted effects on all body systems. Levels of vitamins, minerals, and amino acids will be affected. Pharmaceutical-like actions, such as reductions in viral load, may be observed, organ functions may be affected, and mental and emotional status may be influenced. The whole body will be affected. It is difficult to measure the impact because the action will be very broad as well as pharmacologically powerful.

- The use of radical dietary therapy will also bring about changes in overall body function and metabolism.

- Acupuncture will affect the energetic profiles of patients and is prescribed in accordance with metaphysical principles. Mode of action remains biologically obscure but can be powerful.

- Homeopathy is also a form of energetic medicine, seeking to provoke powerful changes in body function through the introduction of highly dilute substances to effect a specific response.

- Qi Gong, yoga, meditation, and other mind-body-spirit activities also use energetic principles to meet medical needs. There is usually a spiritual element within these practices. Wide and fundamental issues may be addressed through these modes of treatment. Benefits to quality of life are often patently obvious to people who use these methods but very hard to measure.

Reference

1. Management of hepatitis C: clinical audit of biopsy based management algorithm. Foster GR et al. *BMJ*, 315 (7106):453–8, Aug 23, 1997.

14

Conventional Treatments and Hepatitis

Overview

Patients' experience of conventional medicine varies. For a few it provides a cure or something close to it; for others conventional therapy causes only frustration and even makes them more ill. Many routine symptoms of HCV are not addressed by generally available mainstream treatment, which tends to focus on the viral cause.

Although there are many different treatments that could be classified as "conventional" and are applicable to hepatitis C, the emphasis is firmly on drug therapy to eliminate the virus, or surgical intervention to save patients where the disease is life-threatening. It can be very hard to gain access to some of the other useful treatments listed in this chapter. Prior to the identification of the virus, many patients were diagnosed and treated for conditions that are now accepted as being related. Because the research into related conditions is so recent and because so few general practice doctors are aware of the wider pattern of symptoms, patients are frequently misdiagnosed or not diagnosed at all.

Where patients are correctly diagnosed, economic factors are playing an increasingly important role in influencing access to expensive treatments; several papers have been published on the cost/benefit ratio of interferon therapy for HCV patients. Prioritization is effectively already a reality. Where health insurance schemes are operating, there are instances of insurers refusing to finance interferon treatment. Other patients seeking interferon treatment have been offered it free of charge because they happen to qualify for trials. There are significant inconsistencies in the way patients are treated from one area to the next. Some patients will not even be referred to specialists, although this can be due to the ignorance of local doctors as well as financial factors.

Knowledge of hepatitis C is concentrated in a few specialist hepatologists, gastroenterologists, and virologists. These men and women are usually highly motivated and competent, although they can be disparaging about other traditions of medicine. Patients with complications that are not related to the liver are likely to be referred to relevant specialists, many of whom will be new to HCV.

Conventional medicine tends to be reductionist, focusing on the minutiae of the disease, in this case the virus, rather than the patient. Practitioners are more interested in clinical indicators and test results than the actual range of symptoms experienced by patients. They find HCV very frustrating because many of these tests are poor indicators of patients' overall status.

Because of this narrow focus, mainstream medicine is not good at picking up subtle patterns of symptoms and prescribing preventative treatments. For instance, although they advise liver patients to eat well, they do not prescribe appetite stimulants and high-quality vitamins or food supplements to patients, even though there is a profile of digestive problems and likely amino acid and vitamin deficiency. They are slow to pick up on wider patterns of illness and reluctant to concede the existence of links that they cannot currently explain. They are often reluctant to admit that they "don't know." They are generally regarded as being better at acute intervention than treating chronic disease.

The Life Cycle of HCV

Antiviral drug therapy focuses on specific stages in the replication of HCV. These phases can be broken down as follows:

1. The virus attaches itself to host cells.

2. The virus "uncoats" within the target cell.

3. The virus synthesizes its RNA.

4. The virus translates its RNA.

5. The virus replicates its RNA.

6. The virus particles are assembled.

7. The virus "buds," releasing a new generation of HCV virions.

For further details refer to chapter 1 and the technical notes on HCV replication in part 5. Present and impending drug therapy focuses on specific phases in this process.

There are two approaches: *immunological* drugs aim to promote an immune response sufficient to disrupt this process; the *virological* approach involves the design of agents that are directly active against certain phases in HCV replication. The immunological approach can be further classified as treatments that promote a *humoral* immune response (that is, they stimulate the production of antibodies that are active in plasma), and those that stimulate a *cellular* response (that is, they boost antiviral activity within infected cells). Other agents, particularly herbs known to have antiviral properties, can also be classified in this way, although their actions are more complex and difficult to understand.

Interferon

Unlike a number of other frightening "modern" diseases, hepatitis C is not invariably incurable. Although there is more than one treatment that can achieve improved liver function, better qualitative experience of health, and thereby an assumed probability of improved long-term prognosis, only drug therapy has been shown to have achieved long-term suppression or elimination of HCV on a statistically significant scale. With hindsight it is apparent that some patients were successfully treated for hepatitis C before the virus was discovered. So far these results can only be shown to have been achieved where interferon-based therapy has been used.

Essentially this drug refocuses the immune system; antiviral activity within cells is increased, while the activity of other arms of the immune system, such as white blood cells, is decreased. This shift of focus is thought to result in a blocking of the synthesis and translation phases of HCV replication. Vulnerable cells may be prevented from being infected, and the drug is also thought to enhance the elimination of cells that are already infected.

Recombinant interferon alpha is a synthetic version of one of the interferons produced in the body as part of the immune response mechanism. (It is self-administered via subcutaneous injection by patients themselves—it has to be taken this way because if it was taken orally, it would be destroyed by stomach enzymes.) The subject is covered in the "Immune System and HCV" notes in part 5. It is sufficient to note that interferons are "chemical messengers" that communicate the fact of an antigen's presence and trigger the release of substances, called "antiviral proteins" that attempt to "interfere" with the process of viral replication within infected cells.

History of Interferon Development and Use

In the late '70s scientists developed the ability to refine interferon from blood. It was extremely expensive, requiring more than 100,000 pints of blood to produce a fraction of an ounce. A single dose cost around $1,000. However, many in the scientific community, particularly the large drug companies who had spent millions on the project, felt that this was a major breakthrough in the treatment of human disease.

There then followed a series of "miracle drug" stories in the media. In 1980 *Time* magazine hailed interferon as the new miracle drug capable of preventing the development of cancerous tumors (at the time it was felt that viruses were responsible for the development of tumors). Not surprisingly, large numbers of cancer patients besieged their doctors demanding to be treated with this miraculous new drug. However, it was not long before the claims being made for interferon as a cancer cure were comprehensively discredited. Although interferon is still used along with other drugs in the treatment of certain types of cancer, it is no longer a mainstream drug.

Despite the disappointment surrounding the initial hopes for interferon, some drug companies continued their research. They managed to clone the gene for alpha-interferon and insert it into the

E. coli bacteria, allowing the production of large quantities at greatly reduced cost. The price of interferon has fallen significantly over the last few years as a result of this technique and the arrival of new competition in the market.

Initially two companies—Schering-Plough and Roche Biocare—persevered in their marketing of the drug and providing support for clinical research into its efficacy in the treatment of a range of conditions. One of the conditions that attracted their attention was chronic non-A non-B hepatitis. The drug was tried on ten American patients in 1986— six of them showed improved liver function. On this basis larger, randomized trials were carried out. Since the discovery of HCV, interferon has been used to treat thousands of patients in the U.S., Europe, and Japan. Although doctors are still not entirely sure exactly how interferon helps to treat HCV, experience of treatment is now quite "well understood," and coherent strategies are being developed.

Several interferon-based products are now available; Amgen and Glaxo Wellcome have introduced products containing a wider recombinant range of the interferons produced naturally in the human body: alpha, beta, and gamma interferons. These are known as "consensus interferon" products (see below). There are a few other new arrivals as well, such as Interferon Sciences, Biogen Corp., and Genentech. Most of these products are differentiated according to variations in the manufacturing process. Schering-Plough and Roche Biocare have developed their products by adding other agents to create new combination therapies that effectively amount to new forms of treatment (see below for further details on these).

The Efficacy of Recombinant Interferon Alpha

In general, the beneficial effect of interferon-based therapy upon chronic hepatitis C is measured according to two parameters: suppression of detectable HCV and positive changes in the health of the liver that indicate a reduced likelihood of "end stage" liver disease. These parameters are known as

- **Virological response** relates to the level of virus in plasma.
- **Biochemical** or **histological response** relates to changes in the biology and histology of the liver.

Thus the aim of therapy is twofold. Both classes of response are further classified:

- **Sustained response** has previously been defined as HCV RNA remaining undetectable in the blood of patients for six or twelve months following the end of treatment.

- **Temporary response** means that liver function improves and HCV is undetectable for the duration of treatment, but that function deteriorates and the virus reappears shortly after the cessation of therapy.

- **Nonresponse** means that patients demonstrate little or no improvement in liver function and viral persistence despite therapy.

While response of a temporary or sustained nature still occurs in about 50% of selected and treated patients who comply with the regime, it is now apparent that the longer-term sustained virological response rates to interferon alpha therapy on its own are disappointing. The reasons for this are still not fully understood. However, this may relate to the persistence of HCV in certain peripheral blood cells.[1] It is also known that even if replication is halted, HCV RNA can linger in body tissue for lengthy periods. Thus it appears that quite a significant proportion of those with sustained virological response at six months relapse in the subsequent three years or so. Some patients I spoke to claimed that the virus appeared and disappeared several times at very low concentrations before they were classed as "complete responders."

Recent prospective studies demonstrate sustained virological response rates of between 5%[2] and 30%, with an average rate of less than 20%. Since only selected or "indicated" patients were put onto this therapy, the relevance to the overall patient population is dubious anyway. Patients who develop dangerous side effects are also excluded from the final figures. With the benefit of hindsight and the more recent ability to compare and contrast figures from different patient groups and those treated with newer forms of therapy, the reasons for these results are becoming increasingly clear.

For patients or their medical advisors reading this book, the overall figures are relatively meaningless. It is now obvious that the likelihood of obtaining a net benefit from this type of therapy needs to be assessed on an individual basis. The appearance of new licensed therapeutic options also changes the situation. Factors influencing the likelihood of response and the ability of the patient to tolerate the regime are both important.

A note about biochemical or histological response: The case for taking interferon even if the response is "unsustained."

Some hepatologists think that a course of interferon treatment may be good for patients even if they do not have a sustained response. This is because there is some evidence that the heterogeneity of the HCV strains present in treated patients declines after a course of interferon. Heterogeneity—that is the presence of more than one strain or the mutation of the original strain into a number of subtypes—is associated with poorer prognosis and greater resistance to therapy.

Others argue that it gives the livers of "partial responders" a rest from attack and a chance to regenerate. Thus the long-term outcome may be more favorable even for relapsing patients. There are also the theoretically anticarcinogenic qualities of interferon treatment— it helps to modulate the overproduction of oncogenes, which are substances associated with cancer—which may justify its use even where the virus persists.

Factors Believed to Influence Likelihood of Response to Interferon

- **Viral load,** that is the amount of virus circulating in the blood, lower levels being more favorable to the outcome of therapy. Viral loads tend to fluctuate, but not to the same degree as liver enzymes. PCR tests tend to be more sensitive to some strains than others, so it is impossible to define a threshold figure determining the likelihood of response, although a figure of 4 million copies per ml has been suggested.[3] The viral load within liver cells is also thought to have a bearing on response.

- **Genotype.** It is now apparent that one reason for wide discrepancies in response rates from one country to the other is related to genotype prevalence. Thus higher rates of response in countries such as Australia compared to the U.S. can be neatly correlated to the relatively high numbers of patients with genotype 3 in Australia. Thus the genotype of the virus is thought by many virologists and hepatologists to be a very important factor.

Type 1 (particularly 1b), which is prevalent in the U.S. and Canada, appears to be a much tougher nut to crack. One recent report summarized the situation in the U.S. as follows:

> Fifty-eight percent of patients had genotype 1a, 21% had 1b, 2% had 2a, 13% had 2b, 5% had 3a and 1% had 4a.... Twenty-eight percent of patients with genotype 1a and 26% of patients with genotype 1b had a complete biochemical response to treatment with interferon-alpha for six months. In contrast, 71% of patients with genotype 2a or 2b had a complete response to interferon therapy. This study confirms that 1a and 1b are the most predominant hepatitis C virus genotypes in the United States and that patients infected with these viral genotypes generally have more severe liver disease and lower rates of response to interferon therapy than patients infected with genotypes 2a or 2b.[4]

Type 4, which is prevalent in the Middle East, also tends to be unresponsive to interferon. Clinicians are experimenting with new dosage regimes and combination therapy to try to address this (see below). Types 2 and 3 appear to be more likely to be cleared by interferon treatment than types 1 and 4. However, some doctors believe that the apparent influence of genotype may reflect

- **The duration of the infection.** Because type 1b is "older" in many countries, it may be that patients infected with this strain have simply had more time to progress. The time the virus has been present is known to influence the degree to which disease has progressed. It may also have a bearing on viral heterogeneity.

- **Viral heterogeneity.** The longer HCV has been present, the more likely it is to have mutated into viable quasi species, making it

into a more difficult target for drug therapy. Thus the time elaps-
ing after initial exposure to initiation of treatment is also a factor. Patients who have been infected with multiple strains to
begin with are also thought to have a lower response rate.

- **The age of the patient** is also thought to be a factor; the younger,
  the better. The study of thalassaemia patients earlier in the book
  suggests the importance of youth. In turn this means that there
  is a powerful argument for health authorities to instigate ini-
  tiatives to diagnose hepatitis C.

- **Health of the liver.** Good liver function and the absence of cirrhosis and fibrosis are good signs, both for tolerability of interferon and response.

- **The general fitness of the patient** is also thought to have a bearing by many doctors. Patients who are significantly overweight
  have been observed to have lower response rates.

- **Iron levels in liver cells** also have a bearing; the lower, the better. In the past it was thought that women had better response
  rates than men. This is likely to have been caused by the fact
  that menstruation drains off excess iron. Patients with a history of heavy drinking tend to have higher levels of iron deposition in their liver cells.

Hepatologists are particularly interested in the relative importance of viral load compared to genotype, thought by many to be
the two key factors. This debate spills over into the funding question, with the implications of expense for genotype tests. It is still
hard to define an individual patient's exact likelihood of response.

Factors Influencing the Tolerability of Interferon

Apart from the manifestation of side effects, there are some factors
that are thought to influence the advisability of taking up this option.

- **Motivation** is regarded as an important factor by many doctors with experience of treating patients with interferon. It is
  particularly important when side effects begin to build up.

- **A history of depression,** particularly depression interrelated to chemical dependency, is a very important consideration. The adverse consequences of a relapse into chemical dependency can easily outweigh the benefits of response to drug therapy. This is difficult to assess. The subject is covered in more detail in chapter 12.

- **Social stability** and **access to peer support** are thought to be extremely helpful.

General Contraindications for Interferon Treatment

(Many of these are subject to the prescribing doctor's discretion.)

- Decompensated liver disease
- Pregnant, or likely to become so
- Enlarged spleen
- Hyperthyroidism (this can be manageable)
- History of psychiatric illness, particularly clinical depression
- Significant cytopenia (reduced white cells or platelets) or anemia
- Severe autoimmune disorders/patients undergoing corticosteroid treatment
- History of sensitivity to interferon treatment
- Severe renal disease
- Compromised central nervous system or epilepsy
- Heart disease or history of cardiac problems
- General autoimmune disorders

In addition patients who fall into the following categories are often regarded as unsuitable, but may be treated depending on discretion of the doctor:

- Currently using illegal drugs (some clinics stipulate that patients should be drug free for at least three months prior to treatment) or abusing alcohol. There are reports that interferon increases the likelihood of opiate overdose. This is a big question and research is urgently required. It is known that some patients on methadone maintenance have undergone interferon treatment without such problems.

Both men and women must practice contraception if taking ribavirin and continue to do so for six months after the end of treatment.

Dosage, Duration, and Alternative Drug Delivery Strategies

In terms of treatment strategies, doctors are now agreed that the higher the dose of interferon and the longer it is sustained, the better the prospect of viral clearance. When interferon was first used the dose was 3 million units (mu) every other day for six months. It is now accepted that this was not very effective[5] and that therapy should be continued for at least a year, at a dose of 4.5 or 6 mu three times per week. Unfortunately the higher the dose and the longer the duration of treatment, the greater the chance of more serious side effects developing.

Recent efforts aimed at adjusting the dosage of interferon therapy have largely been concentrated on trying to make headway against the type 1 strains of HCV so prevalent in the U.S. It is thought that the action of interferon against HCV type 1 may fail to reach critical mass and keep pace with replication. Two strategies have been tried:

1. High-dose induction therapy, which lasts for up to two weeks and contains dosages of up to three times the normal regime

2. Daily dosage instead of three times weekly dosages

These strategies are now yielding better results for patients with type 1 genotypes, though response is still markedly lower than for types 2 and 3. It should also be noted that a few patients respond completely to much smaller doses of interferon, as low as 1 mu three times per week.

Other approaches include the use of "time release" interferon, "PEGulated" as it is known, which only requires administration once per week. Combination drug therapy is also seen as being promising (see the "Other Treatments" section below). A company called Amarillo Biosciences has also produced an oral form of interferon that is licensed to treat hepatitis B in some developing countries. A company called Powderject has developed a high velocity "hassle free" alternative to the hypodermic syringe, which is widely acclaimed as being a superior and relatively pain-free drug delivery option. This technology may also yield benefits in harm reduction.

Early Indicators of Response

Given the side effects and expense of drug therapy, some doctors and patients believe that it would be beneficial to all concerned if those who were unlikely to respond were taken off therapy as early as possible. Doctors have also noticed that patients undergoing interferon therapy tend to sort themselves into the categories of "responders" and "nonresponders" quite quickly. Current practice in a number of hospitals is to discontinue treatment in those patients clearly not responding after six to twelve weeks. This practice is seen as being more ethically defensible than denying patients treatment on the basis of the likely indicators listed above; these are not conclusive.

There are now a number of studies that seem to indicate the likelihood of response within the first few days or weeks of starting therapy. For example, Japanese researchers have found that the clearance of detectable HCV RNA within the first two weeks of therapy is a very reliable indicator of sustained response. A recent American study reveals that an accurate assessment of antiviral response can be determined within forty-eight hours of commencement.

Why Interferon Is Thought to Fail

Where it fails several factors are implicated. The virus may replicate in sites protected from the antiviral effects of interferon (see "Models of Viral Persistence" in part 5); the immune system may generate anti-interferon antibodies that neutralize the effect of interferon. Some specialists suspect that an element of genetic disposition may influence the likelihood of response.

Summary of Interferon

The paradox of interferon and hepatitis C is that those patients who are most likely to respond are also the least likely to need immediate treatment. Not enough is known about the natural history of HCV to be able to state categorically that this group of patients will definitely develop more serious liver damage later in life, so they cannot be confidently advised that this is the best course of action for them.

Many doctors will support patients seeking the chance of successful treatment, even if the odds are against the treatment working.

Pretreatment factors and early response readings mean that this therapy can be quite well targeted. However, none of these indicators are yet absolute, so there will still be an element of unpredictability.

Figures that are now available suggest that interferon alpha 2 therapy on its own has a very disappointing level of success in terms of sustained virological response, being particularly poor for type 1 genotypes. This is the basis for combination therapies.

Other Interferon-Based Treatments

Ribavirin Interferon

This combination therapy is regarded as a breakthrough in the treatment of HCV by many doctors. Ribavirin has been used to treat lassa fever successfully and is also prescribed for respiratory syncitial virus. Ribavirin is classed as a "guanosine analogue"—this means that it has the effect of disrupting the process of viral replication by providing a building block substance that is assimilated instead of the real thing; the idea is that this "fooling" process prevents the virus from assembling the proper set of genetic material, thereby halting replication. It is also described as a "nucleoside analogue."

It is taken orally. Despite the sophistication of this drug it is relatively cheap, and there are also a number of generic imports available. Side effects are usually milder than interferon; they include a drop in red blood cell count, flulike symptoms, indigestion, and insomnia.

Trials of ribavirin as a sole treatment for hepatitis C have been only mildly encouraging. It seems to improve some patients but does not reduce viral load. Liver enzyme tests show some improvement in function, while HCV RNA levels in the blood tend to remain constant.[6] It has been largely abandoned as a single therapy, although recent research suggests that it may be effective for clearing HCV from the lymphatic system and also be a useful option for posttransplant patients.

Schering-Plough now holds the license for ribavirin in America and has nonexclusive rights in Europe. They have branded their set of hepatitis treatments as Intron A (interferon 2b), Rebetol (ribavirin), and Rebetron (combined interferon and ribavirin). The company has conducted a number of trials of combined interferon-ribavirin therapy for hepatitis C.

The results of these trials show that this combination therapy can convert a number of people who were previously only partial or temporary responders into complete responders. Indeed it now appears that between 40% and 60% of patients deemed suitable for therapy can achieve a sustained virological and histological response to this therapy. Interim results from a small Canadian study suggest a histological response in 43% of previous nonresponders. These results will need to be reassessed at a future date for confirmation of long-term efficacy. Schering-Plough appears to be confident that response rates will hold up.

Therefore the situation is significantly improved for those patients who have good pretreatment indicators, particularly with regard to genotype. There is also some hope for those who have not responded in the past. Those with higher viral loads have also been shown to become responsive where they otherwise would not. This aspect of therapy is reflected in the licensing of the product, which only allows it to be used on patients who are not responding after the first twelve weeks of interferon therapy alone.

The bad news is that those with poor response indicators are still, on balance, unlikely to benefit in terms of viral load. It is also apparent that quite a number of patients have to be taken off the drug or have the dose reduced due to the development of dangerously low red blood cell counts. While the overall level of side effects are only marginally greater than with interferon alone, it is still a further burden for patients to bear. It is also clear that contraindications for ribavirin combination therapy, such as the existence of heart disease in men over fifty and the presence of kidney disease, make this therapy inaccessible to a number of patients.

A further criticism, which has been voiced by doctors in the U.S., is that the therapy is packaged in a rigid manner that makes it difficult for them to adjust the dose in response to patients' individual situations. This is being addressed by making variable-dose packs available.

The low blood count effect can theoretically be addressed by the application of certain herbs, which are known to offset bone marrow deficiency. However, it has proved very difficult to have such treatments incorporated into mainstream options. This combination regime reduces relapse rates and is therefore a positive contribution, but is still unlikely to be suitable or satisfactory for many patients.

Interferon-Amantadine and Amantadine as Monotherapy

This combination is being investigated by Roche Biocare, who produces interferon alpha 2a, brand name Roferon. The intention here seems to be to enhance efficacy but also improve tolerability. Amantadine hydrochloride is thought to be active against the viral uncoating phase of the HCV replication process. A pilot study at St. Mary's and Charing Cross Hospitals in London has yielded very encouraging results. A number of larger trials are currently underway.

Amantadine has also been used as a single therapy for HCV and has been reported to have brought about a reduction in HCV viral load and improvement in the liver enzyme profiles of interferon relapsers.[7]

Dr. Jill Smith, who has pioneered the application of amantadine in hepatitis C treatment, describes the drug as follows:

> Amantadine is an oral antiviral agent that was developed three decades ago for the treatment of influenza. Since the advent of flu vaccinations, many have forgotten about the antiviral applications of amantadine, and its use for the past thirty years has primarily been for Parkinson's disease. In a pilot study includ-

ing twenty-two patients who have previously failed interferon therapy, amantadine was shown to significantly decrease ALT values in 64% of patients receiving this drug at 100 mg twice daily by mouth for six months. Approximately one-third of the patients had normalization of ALT values and loss of HCV RNA after six months with an overall sustained response to therapy of 18% after discontinuation of amantadine. Response was not related to pretreatment ALT levels, histology, or gender. Patients who responded to amantadine therapy had significantly lower hepatitis C RNA levels than the nonresponders. Presently a larger double-blind placebo-controlled trial is being conducted to evaluate the response to six versus twelve months of therapy. Efficacy is also being evaluated in patients who have not previously received interferon and in children.

Amantadine offers several advantages over interferon therapy including the following: fewer side effects, oral administration, less costly, and no adverse effects on the bone marrow. Amantadine does not significantly augment the immune system; hence its potential for use in patients with autoimmune disorders or who have had transplants warrants investigation. Since this medication is available in a liquid formulation, it may be administered to young children. Patients with low platelet and white blood cell counts are not eligible for interferon therapy; however, since amantadine has no adverse effects on platelet or white blood cell levels, it may be advantageous for patients with these disorders. Lastly, significant information is available regarding the chronic use of amantadine in patients with Parkinson's disease. Since hepatitis C is a chronic infection which is difficult to eradicate in some patients, amantadine could potentially be used for chronic suppressive therapy.

Patients who have tried amantadine report that it tends to improve their energy levels, although it may induce a "frenetic" state of mind; thus a balanced mental disposition may be a safety factor for this drug.

Interferon + Zinc-Containing Salts and Zinc Complexes

A Japanese company, Otsuka Pharmaceuticals, has claimed an excellent rate of response among patients with high viral loads undergoing the above combination. Exact details are not yet available, being currently subject to patenting procedures. This, together with technical reviews of HCV treatments, is written up in "Anti-infectives update, developments in hepatitis C during 1996–1997," Berwyn Clarke and Martin Slater, *Exp. Opin. Ther. Patents,* 7(9):979–987, 1997.

Consensus Interferon

These products contain a wider range of the chemical messengers that regulate intracellular immune response; instead of just containing interferon alpha 2, they contain a selection of interferons. Two companies, Glaxo Wellcome (Wellferon) and Amgen (Infergen), have taken up this therapeutic approach.

In one large-scale Australian study that pitted Infergen against Intron, it was evident that there was a higher rate of sustained response in the consensus-treated group.[8] Both biochemical and virological response was about 40% better. Again nonresponders were not helped.

Most of these products are being positioned for treatment of relapsers from standard interferon. More work is being done on producing variations of interferon, which has yet to be properly optimized for action against HCV. Expect superior variations to emerge in the near future.

For further information on these treatments, affordability, and their providers, refer to chapter 11 and the Resources.

Side Effects of Interferon and Their Management

In general, the side effects of interferon are exaggerations of typical hepatitis C symptoms, both clinical and subjective, listed in chapter 1, pages 9–10, 26, and 45–46. It seems possible that interferon treatment triggers an accentuation of a number of these symptoms, and therefore that a number of patients who are symptomatic will find

Common Side Effects of Alpha Interferon
Usually Not Requiring Dose Modulation

Influenza-like: fatigue, fever, myalgia, malaise, poor appetite, tachycardia, chills, headache, arthralgias

Neuropsychiatric: apathy, irritability, mood changes, insomnia, cognitive changes

Miscellaneous: diarrhea, nausea, abdominal pain, back pain, pruritis, alopecia, rhinorrhea

Laboratory: decrease in granulocytes, platelet counts, and red blood cell counts; increase in serum triglyceride concentrations; proteinuria; increases in serum alanine and aspartate aminotransferases

---

Serious Adverse Events Reported
with Alpha Interferon Therapy

Neuropsychiatric: psychosis, depression/suicide, delirium, confusion, extrapyramidal ataxia, paresthesia, seizures, relapse in substance abuse

Immune disorders: autoimmune thyroid disease, autoimmune hepatitis, systemic lupus erythematosis, primary biliary cirrhosis, septicemia, graft rejection

Skin: psoriasis, erythema multiforme

Systemic: hepatic decompensation, bleeding, cardiac arrhythmias, sudden death, dilated cardiomyopathy, hypotension, acute renal failure

Other: retinopathy, hearing loss, pulmonary interstitial fibrosis

Laboratory: granulocytopenia, thrombocytopenia, anemia, hyperthyroidism, hypothyroidism

that the "side effects" are little worse than their day-to-day experience of HCV. It may therefore be logical to seek treatment for symptoms prior to commencing drug therapy. Their extent varies drastically from one person to another. For some patients, treatment is easily tolerable and even unnoticeable for long periods of time; for others, it can be a nightmare, with severely debilitating consequences that may persist after the end of treatment.

Some patients cannot tolerate the therapy and come off quite soon after commencement. Others, having assessed the facts, reject this approach. It has been suggested that hepatitis C patients with a sensitive disposition are less likely to be able to tolerate this therapy. Most doctors tend to encourage patients to look on the bright side, which means that the more debilitating side effects are often not mentioned. There do not seem to be any reliable ways of predicting who is likely to suffer the more severe side effects.

In general, the physical side effects diminish over time, while the mental and emotional side effects become more pronounced toward the end of therapy. Depression, loss of mental clarity, and fatigue are the symptoms found to be most difficult by many patients. If you wish to follow up some interferon-related side effects in detail, see the references at the end of this chapter.[9]

There is also a phenomenon, known as *post interferon syndrome,* that can catch some patients by surprise. This is well described by Kathy, who was taken off interferon and ribavirin combination therapy due to nonresponse:

> During the first week after stopping, I experienced muscle and bone pains, especially in my back and limbs, a piercing headache, extreme depression and lethargy, lack of appetite and nausea, and suddenly feeling boiling hot or freezing cold. I also found it hard to sleep because of the pains in my body. These "withdrawal" symptoms gradually lessened and, apart from the fatigue and depression, abated over a period of six weeks. It is now six weeks since I stopped the treatment. I still feel extremely depressed and have had to take two weeks off work. Before this I had only three days off work due to sickness in the last five and a half years.

Clearly it is vital to be closely monitored both during and in the period immediately after the cessation of treatment. It appears that some sort of reaction may set in when interferon is withdrawn. Whatever the cause, it is vital to obtain assurances from your doctors that you will be carefully monitored, particularly at this point. Post interferon syndrome might be alleviated by a gradual tapering of the dose at the end of therapy, which is regarded as good practice by some doctors.

For most patients interferon treatment is an uncomfortable but tolerable ordeal. Some manage to work throughout treatment, while others require special care. Depression is the most commonly reported side effect among patients I have spoken to—some hepatologists prescribe antidepressants throughout therapy. The precipitation of thyroid disease was also a commonly reported side effect, and the relative frequency of this is substantiated by a number of reports. On the whole the reported standard of care is excellent.

One worrying aspect of interferon treatment is that it may occasionally precipitate M.E. There are anecdotal reports that some patients successfully treated for HCV have suffered significant fatigue-related symptoms following the end of treatment; this may be post interferon syndrome.

Nigel Hughes, a registered nurse who has considerable experience of patient management through drug therapy, summarizes the situation as follows:

> Side effects may be reversible and dose modulation may successfully reduce the occurrence of side effects while maintaining therapy. Administration prior to sleep, in the evening with a predose of 500–1,000 mg of Paracetamol (acetaminophen) in the initial few weeks of treatment may reduce the "flulike" symptoms associated with initial interferon therapy.
>
> These symptoms are often characterized by the onset of chills, fevers, arthralgias and myalgias, and fatigue with headaches and nausea four to six hours after initial dosage, reducing in severity and incidence within the first month of therapy in the majority of patients. Adequate hydration and appropriate rest are beneficial, as is continued support by significant

others and treatment services. Due to the phenomena of tachyphylaxis (decreasing response to repeated dosing of the same medication), characteristic of interferon therapy, these side effects should be self-limiting and naturally decline over time.

The above side effects may result in significant alteration of therapy, or possible cessation of treatment, with follow-up and monitoring in 2–10% of patients. There is a documented association with higher doses of interferon (above 5 million units three times weekly) and frequency of side effects. It would be beneficial and safer for the patient if prescribing services were specialist in the use of interferon therapy and willing to maintain clinical responsibility.

Other Methods Reported by Patients To Be Helpful Include:

- Taking **adjunct herbal therapy** can alleviate side effects and perhaps even improve efficacy. TCM practitioners may be able to help, but only qualified professionals with extensive experience should be consulted. A Chinese herbal formulation called "Adjunct" is currently being proposed for testing at two hospitals in London.

- **Ear** and **body acupuncture** is commonly reported to be helpful by patients.

Interferon Nurses

The introduction of interferon nurses at some hospitals is a notable and significant improvement in the quality of care available to patients. They are able to provide the ongoing support and monitoring that hard-pressed consultants cannot. A number of patients have commented that they do feel that they are being more professionally looked after as a result. Experienced doctors regard this resource as being critical to the effective management of interferon-based therapy in hepatitis C.

Other Treatments

Acyclovir has been tested. Results are poor. This drug is normally used to treat herpes viruses.

Augmentative immunotherapy (AI) may be an excellent treatment for patients who cannot present a strong immune response to HCV, or posttransplant patients who have to take immunosuppressants. AI involves the transfer of certain immunoactive blood components from an immunocompetent HCV patient to one who is not. In this context "immunocompetent" means that the patient has the ability to present an effective response to HCV. Thus the aim is to confer the ability to manage the virus onto patients who currently lack it; AI can be classified as a humoral immunological approach.

It has been observed that patients diagnosed with hepatitis B prior to the development of HCV tests who underwent transplants and received AI to overcome complications had improved prognoses. Some of these patients have been subsequently found to have HCV, as were their AI blood donors. It is therefore inferred that AI may have triggered a more effective response to HCV as well as HBV.

AI has been used to treat HIV. The main drawback is that it is expensive. This is being addressed by some current work on chimpanzees, which may enable the inexpensive production of as much immunoglobulin-bearing plasma as is required. Dr. Graham Alexander reports that five "constant region antibodies" have been identified; these are key antibodies that retain action against the virus even if it mutates. This means that AI can be delivered with a high degree of precision. The next step would be to give plasma bearing these key antibodies to "at-risk" patients, such as those who have just had liver transplants, and then monitor them for signs of improved survival and modified antiviral response.

This approach, which amounts to a postexposure vaccination, is clearly a very promising option particularly for the most vulnerable patients. As with many other nonpharmaceutical treatments, doctors who have championed this approach have sometimes found themselves professionally isolated.

Colchicine is an extract from the bulb of the meadow saffron plant *(Colchicum autumnale)* and has been tested in combination with interferon in Italy by doctors at the University of Pisa in Italy. They concluded that its use was "associated with a lesser rebound of viremia." In other words it may help partial responders to become sustained responders.

Gene supplementation. If it is true that many patients lack the necessary immunological equipment to combat HCV, then immune supplementation and augmentation would seem to be a logical avenue of approach for future research. Some biotechnology companies are looking at the possibility of inserting benign immunological genes into patients who lack them. This approach may offer the possibility of an effective immunization as well as a cure. No one has tried this yet.

Hemodialysis has been shown to reduce circulating viral load in patients studied in Japan. Doctors there reckon this treatment should be studied with a view to viral elimination and alteration of the course of disease.

Interleukins are a family of cytokines and can now be synthesized in much the same way as alpha interferon. Interleukin 12 has been used to treat HIV. Results of trials suggest that it is not such a promising approach to HCV. Side effects are similar to interferon.

Maxamine is a new cellular immunological approach that combines interleukin 2 with histamine. A small preliminary trial is underway; no results are available as yet.

MTH-68/B is a refined form of bursal disease virus (BDV), which affects certain birds but does not cause disease in humans. It has been observed that the introduction of certain viruses can modify the behavior of the immune system in humans, or even have a direct impact on other pathogens. This line of thought has been regarded as being most promising by Eastern European medical researchers. It could be described as a kind of postexposure vaccination that aims to increase rates of viral clearance and reduce rates of progression toward end stage liver disease. It could also be described as a form of biochemical homeopathy.

Publication of a study in early 1998 was somehow interpreted as "The Cure" for hepatitis C in certain parts of the media and on the Internet.[10] What this study claimed to show was that treated patients had lower rates of progression into chronic hepatitis C and a higher rate of remission; however, what it actually showed is debatable, with some signs that the researchers lacked access to the necessary tests to generate good data for hepatitis C.

Having said this, the general approach is promising, with a number of animal studies showing success against other viruses. It remains to be seen whether this therapeutic approach will receive the necessary research funding.

N-acetyl cysteine has been shown to enhance the biochemical response to interferon but is rarely used in combination therapy. See chapter 18 for details.

Pentoxifylline has been tried in combination with interferon in New York. This drug enhances natural interferon production and reduces levels of tumor necrosis factor (TNF), which is associated with liver cell damage. It appears that this drug may enhance response to a similar extent as ribavirin. Trials are still ongoing, and it is too early to make any firm conclusions.

Phlebotomy, also known as iron reduction therapy, is used to counteract the overconcentration of iron deposits in liver cells noted in some patients (see "Cancer" section in chapter 1 and chapter 18). It is not an antiviral treatment, but aims to minimize liver disease, particularly the prospect of tumors developing. It usually involves phlebotomy—which actually means bleeding, as in the medieval "cure all." Some Japanese doctors are enthusiastic about the benefits of this treatment.

Because the prospect of response to interferon is higher in patients with lower levels of iron in liver cells, iron reduction therapy is sometimes prescribed before the start of drug therapy. The treatment consists of taking a pint of blood from patients once a week.

Thymic extracts are really an alternative therapy. It is a branch of live cell therapy, a treatment approach that is popular for cancer in Germany and involves the injection of live cells from certain parts of particular animals—cattle thymus and shark cartilage are the usual candidates—into the blood of patients. A number of preparations are available. The general idea is to reinvigorate the immune system. There are no accurate reports on its efficacy for hepatitis C as yet.

Thymomodulin has been used to boost phagocytosis in elderly patients.[11] Some reports suggest that elderly patients succumb to liver disease much faster than younger patients. This may be because they have less vigorous immune defenses in the liver. This substance may help them to counter HCV.

Thymosin has been used with interferon in one recent trial; the results suggest that overall viral clearance was significantly improved by this combination of therapy [Thymosin alpha 1 + interferon, Sherman KE et al., paper presented at the American Association for the Study of Liver Diseases, Chicago, 1996]. Thymostimulin may also help to invigorate the immune system. Thymic factor D can be effective in boosting levels of glutathione (see chapter 18).

Ursodeoxycholic acid has been used with interferon with little apparent clinical benefit in terms of viral clearance, but with improved liver function test results. It may help some patients to feel better and might provide more subtle benefits. It is a cholagogue, which means that it induces increased bile flow. This may have an anti-carcinogenic effect. It may decrease fat content in liver cells and reduce cholesterol levels. It can improve liver enzyme profiles. As a single treatment it doesn't seem to have any impact on HCV RNA. It may be more beneficial to patients with a history of high alcohol consumption.

Zidovidine, also known as AZT and Retrovir, is being tried in the U.S.; used extensively to treat HIV, its efficacy in HCV is unknown at present. Like ribavirin, it is a nucleoside analogue. This is one of the drugs whose use in combination to treat HIV has attracted so much attention recently.

Treatments to Prevent Progression from Cirrhosis to Liver Cancer

This is an important aspect of treatment for many patients.

There are claims that interferon treatment helps to prevent liver cancer in cirrhotic patients. However, studies on which these claims are based are conflicting and inconclusive; for instance, some studies present comparisons between treated and untreated (by interferon) groups of patients showing higher numbers of cancers in the untreated group, or higher rates of incidence per year. However, these are meaningless because only patients with better prognoses are usually selected for drug treatment; such studies also omit key factors such as alcohol consumption, even where "matched pairing" has been employed. There is some good evidence to suggest that total responders are less likely to develop HCC, though, somewhat disconcertingly, some do. It is possible that some kind of refractory effect is taking place where total responders have better prognoses, while nonresponders have worse ones. This would suggest that the ability to predict response is very important.

Because some doctors believe that cirrhosis is a contraindication for interferon treatment or a reliable indicator of a poor likelihood of response, the relevance of this debate is questionable.

The only treatment that has been specifically tested for the ability to reduce the chances of cirrhotic patients developing HCC is called SNMC, which stands for Stronger Neo-Minophagen C. This product is a highly concentrated extract from the roots of two species of licorice. It also contains cysteine and glycine. It is taken by injection. Studies have shown that it is good treatment for chronic hepatitis, lowering liver enzymes, and helping to prevent immune-response-related liver cell damage.[12] Traditionally licorice root is used as an antiviral treatment in the Far East, and some recent research suggests that it is active against some viruses.[13]

A long-term study in Japan found that cirrhotic HCV patients who were administered SNMC had lower rates of HCC incidence than those who were not; untreated patients were 2.5 times more likely to develop HCC compared to those who were given the treatment.[14] Unfortunately no Western pharmaceutical company is backing this product, which means that it is not being made available to "mainstream" doctors. If you are interested in SNMC, contact some HIV organizations; they may be able to help.

Treatments for Liver Cancer

Conventional treatments for primary liver cancer have poor rates of success, with less than 10% of patients responding at best. Radiotherapy is highly toxic to the liver. Surgery can help a few, but only 10% of tumors are removable as the liver is almost always cirrhotic and does not regenerate itself. The delivery of chemotherapy directly to the liver via the hepatic artery is the main hope at present; a cocktail of cytotoxic drugs can shrink some tumors, sometimes making them removable and perhaps extending life.

Focal destruction of the tumor by local injections of alcohol and tumor destruction by freezing or heating by laser beam are other approaches to palliation. Liver transplantation is often needed.

Recent advances in the understanding of the development of liver cancer in hepatitis C together with genetic technology may be the most promising avenue of approach. It has been found that HCV may cause a cellular imbalance that favors the proliferation of hepatocytes that are vulnerable to becoming cancerous. The promise of gene therapy is that it may enable the implanting of liver cells that are resistant to becoming cancerous. Such cells could be cultivated in the laboratory or grown in other animals. Thus the imbalance could be redressed. Therefore gene therapy is promising both as a preventative treatment and for cancer itself.

Liver Transplants

This is a major operation, pioneered during the 1960s in the U.S. and the U.K. Some patients will need liver transplants, especially those with small hepatocellular cancers and those with liver failure. Although HCV is known to reinfect newly transplanted livers, the generally slow rate of ongoing damage is such that natural causes are a more likely cause of death than HCV-related liver damage to the graft (the transplanted organ).

Currently about 80% of transplant patients survive for at least five years. A lot of work is now being done to increase this already remarkable figure. The main problem seems to be that transplanted livers are often rejected by their new hosts. Doctors are increasingly able to address these immunological problems. However, there do seem to be some reports of HCV patients suffering particular complications immediately following transplant, and the figures are not so impressive for HCV. Sometimes the new liver is rapidly damaged by HCV; this may be connected to the use of immunosuppressants to assist the acceptance of the new liver. Ribavirin and hypericin have both been suggested as suitable posttransplant medications for hepatitis C patients.

Xenotransplantation holds some promise. This is the process where genetically engineered animals—most probably pigs in this case—are bred to produce livers suitable for transplantation into humans. Unfortunately it is believed that we are at least twenty years away from such a treatment becoming available. There are a number of safety concerns vis-à-vis the possibility of introducing new viruses into the human population, and there are some ethical concerns as well.

An intermediate step is for patients with advanced liver disease to be linked up to animal livers. A company called Imutran, based in Cambridge, U.K., claims to be ready to test this in human patients now. Apparently confident that immunological problems have been overcome, they are now seeking ethical approval to go ahead with treatment for human beings.

A Note about Anti-Inflammatory Drugs

These substances are often prescribed to HCV patients presenting with some of the common secondary symptoms, such as kidney disease or arthritis. Some commentators feel that it is dangerous to prescribe these to patients because they are immunosuppressants and may weaken the ability to counter the pathogenesis of HCV.

Future Treatments for Hepatitis C

It is very likely that new treatments for HCV will become available in the near future. They may make existing therapy look clumsy or inadequate. Patients with reasonable levels of health or with contraindications to treatment are sometimes advised by their specialists to await new developments while exploring complementary approaches and maintaining a healthy lifestyle in the meantime.

Protease Inhibitors, Helicase Inhibitors, and Other Drugs

One senior consultant interviewed for this book was entirely confident that a large number of high-profile pharmaceutical companies are currently working on treatments for HCV. The size of the patient population, or the market to them, is a powerful incentive. Because of the nature of commercial competition within the industry, it is also true that none of these organizations are keen to publicize any aspect of their work. An atmosphere of intense confidentiality prevails.

A very important step in the development of antiviral agents is the ability to cultivate live HCV cell lines in the laboratory. This is vital because scientists taking this approach need to be able to break down all aspects of the virus's structure and replication behavior into component parts. Once this is achieved, it will be possible to develop HCV-specific virological treatments. There are two possibilities that will arise once this task is accomplished.

The first is that once a cell line is available the researchers concerned will simply "fire" all known pharmaceutical agents and combinations thereof at the infected cell lines until one with detectable antiviral action is found. Well-equipped laboratories can "fire" up to 1,000 agents a day at such cell lines. If action is found, then the company concerned will secretly try to buy up the licenses for these agents as treatments for HCV. Then they will proceed to testing in animals, and, if found safe, to trials in HCV patients.

The second course of action is that researchers will develop the ability to accurately model the detailed structure of the virus so that new drugs can be designed to address HCV. This is where protease and helicase inhibitors, which aim to disrupt the attachment phase of viral replication, come in.

Dr. Graham Alexander, who is interested in the possibilities for this approach and whose office is conveniently located opposite the University of Cambridge molecular biology faculty, explains the strategy as follows:

> Protease and helicase are two enzymes which are integral to the reproduction process. In order to reproduce the viral structure it is necessary for these substances to "cut" the current structure, which has specific sites where this takes place. If the structure of the virus is accurately and explicitly defined, it will be feasible to design substances which will preferentially bind to these receptor sites. In other words, when the enzymes try to reach their destined site, they will find that it is already occupied, and they will not be able to play their critical role in the replication process. Thus these "inhibitors" will prevent viral

replication. They will not necessarily be a cure because the viral RNA will hang around in tissue for lengthy periods. However, by arresting replication, they will effectively halt ongoing damage.

Thus these substances can be seen as "designer wrenches" that can be thrown with accuracy into specific points in the "replicative works" of HCV. With the help of sophisticated 3D modeling techniques, researchers should be able to design exact fits for these sites. There are some signs that progress has already been made. HCV protease has been crystallized. Other scientists, unable to cultivate HCV itself, have managed to trick other cells into behaving as though they were HCV infected. Some doctors are also using HCV-infected cells from biopsies to try to test antiviral substances, though this is quite crude. There are also reports of a very similar virus being discovered in a remote colony of monkeys; several pharmaceutical companies are attempting to obtain samples of infected tissue and plasma to further their research.

The tolerability of such drugs will depend upon the extent to which HCV helicases and proteases differ from those in normal human cells. If they are too similar, then multiple adverse effects will occur as the inhibitors disrupt normal biological functions. HIV protease inhibitors do have a range of side effects; disturbingly the most serious of these are most commonly found in patients who also have liver disease. Other common side effects of protease inhibitors are lipid redistribution (i.e., patients accumulate fat in various parts of the body) and a kind of humpback syndrome. Bloating and indigestion are also reported.

Berwyn Clarke, an experienced pharmaceutical research manager with an interest in hepatitis C, is optimistic about the prospects for the development of new and effective treatments. However, he is extremely respectful of the difficulties the virus presents; among his comments are the following:

> In many ways HCV is more difficult than HIV; the fact that it lacks retroviral qualities does not simplify the challenge. HCV has several completely novel characteristics which make targeting problematic. The receptor sites are relatively few, but

they are open ended and at least one of the key proteins runs through the entire structure, something we have not seen before. Thus it may be difficult to block access to receptors, meaning that specific virological treatments may be difficult to isolate. Those that do emerge are likely to be combined with interferon treatment in the first instance and may include polymerase inhibitors. We may see triple or quadruple therapies becoming available.

I suspect that a decisive solution is more likely to emerge from an immunological approach. Because HCV escapes from CD4 and CD8 responses, which are often pronounced, we will need a very specific immune stimulant. Once we understand the exact mechanism involved, we already have a large inventory of peptide molecules that could be applied. I would expect a DNA-based therapeutic vaccine to emerge in the next five years. Such a treatment would be taken orally and may not have to be prolonged.

Chiron Corporation is currently working on vaccines that could be used as both preventatives and postexposure treatments.

Phytopharmaceuticals

A second promising approach is to take sets of biological agents already known to be helpful in the treatment of liver disease and turn them into generally available medical products that can be shown to have a very high degree of consistent and specific action against HCV or related disease.

The renowned scientist and molecular biologist John Babish has developed a procedure known as Bioprinting, which will deliver the basis for identifying, quantifying, and guaranteeing a specific effect using "signal transduction technology." He explains the technology and its implications with regard to HCV as follows:

A popular route in the development of antiviral therapeutics is to identify specific inhibitors of essential viral enzymes such as the proteases, which are necessary for final processing of the viral particle. Another course of action is to limit the ability of the virus to usurp cellular processes for its benefit. Since the number of functional proteins coded by viruses is extremely limited, these organisms have evolved unique ways of fooling the cell to perform the more elaborate reproductive proteins for them. Understanding the signal transduction processes involved in these critical host-virus interactions enables researchers to develop efficient countermeasures.

"Signal transduction" is a term used to describe the constant flux of protein structure that underscores all cellular processes. Since protein function is dictated by structure, modification of structure will, in turn, modify function.

Over the last three years, research has described several characteristic alterations in signal transduction pathways in HCV-infected cells. For example, HCV core protein can bind to a specific DNA sequence of the regulatory region of the p21WAF1 gene and inhibit the transcription of that gene. Since this gene functions to inhibit cell cycle progression, loss of p21WAF1 results in the promotion of cellular proliferation.[15] These observations suggest that HCV infection may increase the risk of hepatocellular carcinoma through increased and abnormal proliferative signalling.

A method to study the pattern of protein expression and modification in whole cells has been developed and is termed "Bioprinting." The process allows for an analysis of multiple signalling pathways simultaneously. Using a cultured cell in a petri dish, the condition of interest is reproduced and a two-dimensional characterization of the protein complexes or degree of protein phosphorylation is obtained. This two-dimensional representation is called a "Bioprint." Using the earlier example of the inhibition of p21WAF1 expression by HCV core protein, the specific condition can be reproduced in a petri dish by using a liver cell line with a mutated p53 gene. Expression of nonfunctional p53 results in failure of the cell to express p21WAF1. This, as with HCV core protein expression, results in the loss of G1/S regulation in the affected cells.

Similarly, the HCV core protein may be transfected into liver cells in culture with and without functional p53. Bioprints of the signalling pathways affected identify changes in signal transduction pathways occurring with HCV core protein expression. Treatment of the cells with agents capable of inhibiting protein phosphorylation at specific sites provides important information concerning the mechanism of action of HCV core protein. Thus, it is possible to recreate HCV-mediated cellular pathologies without the need to culture the virus. These data can be used to refine the search for compounds that may intercept the signal transduction pathways necessary for HCV reproduction or HCV-mediated pathologies.

Like the modeling procedures used in enzyme inhibitor design, this approach breaks down and identifies the "messages" corresponding to stages in HCV behavior, such as those associated with the entry of HCV into cells. In this approach it is not necessary to cultivate cell lines; creating cells that behave as though they were HCV is sufficient. Specific biological agents, particularly Chinese herbs, will be identified and matched to patterns of action. Combinations of herbs, or extracts thereof, that effectively block HCV pathways and have an impact on particular pathologies can then be consistently profiled. Each batch of herbal medicine can then be quantified for this effect, thus guaranteeing the desired response. Such actions do not have to be confined to antiviral activity. Any measurable effect, such as improvements in liver cell function or enhanced levels of energy, can be profiled in this way.

The advantage of this approach is that a range of ingredients can be added, since it is the effect, not the components, that is of primary interest. Thus medicines that combine herbs, vitamins, or even drugs can be compounded and produced on a consistent basis. Such an approach might yield a family of specialized biological agents that could be deployed in the treatment of all aspects of HCV. It is also widely thought that such broad-range medicines are less likely to generate difficult side effects in comparison to highly abstracted pharmaceutical agents. It is also entirely feasible that this approach could yield a composite of both plants and drugs, rendering the division between plant- and pharmaceutical-based medicines obsolete.

Another very important implication of this process is that multi-ingredient phytopharmaceutical medicines will become patentable.

If this proves to be the case, then the entire pharmaceutical industry could be revolutionized. Investors in the industry would no longer be deterred by the inability to protect such products. The attraction of the additional power and tolerability of synergistic medicines would quickly cause a major refocusing of this industry, allowing patients to benefit from a wider choice from within the mainstream medical system.

Patients' Experiences of Interferon Treatment

Steve underwent a one-year course of interferon in 1994. This is his experience:

> After a rough start the physical side effects began to decline. I found that the mental side effects were by far the hardest thing to deal with. I really knew that I was taking a powerful drug. A sense of depression and negativity set in, which I found really hard to cope with over such a long period of time. I knew what was going on and why I felt depressed, but that didn't make it any easier. I found my self-confidence and belief dissipating, which was hard because I was setting up a business at that time.
>
> The doctors were absolutely brilliant—they monitored my situation very closely. I've got no complaints about them. They told me that my thyroid was showing signs of deterioration and asked me whether I wanted to stop the treatment. Because I had gone HCV negative, I decided to go through with it. It was a terrible blow when they told me that it had come back three months after the treatment ended.

Sue underwent a one-year course of interferon during 1995/96:

> I felt terribly ill to begin with and was kept in the hospital for several days. After I went home I began to feel a bit better, but I came to dread the injection and would take paracetamol to lessen the effects. After a few months I began to put on a lot of weight and looked like I was pregnant. I found I could just about function and work part-time. Going to a support group really helped. The doctors were really supportive.

I felt terrible when the treatment finished—worse than at any point during it—and my liver counts climbed dramatically. There was very little in the way of follow-up care, and I felt very isolated at that time. The HCV went while I was on interferon, seemed to come back at the end of treatment, and then disappeared completely. I've had a couple of negative PCR tests since. They consider me cured. I do feel a lot better, although I'm still overweight—that's probably due to the thyroid. I've got color in my cheeks for the first time for years.

Joanne took interferon for six weeks in early 1996:

Despite my history of depression, my doctor agreed to put me on interferon after I begged him to. I really wanted the chance of a cure.

Pretty soon I began to go into a really deep dark depression. I couldn't sleep properly although I was exhausted. I found that I couldn't eat and became anorexic. My moods swung without warning, and I felt that I was going stark raving mad. I would burst into tears for no apparent reason. Then my hair started to fall out. After a while I just couldn't take it any more and stopped the treatment.

Peter, a sixty-four-year-old hemophiliac, took interferon-ribavirin therapy:

The hospital contacted me and, after a series of tests, ascertained that I had HCV (no doubt via blood products) and proposed with my consent to give me combination drug treatment, using interferon and ribavirin over a period of one year. This started in May '96, and I visited them monthly during the course for checks on blood and general health. After about four months the doctor monitoring me said he was very optimistic, and the tests were positive with regard to HCV.

During the period May '96–'97 and two or three months afterwards I experienced extreme tiredness, irritability, and lack of concentration. My cousin aged fifty was on the same course but stopped after three months as a result of these symptoms. He was still working, whereas I had retired, and this no doubt affected him more so. The period May '96 –'97 was effectively a lost year, as I did nothing (hobbies, etc.) although normally I am very active. My appetite remained, but a complete lack of energy ensured the physical side of my life was virtually non-existent. The blood tests subsequent to the course (one, three, six months) have been HCV clear, so I am very pleased and consider the treatment a great success.

During the course I developed a throat irritation which is still not completely gone, but is receding. The symptoms are not being able to clear my throat completely, but as I said, it is improving and is a small problem in relation to HCV. I consider myself in good health now, enjoy my food and drink, and am currently working on my retirement hobby (rebuilding from scratch a 1937 Austin 7).

Marty, a fifty-year-old female, is currently taking interferon; she reports side effects and coping techniques:

The interferon has really slowed my life down, something I now feel I needed to allow my liver to heal. If you can, I suggest you take the year off while under treatment. Your body will need the rest as it is working very hard to fight the virus. I am now at week thirty with eighteen more to go. The worse part of the treatment for me thus far was and is:

My highly activated immune system attacked my thyroid. It is now necessary to take thyroid medication, perhaps for life.... I have lost about half the volume of my hair. They assure me that I won't go bald and will thicken back up when I go off the medication.... Headaches, fatigue, and muscle weakness have been prevalent throughout, however there are more days now when I feel normal.... Dry eyes, mouth, and bladder all through the night interrupt my sleep.... Regarding libido I now know why they call it interferon!

These symptoms may sound pretty bad, but they are tolerable. I feel that they are worth enduring for the chance of a sustained cure.... Here are a list of the other therapies I am trying. I feel they help me to tolerate the medication and promote healing:

Acupuncture twice a month to support the body. The style of acupuncture I receive is also geared to enhance awareness.... Massage once a month really feels good to those sore muscles.... I do relaxation and visualization every day.... Crystal healing and meditation ... I find the group very supportive and loving, and I always feel better afterwards.

Just a couple of last suggestions: Try not to focus too much on the physical. Keep the quality of your life high. Laugh as much as you can. Don't push yourself to do too much, take it slow and easy, rest as much as you can, reserve your energy for your healing. Use your quiet time to meditate—healing occurs in that quiet space.

Remember, no alcohol, and a low-fat, high-fiber diet helps as do vitamins and minerals.

References

1. Hepatic and extrahepatic HCV replication in response to interferon therapy. Saleh SM et al. *Hepatology,* 20(6):1399–1403, 1994.

2. Durability of serological remission in chronic hepatitis C treated with interferon-alpha-2B. Sim H et al. *Am J Gastroenterol,* 93(1):39–43, Jan 1998.

Also see comments by Gary Davis reported by Brenda C. Coleman. The Associated Press, Chicago, Nov. 10, 1997.

3. Factors affecting treatment responses to interferon alpha in chronic hepatitis C. Pawlotsky J-M et al. *Journal of Infectious Diseases,* 174:1–7, 1996.

4. Hepatitis C virus genotype in the United States: epidemiology, pathogenicity, and response to interferon therapy. Zein N et al. *Annals of Internal Medicine,* 125:634–639, 1996.

5. Therapy for chronic hepatitis C. Davis et al. *Gastroenterology Clinics of North America.* 23(3):603–615, 1994.

6. Hepatitis C viral RNA titres in serum prior to, during, and after oral treatment with ribavirin for chronic hepatitis C. *Journal of Medical Virology,* 41(2):99–102, Oct 1993.

Ten patients with biopsy verified chronic hepatitis C virus (HCV) infection were treated with oral ribavirin at a dose of 1,000–1,200 mg per day in two divided doses for 12 weeks. ALT levels decreased significantly in all patients during therapy. Hereafter, relapse to pretreatment levels was seen within 12 weeks after treatment stop. The hepatitis C viral RNA levels decreased from a mean 10 log titre of 4.1 (range 1–6) before treatment to 3.4 (range 1–5) at treatment stop. Five patients did not change their HCV RNA titres during treatment. Twelve weeks post treatment only 3 patients had lower titres than prior to treatment. We conclude that oral ribavirin seems to reduce the viral load, at least temporarily, in some patients with chronic viraemic HCV infection.

7. Issue 10 of *Birchgrove*, a U.K. hemophilia magazine. Probably referring to Dr. J Smith's open label pilot study. *Dig Dis Sci*, 42:1681–1687, 1997.

8. Lymphoblastoid interferon alfa-n1 improves the long-term response to a six-month course of treatment in chronic hepatitis C compared with recombinant interferon alfa-2b: results of an international randomized controlled trial. Farrell GC et al. *Hepatology*, 27(4):1121–1127, Apr 1998.

9. Endocrine-mediated mechanisms of fatigue during treatment with interferon-alpha. Jones TH et al. *Semin Oncol*, 25 (1 Suppl 1):54–63, Feb 1998.

Mood and cognitive side effects of interferon-alpha therapy. Valentine AD et al. *Semin Oncol*, 25(1 Suppl 1):39–47, Feb 1998.

Interferon-alpha therapy may induce insulin autoantibody development in patients with chronic viral hepatitis. di Cesare E. *Dig Dis Sci*, 41(8): 1672–1677, Aug 1996.

Bilateral transient visual obscurations with headaches during alpha-II interferon therapy: a case report. Detry-Morel M. *Eur J Ophthalmol*, 5(4):271–274, Oct 1995.

Also refer to references on pages 179–180.

10. Preliminary report of a controlled trial of MTH-68/B virus vaccine treatment in acute B and C hepatitis: a phase II study. Csatary LK et al. *Anticancer research*, 18, 1998.

11. Restoration of polymorphonuclear leucocyte function in elderly subjects by thymomodulin. Braga et al. *Journal of Chemotherapy*, 6(5): 354–9, Oct 1994.

12. Effects of glycyrrhizin on immune-mediated cytotoxicity. Yoshikawa M et al. *J Gastroenterol*, 12(3):243–248, Mar 1997.

13. Effects of glycyrrhizin (SNMC) in hemophilia patients with HIV infection. Mori K et al. *Tohuku Journal of Experimental Medicine*, 158 (20):35, 1989.

14. The long term efficacy of glycyrrhizin in chronic hepatitis C patients. Arase Y et al. *Cancer*, 79(8):1494–1500, Apr 15, 1997.

15. Ray et al. *Gene*, 208(2):331–336, 1998.

Farinati et al. *Hepatology*, 2396:1468–1475, 1996.

15

Traditional Chinese Medicine
and Hepatitis C

TCM Overview

TRADITIONAL CHINESE MEDICINE (TCM) has been evolving for over 3,000 years. Hepatitis and other liver health issues are endemic in the East; therefore there is a massive reservoir of relevant experience in this tradition that is lacking in Western medicine. Like Western medicine TCM has a sophisticated and internally logical methodology that allows the processes of diagnosis and treatment to be applied systematically. Although there may be problems with the control of unqualified practitioners in the West, it is a heavyweight contender for the attention of HCV patients. Indeed it could be forcefully argued that any discussion of the treatment of liver disease that ignores this approach is guilty of a serious error of omission.

Although aspects of its practice were suppressed in China itself following the Cultural Revolution, the great numbers and geographical dispersion of the Chinese peoples means that the accumulated experience gained over millennia is available to us today. Although there are a number of traditional medicinal systems available, none of them approach TCM in terms of the sophistication of their diagnostic systems or in the scale and subtlety of the combination of treatments available.

According to John Tindall, an experienced practitioner, "To understand what TCM is about, it is actually much easier if you know nothing about Western medicine at all, if you have no scientific background whatsoever. Chinese medicine is a very logical subject, but if you go into it with a Western medical model, you will find that some things don't fit."

The traditional Chinese "Five Element" system is applied in medicine to identify patterns of imbalance both within and between the main energy centers of the body. The energy centers are associated with certain organs, although they may not be literally and solely linked to these biological entities. Disease occurs when there is an imbalance between or within the energy of these centers. The emphasis here is on process and balance rather than on distinct structure. It is a feature of this system that organs do not function in isolation and that therefore any dietary or other prescriptions have to take into account the processes of interaction within a dynamic context.

These centers are linked with identifiable "symptoms" of health and disease that may embrace physical, mental, emotional, and esoteric characteristics. Each energy center is also allocated a season with which it is linked. It is often thought that these times of year are particularly opportune for taking action to improve the energy or Qi of the associated organ. The five energy centers are as follows:

The Wood Element

Associated with the liver and spring. Described as the "emperor" of the other elements.

Poor health is associated with the emotional or mental symptoms of anger, denial, depression, emotional repression, impatience, wilfulness, arrogance, negativity, and nervousness.

Physical presentations include indigestion, eye disease, "floaters," red face, headaches, insomnia, allergies, distended abdomen, menstrual problems, fatigue, rigid inflexible body, skin disorders, weak ligaments and tendons, and dizziness.

Good health associated with a free flow of smooth energy, leadership qualities, openness, able to change, generosity, kindness, charisma, and an absence of the above symptoms.

The Fire Element

Associated with the heart and summer. Also "rules" the small intestine and closely linked to the mind. Closely linked to Chinese concept of "Shen."

Poor health is associated with emotional or mental symptoms of lack of focus, weak spirit, mental illness, amnesia, lack of laughter, speech problems, and a poor level of personal integration.

Physical presentations may include poor circulation, hardening of the arteries, chest pains, aversion to heat, palpitations, and irregular heartbeat.

Good health associated with good mind-spirit connection, a sense of joy, and an absence of the above symptoms.

The Earth Element

Associated with the spleen-pancreas, stomach, and late summer.

Poor health is associated with emotional or mental symptoms of mental stagnation, repetitive behavior, lack of creative completion, sloppy appearance, chaotic lifestyle, and a tendency to accumulate useless possessions!

Physical presentations may include weak digestion, chronic fatigue, nausea, poor appetite, weight problems, and blood sugar disorders such as diabetes.

Good health associated with being hard working, responsible, orderly, active, creative, and an absence of the above symptoms.

The Metal Element

Associated with the lungs and autumn. Also linked to the colon.

Poor health is associated with emotional or mental symptoms of prolonged grief, overattachment, and problems with "letting go."

Physical presentations may include lung disorders, throat and nose problems, colon disease, skin disease, pallor, too much or too little mucus, frequent infections, and colds (lungs are linked to immune function).

Good health associated with light moist mucous membrane coating, healthy "glowing" skin, lustrous hair, rapid resolution of negative emotion, and a lack of the above symptoms.

The Water Element

Associated with the kidneys and winter. Also linked to the concept of "Jing" which means essence and relates to the quality of well-rooted vitality.

Poor health is associated with the emotional or mental symptoms of excessive fear and insecurity and impaired development.

Physical presentations may include bone problems, particularly of knees and lower back, hearing disorders, premature ageing, and urinary, sexual, and reproductive imbalances.

Further Key Concepts

Shen can be translated as spirit and relates to an individual's connection with the universe (see the section on "Shen Qi" for further details).

Yi can be translated as mind, which embraces consciousness, belief systems, and attitudes.

Qi can be translated as energy and is a central concept in practical health delivery, particularly with regard to herbal medicine. Disease can be analyzed in terms of patterns of presentation that are governed by Qi balances within and between the elements.

Qi is also a metaphysical concept that, according to the ancient Chinese, flows through the entire universe; without this energy nothing material would exist. Qi also runs through the bodies of all living beings. TCM practitioners over the centuries have developed a body map of the channels for Qi energy in the human body—these channels are called *meridians*. A primary aim of treatment is to keep this energy flowing smoothly—if the Qi stops moving, the patient will die; if Qi movement is obstructed or becomes stagnant, illness will result.

Imbalances between the five organ centers mentioned above relate directly to patterns of Qi movement and control. For instance water, which relates to the kidneys, controls fire, which relates to the heart. Or the wood organs, the liver and gallbladder, assist the earth organs, the spleen and stomach, in digesting food. Thus a poorly functioning liver, which is common in hepatitis C cases, often correlates with poor digestion, a link that is not always made in mainstream medicine.

Xue can be translated as blood. Xue is intimately related to Qi. Acupuncture and herbal diagnosis and treatment will often have its primary objective as "moving" the blood.

Yin and **Yang.** Qi energy will manifest in either Yin or Yang forms. Yin was envisaged as the dark side of a mountain, while Yang was the sunlit side. Words that can be used to describe Yin qualities include female, dark, solid, cool, and downward moving. Yang qualities are the reverse—masculine, light, warm, positive, tending to move upward. Yin and Yang are relative terms, so a given object can be Yin in the context of comparison to a Yang object, or Yang when compared to an object with Yin qualities.

In TCM, diagnoses are made by looking at the tongue, by taking the "Qi pulse" of the five organs (a highly skilled procedure), by examining the patient, and by asking questions and listening carefully to what the patient has to say.

Treatment usually consists of a combination of acupuncture, herbs, dietary adjustment, massage, and practice of Qi Gong (see later section). Acupuncture and herbs are the most common combination. See below for details of how these treatments work and how they relate to hepatitis C specifically.

The Appeal of TCM to HCV Patients

There are a number of reasons why TCM is an attractive treatment option to many HCV patients. Most importantly it has a strong reputation for being able to deliver effective and satisfactory treatment to hepatitis patients. This is not controversial in China—doctors there conservatively estimate that around 50% of chronic hepatitis sufferers are relieved of their symptoms following a course of TCM treatment. There has been no research into whether this means that the hepatitis C virus actually leaves the bodies of these patients. Appropriately specialized clinics in the West appear to be able to replicate this success (refer to the section in "Preliminary Report into Efficacy" at the end of this chapter for details). TCM is also a generally supportive approach that may spare patients from the side effects of some other forms of hepatitis C treatment.

Although health is seen as a function of a good balance between the various organs (heart, liver, spleen, kidneys, and lungs) and the elements they represent, the liver is regarded as the "general" in this system and is seen as being of primary importance; it is recognized that problems in the liver can lead to an "invasion" of the other organs and disruption of their functions. Thus Chinese doctors are particularly interested in, and sensitive to, liver disorders and their treatment.

There are currently estimated to be around 120 million people with hepatitis of one type or another in China. It appears to have been a major health hazard for thousands of years not just in China but throughout the East. The characteristics of hepatitis and recommendations for its treatment were described thousands of years ago.

Patients who have used TCM report that practitioners often appear to understand and affirm the emotional and subtle physiological effects of HCV. This may be because it is a holistic system that appreciates that a problem in one area can lead to "knock on" effects elsewhere in the body. Certain emotions are also associated with particular organs, so TCM practitioners can be quick to recognize a wider pattern of symptoms and react affirmatively rather than dismissively as some conventional doctors do. Indeed the emotional experience of patients can be important in the process of diagnosis.

The Pathogenesis of Hepatitis C: The TCM Perspective

It is apparent that TCM has, in some respects, a superior ability to clearly identify and explain what is happening to people who have hepatitis C. In particular, the wide range of symptoms and clinical disease associated with chronic conditions can be incorporated into a convincing and affirmative model. Such models of disease progression are strikingly similar to those used by modern systems analysts; they are interested in the processes and the patterns of illness more than the minutiae such as a viral "cause"—in fact there is no concept of a virus in TCM. John Tindall has put forward the following analysis:

The virus, an "external pathogen," enters the body from the outside; it takes up residence in the body if it is not expelled, becoming a "latent pathogen." The virus invades the cells and replicates—creating damp heat toxins that consume Qi, Xue, and body fluids—and it blocks the production of new substances and prevents the elimination of waste materials. If the constitution of the person and the strain of virus produces more damp than heat (which block the liver Qi's free-flowing function), this tends to affect the earth element primarily, that is, wood invades earth, and this will cause symptoms of nausea, vomiting, an acid, bitter taste in the mouth, loose stools or alternating loose and hard or incomplete stools, halitosis, and mouth ulcers.

As the earth element function, that is, Qi, Xue, and body fluid production, is affected, the person becomes pale, often has cold hands and feet, lethargy, lassitude, and tiredness.

Over time the body seeks to prevent damage to the internal organs and stores the damp heat toxin in the secondary defense channels of the earth element such as in the muscles, leading to a heavy feeling, aching, and a woolly sensation all over. The earth element then draws on its mother, the fire element, for help, thus compounding the paleness, tiredness with palpitations, poor sleep, vivid dreams, depression, and so on.

This pathology, continued viral activity, mental and emotional frustration becomes a vicious circle. The tissues related to the liver are affected, causing joints to ache, especially elbows and knees, as these are plane joints primarily supported by the ligaments and tendons which are nourished by the liver blood. The eyes are tired and ache, hair lacks luster, and nails are brittle and skin is dry, the mood fluctuates between depression and anger. Gynecological disorders, especially PMS and other bleeding disorders, may occur.

This general pattern tends to consume the kidney Yang and over the years these factors can all continue and cause stagnation of Qi, Xue, and body fluids, resulting in fibrosis and hardening of the liver, kidney, spleen, and pancreas and possibly cancer.

If the constitution of the person and the strain of the virus produce more heat than damp, this consumes the Qi, Xue, Yin, and body fluids of the liver, and it subsequently calls on the root of Yin in the kidney for help.

This pattern develops over a long period of time—kidney Yin becomes deficient and cannot nurture liver Yin or control heart fire. The general Yin deficiency symptoms will be night sweats, hot flushes, thirst, dry mouth, restless mind, constipation, dark urine, hot restless hands and feet, and bleeding disorders. The kidney Yin Xue symptoms will be backache, bone and big joint pains, which tend to be hot and swollen, infertility, lack of libido, impotence, poor memory, anemia, fear, paranoia, toothache, tinnitus, deafness, ascites, adrenal dysfunction, vertigo, dizziness, recurrent urine infections, kidney stones, cataracts, glaucoma, and diabetes.

The liver Yin Xue symptoms will be headache, migraine, floaters, tired eyes, ridged nails with red or dark lines, liver pain, twitching, flanks painful, hardening of the liver, ligament and tendon pain, anger, depression, frustration, bruxism.

Gynecological problems—heavy bleeding, painful and clotted periods, clotting disruptions, cirrhosis, fibrosis, spider nevi, hot, dry red skin.

The Heart Yin Xue symptoms will be insomnia, dream disturbed sleep, palpitations, pains in the chest, short of breath on exertion, thyroid dysfunction, depression, poor circulation, poor concentration, mania, hysteria, angina, phlebitis, varicosity.

Over the years the consumption of the Qi, Yin, Xue, and body fluids creates a drying and hardening, thirsting and wasting of the body generally and may lead to cirrhosis and cancer.

All of these possibilities could be prevented, and, provided all the necessary measures are taken, they may also be reversed, even when they are well advanced.

Thus we can see that some difficult aspects of HCV pathogenesis can be explained in a single model. For instance the autoimmune diseases, which are a common feature in HCV and are still described as "coincidental" by some doctors, are a definite feature of progression in the TCM model. These symptoms are seen as a pattern of wider disharmony and stagnant heat. Also the way in which there are a preponderance of kidney problems in female HCV patients, while males tend to suffer more severe liver disease, is entirely rational in TCM—menstruation contributes to a Yin deficiency, which weakens the Yin organs, such as the kidneys; because men do not lose blood and are generally less inclined to let off emotional steam, they are more likely to develop stagnant liver Qi conditions, such as cirrhosis.

TCM treatments will vary according to the state of the individual patient. Although there are "broad band" herbal formulae for general complaints (see below for hepatitis C formulae), TCM practitioners will usually prescribe treatments on the basis of the exact state of the patient as he or she presents. It is probably for this reason that TCM is becoming increasingly popular as a complementary form of medicine in a number of illnesses. For instance, cancer patients can receive treatment not only for their condition but also for the side effects of any chemotherapy they may be undergoing. Indeed some of the best results in cancer treatment seem to be obtained by combining mainstream medicine with TCM. This also applies to HCV, where a number of patients are now using both sets of resources simultaneously.

Patients may also receive treatments aimed at parts of their bodies other than the liver because the restoration of overall balance is the aim. The approach of the Gateway Clinic, a pioneer in the application of TCM to hepatitis C, is to first build the patient up using tonic herbs and appetite stimulants. The health of the digestive system needs to be bolstered right at the beginning of treatment.

One TCM specialist interviewed for this book stated that whenever liver problems had existed for any length of time it was almost inevitable that other systems would have been affected, typically the spleen, which, in TCM, governs digestion and the conversion of food into energy. Since hepatitis C is almost always chronic and has usually only been detected years after infection, it is highly likely that the liver is not the only area affected. Indeed the latest conventional medical research clearly indicates that HCV physically invades other organs and blood cells (see chapters 1 and 14).

Because patients often have a number of secondary conditions, some of which can be serious in their own right, TCM is well placed to address an entire matrix of illness in a "one stop" consultation. This is in stark contrast to conventional medicine, where consultations with a number of different specialists would be necessary. The treatments prescribed by these specialists often conflict with each other and can cause further problems. Thus TCM is a practical and highly economical option to those who manage health delivery services.

There has been very little research into the efficacy of combining TCM with mainstream medicine. The medical profession seems generally resistant to this avenue of approach and appears to be reluctant to conduct clinical trials. This may be partly due to the cost and the fact that herbalists are not in a financial position to underwrite such trials in the same way that drug companies do for their medicines. However, there are some encouraging signs: doctors at two central London hospitals are now trying to set up trials into standardized adjunct Chinese herbal therapy for patients taking interferon and interferon plus ribavirin.

Lastly, and perhaps most importantly, TCM stresses the absolute necessity for those suffering from hepatitis C to learn to relax, an aspect of treatment that is often neglected in conventional medicine. In the words of John Tindall, "The first thing we need to do in the treatment of hepatitis C is to relax. Relax, be at ease. If you get tense, worried, uptight, then you generate heat, tension, anxiety ... you're not doing yourself any favors." A good TCM practitioner may incorporate relaxation into treatment.

Details of TCM Treatments for Hepatitis C

As mentioned above, there are usually five "arms" of TCM. This section takes each one in turn and explains both the general principles of the technique and its likely application to hepatitis C patients.

Acupuncture

General Purpose

To move Qi, unblock the meridians, and restore organ function. This is the most common form of TCM and is routinely used in China. It is also becoming more popular in the West with many hospitals now offering acupuncture. It is the most researched of all traditional measures, and it has been shown to work. For instance, regular ear acupuncture will increase the levels of certain cells associated with immune response in the blood.

Typical Role in HCV

Acupuncture involves the insertion of fine metal needles into focal points on the body where the Qi can be adjusted. Over thousands of years the Chinese have observed the interconnection of the energy channels and internal organs of the body and discovered the key locations to effect changes in the internal condition. Key objectives with respect to HCV are the promotion of optimum function of the digestive system, kidney, and liver and to calm the mind and keep the Qi and Xue moving smoothly.

The earliest records of acupuncture principles and practice describe what happens when liver Qi stagnates or becomes unbalanced and how to treat the problems that arise as a result. Typically hepatitis will be characterized by an excess of damp heat, reflecting the presence of the virus (a "latent pathogen" in TCM terminology), along with stagnation in liver Qi, a process that may eventually result in cirrhosis, which is a scarred, blocked liver. As seen above HCV patients may present with an array of varied disharmonies. Liver Yin deficiency is another common symptomatic profile.

Thus acupuncture will be applied according to the relative severity of these symptoms. If the patient has a high temperature, then the practitioner may use a fire point; if the high temperature is less serious, an earth point may be used. Points that clear heat are often on the back of the body, the Yang side. A good practitioner will take care not to completely clear the heat, since this is an indication that the body is actively engaging the pathogen.

If there are signs of stagnant liver Qi, acupuncture will be applied to stimulate the energy and help to clear blockages. As well as keeping the liver cool, the acupuncturist will also aim to keep it moist. John Tindall comments:

> In cases of damp heat in the liver one would clear this by using points in the corresponding channel such as GB34, LIV14, and LIV5. This problem often affects the digestive system, so one would apply treatment to regulate the stomach and spleen (earth energy), such as HC6, SP4, and SP6.
>
> In cases of Yin deficiency it will be necessary to balance the liver (wood) with the kidney (water) energy, using such points as LIV8, LIV3, K3, K6, and CV4."

Ear Acupuncture

Ear acupuncture is a widely accessible treatment that can be administered by trained practitioners. The National Acupuncture Detoxification Association (NADA) network trains ear acupuncturists in a well-known protocol that is known to relieve stress, improve various bodily functions including immune response, and be very helpful in withdrawal from all forms of chemical dependency, ranging from nicotine to crack cocaine. This form will be of benefit to many hep C patients. Even better, an ear acupuncture protocol for hepatitis C has now been developed, which may become widely accessible. In conjunction with standardized herbal formulations, this approach might form the basis of a robust front-line treatment strategy. The "points" are as follows:

- **Hepatitis Point:** 2 mm lateral to the uterus point and slightly above. *Do not use in pregnancy.*

- **Zero Point:** At the lower part of the crus of the helix, for regulating Qi and Xue.

- **Endocrine:** At the bottom of the inter-tragic notch; *Do not use in pregnancy or during periods,* for all hormone functions and regulating metabolism.

- **Liver Yang I:** On the helix above the auricular tubercle, for chronic hepatitis and to lower transaminase.

- **Liver Yang II:** On the helix below the auricular tubercle, for chronic hepatitis and to lower transaminase.

In general, acupuncture treatment remains active for 48–96 hours. Members of the NADA network may be able to apply the hepatitis C protocol. Body acupuncture should only be applied by fully qualified TCM practitioners with experience of hepatitis C.

Contacts for Ear Acupuncture

NADA (U.S.): Phone/fax (360) 260-8621
Email: AcuDetox@AOL.com

NADA (U.K.): 0171 820 9892
NADA U.K. produces a hepatitis C training manual; both branches produce newsletters.

Diet

General Purpose

To promote the right physical conditions for strength and healing is essential. In the first instance the practitioner will focus on the efficiency of the digestive system. This is seen as a vital prerequisite in TCM, as in some other approaches (see chapter 22). Once digestion has been optimized, the diet can be adjusted.

The "Tao of Balanced Diet" underlies much of TCM's approach to the subject; the emphasis is on balance. However, there a number of different Chinese dietary systems, reflecting different interpretations of this philosophy and geography. Foods are classified according to the same principles as herbs—that is, is the food hot or cold, moist or dry? Diet may be individually prescribed along the same lines as herbal prescription. In practice, Western dietary principles and ingredients are often incorporated into recommended diets.

Typical Role in HCV

TCM classifies foods according to their temperature properties: hot, warm, neutral, cool, and cold. Some foods are known to have a therapeutic effect on Qi as well, although herbs are usually used in this respect.

Strictly speaking, diet should be individually prescribed along the same lines as herbal therapy. However, because hepatitis C is a condition typically characterized by "damp heat," and this is seen as being caused by stagnant foods, which are heavy and hard to digest, most TCM specialists will recommend a general diet to counteract this common tendency. Thus fresh, light ingredients will be stressed. This is similar to what most Western dieticians will advise, although the reasoning is somewhat different. (TCM often seems to come up with similar prescriptions to Western science although the logical structure is entirely different.) The usual advice is to avoid fried or processed food.

It is also good to bias the diet in favor of cooling, drying foods to counter the dampening, heating effect of hepatitis. Avoid foods that tend to be hard to digest; many people with HCV find that fried foods can be very hard on the stomach and drain energy. It is important to allow time for digestion after each meal.

Although the TCM practitioner will often provide dietary guidelines, it is quite acceptable for the patient to behave intuitively. After a while you may get to know what suits you, what your system likes, and what it finds difficult to process. Practicing Qi Gong may help people to develop this awareness (see below).

According to the Chinese system some common foods are classified as follows:

- Hot: trout, chili pepper

- Warm: chicken, lamb, cherry, peach, leeks, onions, butter, basil

- Neutral: tuna, herring, rice, beans, grapes, olives, carrots, milk, peas

- Cool: soybean, apples, pears, cucumber, marjoram, barley

- Cold: crab, octopus, watermelon

See chapter 22 for further information on the application of TCM principles to diet.

Herbs

General Purpose

To open, clear, nourish, and strengthen the body. The qualities of a large number of herbs are well known to TCM practitioners. They are often prescribed in complex formulae. They may be taken dried, in pill form, or the patient may be required to boil them up, a process known as *decoction*. Large numbers of people with hepatitis have derived great benefit from their use over millennia. However, in order to access this form of medicine, it is important to follow certain safety guidelines.

Safety, Toxicity, Quality Control, and Other Considerations

Contrary to the impression sometimes given by the media, they are safe if taken in accordance with the instructions of a qualified and experienced TCM herbalist. In general, Chinese herbs are far less likely to cause an adverse reaction in comparison to drug therapy. It has been shown that in Hong Kong, where the use of Chinese herbs is routine, only 0.2% of hospital admissions were due to adverse reactions to Chinese herbs, compared to 4.4% of admissions being caused by adverse reactions to Western pharmaceuticals[1] (refer to this paper for a good overview of this topic).

The traditional Chinese materia medica contains a very large number of medicinal substances. Some of them are toxic and may only be employed on an inpatient basis for serious illnesses by experienced practitioners. Others should only be prescribed for external use. Still more should only be prescribed in certain combinations. Certain herbs need to be prepared in precise ways in order to deliver their intended effect.

Individual ingredients to be avoided:

(Guan) Fang Ji	(Guan) Mu Tong	Ma Huang
Fu Zi	Wu Tou	Cao Wu
Datura Straemonium	Rhus Toxicodedron	Ma Dou Ling
Ma Qian Zi	Zhu Sha	Hei Zi
Ying Su Ke	(Shui) Ban Xia	

In addition, serious problems have been reported with HCV+ people using He Shou Wu (polygonum multiflorum), which is often contained in formulations aimed at treating hair greying or loss.

Formulations that can cause toxicity or adverse consequences:

Niu Huang Jie Du Pian

Tian Wang Bu Xin Dan

Jin Bu Huan

The latter formulation has been implicated in several cases of hepatitis, for example.[2] Any formulations also containing Western drugs must also be avoided.

Adulteration and the presence of incorrect species have also been reported, particularly with prepackaged formulations. Some may also contain unsafe levels of certain trace elements such as mercury and aluminum; corticosteroids and hormones have also been detected.

The upshot of this is the following:

1. It is essential to only take Chinese herbal preparations that are specifically aimed at treating hepatitis C and are manufactured by companies with exhaustive quality control procedures (see below).

2. Or only take herbs that are individually prescribed by fully qualified TCM practitioners with experience of treating HCV who also have access to quality-controlled and extensive herbal pharmacies (see the "Finding a TCM Practitioner" section).

3. If you are in any doubt about the quality, you can take your prescription to a reputable supplier.

The Theory and Practice of Chinese Herbal Medicine

These herbs are pharmacologically complex. In TCM their efficacy is rooted in the "Tao of Forgotten Foods," which stresses that they are to be regarded as foods containing powerful nutrients often absent in the normal diet or only necessary due to a deficiency caused by illness. In TCM their usefulness is rooted in empirical observation, matching the herbal prescription to patterns of illness observed over millennia; their value is based on the pure science of empiricism, and they have been tested not on animals but on millions of human beings.

Recent research confirms that many of these plants do indeed contain obscure and novel pharmacological substances, some of which are of obvious value in the treatment of chronic liver disease (see details below).

There have been some other reports into the efficacy of Chinese herbs,[3] but the subject as a whole has not yet been well researched. This is mainly because these herbs are available to everyone and do not represent huge potential profits to the commercial organizations that fund the vast bulk of medical research. Some drug companies, tacitly acknowledging their effectiveness, have attempted to isolate active ingredients so that these can be patented, packaged, and marketed. Such efforts have usually resulted in failure because of the complexities of these agents.

Chinese herbs can take some time to have an effect. They do not have the instant impact of drugs like aspirin, for instance. Most of the herbs used for hepatitis require regular use for up to two weeks before they have a noticeable effect.

One problem with evaluating the efficacy of Chinese herbs arises out of the fact that TCM has no concept of a virus. The closest it comes is "latent pathogen." This means that a patient may be regarded as being "cured" in TCM while regarded as being still infected by a virologist, even though liver histology and other tests demonstrate improvement.

Some work needs to be done here; both traditions can learn from each other. There are Chinese herbs with more powerful antiviral properties than those normally used in hepatitis. Some of these are being tested for their efficacy against HIV.

Typical Role in HCV

A. *Individually Prescribed*

Herbal prescriptions will vary according to the individual more than any other aspect of treatment. The Chinese have accumulated a vast herbal armory over the centuries and an equally formidable method of prescription, which will vary according to the individual patient's condition.

Dr. Quing Chai Zhang, director of Zhang's Clinic in New York, has reported significant levels of success in treating hepatitis C. He bases his prescriptions on the findings of pharmacological research conducted in China over the last thirty years, as well as traditional wisdom. He describes himself as a practitioner of modern or integrative Chinese medicine. He presents his approach and the thinking behind it:

> Over the past twenty years many new therapeutic methods have been developed by Chinese medical researchers which suppress the HCV virus, regulate immune functions, clear jaundice, normalize liver enzyme levels, heal the inflammation of liver cells, reverse fibrolization, and improve cirrhosis.
>
> In 80% of the patients using this protocol, liver enzymes are normalized within two months, jaundice disappears within three weeks, fatigue is reduced, and poor appetite is improved. In many cases the viral load tests show substantial reduction of viral load in the blood. The liver cell's life span is about eighteen months and the treatment should last two years to ensure the replacement of all inflammation-damaged liver cells with new cells.
>
> *Normalizing liver enzymes, reducing inflammation, and repairing damaged cell membranes:* There is a group of herbs that normalize the liver enzyme levels and reduce the inflammatory changes of liver cells. The most important herb is *Schizandrae fructus chinensis* (Wu Wei Ze). Its active ingredient can reduce 84%–97% of ALT and AST levels and normalize 75% of patients within three to six weeks.
>
> *Immune regulators can promote the elimination of HCV.* Immune regulation and antiviral effects are related and the elimination of the virus is mainly dependent upon the immune system of the host. Extracts from Chinese medicinal herbs, such as *Polyporus umbellatus pers, Sophorae substratae radix, Phyllanthus amarus, Glycyrrhizae radix* (Gan Cao), and *Cordyseps sinensus,* promote cellular and humoral immune reactions that can eliminate the HCV virus. They also help repair damaged immune cells caused by immune dysfunction.
>
> *Once the inflammation is gone the liver cells can regenerate.*

Liver cells have a strong ability to regenerate. This ability is closely related to proper nutrition, including trace elements. *Astragalus radix* (Huang Qi), *Atractylodes macrocephalae rhizoma* (Bai Zhu), *Codonopsis pilosulae radix* (Dang Shen), ginseng (Ren Shen), *Bupleuri radix* (Chai Hu), and *Lycii fructus* (Gou Qi Zi) are rich in sinidium, zinc, and germanium, which promote liver cell regeneration.

Chinese herbal treatments are not a cure for chronic hepatitis. But there is a chance for a lifetime with normal liver enzyme levels, reduced viral loads, and an overall improvement in quality of life.

Dr. Zhang stresses that hepatitis C is a systemic condition whose effective treatment requires the attainment of multiple clinical objectives. He believes that pharmaceutical approaches that concentrate upon viral suppression to the exclusion of other parameters are irrational. He notes that such treatments can cause a more intractable pattern of disease than hepatitis C itself, and stresses the importance of balancing immune function, particularly in the light of recent findings suggesting that most liver damage is immunopathic in the case of HCV. For information about Zhang's protocols, see contacts in the "Finding a TCM Practitioner" section.

While there have been no controlled studies of the impact of Chinese herbal treatment upon viral load, a number of individual patients have reported either dramatic reductions in viral load, or becoming PCR or b-DNA negative for HCV. The case history cited in chapter 6, pages 108–109, is a typical example.

It is not yet known how Chinese herbs are achieving this effect: whether they stimulate humoral or cellular immunity, have a direct inhibitory effect on some phase in HCV replication, or some combination of the three. Not enough research has been done to establish whether or not the action is consistent or can be recreated consistently. What seems to be apparent is that antiviral action is slower but more comfortable compared to drug therapy. It is also apparent that antiviral treatment is not necessarily the top priority, particularly in the case of more advanced patients where stabilization of organ function may take priority.

Some Examples of Commonly Prescribed Chinese Herbs for Hepatitis C

Bai Shao Yao—White Peony Root—*Radix paeoniae alba*

A liver tonic. It often helps to stop night sweats and relieves hypertension. It is also good for purifying and nourishing the blood. It has been observed to reduce learning impairment, relax muscles, exert an antiallergic effect, and reduce edema.[4]

Bai Zhu, Pai Shu—No Equivalent—*Rhizoma attractylodis*

Supports digestion process by stimulating production of enzymes. Diuretic—that is, it promotes the release of excess fluids via the urine, although it is gentle on the kidneys and safe. Lowers blood sugar and helps the liver to retain glycogen.

Ban Lan Gen—Isatis Root—*Baphicacanthi radix*

Eliminates excess heat and toxins from the blood; anti-inflammatory, antipyretic.

Chai Hu, Cai Hu—Chinese Bupleurum—*Radix bupleuri, Bupleurum falcatum*

This is one of the finest herbs for detoxifying the liver. It is an antipyretic—that is, it reduces feverishness and sweating.[5] It is anti-cirrhotic, countering stagnancy of liver Qi. This herb is anti-inflammatory, hepatoprotective, making it a good candidate for simultaneously treating liver disease and autoimmune conditions. This herb is cold in TCM terms and has a bitter taste. It is a key ingredient in SSKT (see below) and contains substances called saikosaponins, thought to be responsible for many of the medicinal actions that have been noted.

Dang Gui, Dong Quai—Angelica Root—*Radix angelicae*

Nourishes blood and improves circulation. This is an antispasmodic and is often prescribed to alleviate PMS or during menopause. It has been observed to increase red blood cell counts, promote sexual activity in female mice, correct certain heart abnormalities, enhance certain liver metabolic functions, and reduce proliferation of smooth muscle cells.[6] It should not be used during pregnancy.

Fang Feng—Sileris—*Ledebouriella divaricata*
Relieves pains in the joints, flu, headaches, chills, and rheumatoid numbness. It is thought to be a tonic to the immune system.

Huang Lian—Coptis Root—*Coptidis rhizoma*
This is an antiviral herb that also has a mild sedative effect. In TCM terminology it helps to eliminate heat and dampness. This herb has sometimes been confused with Hu Huang Lian, which is actually the very useful herb *Rhizoma picrorrhizae,* covered in chapter 17.

Huang Qin—Baikal Skullcap Root—*Scutellariae baicalensis, radix*
Clears heat. Observed to exert anti-inflammatory and antiviral action, inhibits collagen aggregation, and suspected of exerting anticarcinogenic action.[4]

Tai Zi Shen—Pseudostellaria—*Pseudostellariae heterophyllae, radix*
Strengthens the spleen and augments the Qi. Prescribed to address lack of appetite and fatigue, also to help in recovery from febrile diseases.

Wu Wei Zi—Schisandra fruit—*Schisandra chinensis*
Used to "tonify" the kidney and to treat coughs, excessive sweating, chronic diarrhea, insomnia, and poor memory. Also observed to be hepatoprotective, to promote liver detoxification, to enhance antioxidant liver function, to lower death rates in fulminant hepatitis, to exert antidepressant action, to reduce SGPT levels in hepatitis, to act against tumor formation, particularly in the liver and to increase RNA, glycogen, and enzymes in the kidneys.[4]

Zhi Ke—Bitter Orange—*Citrus aurantum*
Softens hardening in the gastrointestinal tract. It is a carminative and helps to prevent dyspepsia (i.e., stomachaches) and constipation.

Note that these are only a few common examples. Your TCM practitioner will prescribe a blend of herbs to meet your individual needs. It is important that you trust their judgment. For further details on selected Chinese and Ayurvedic herbs, refer to chapter 17 and the book *Clinical Applications of Ayurvedic and Chinese Herbs* (see the "Further Reading" section at the end of this chapter.) Or refer to the Chinese materia medica.

B. "Broad Range" Chinese Herbal Formulae
Specifically Designed for Hepatitis C

CH100—produced by Cathay Herbal; an Australian-based standard Chinese herbal treatment for hepatitis C.

This is the first Chinese herbal formulation developed specifically to treat hepatitis C in the West and the only one that has so far been subject to double-blind placebo-controlled trial.[6] Designed as one standard formulation applicable to the broad swathe of patients, the clinical aim is to improve clinical liver function as measured by ALT and AST levels with a view to modifying the course of hepatitis C in favor of a benign outcome. The results of the trial demonstrate improvement in the majority of trialists, even those who were interferon relapsers or nonresponders and who were also using moderate amounts of alcohol, although only one had sustained normalization of liver function after the therapy.

Treatment involved five 360 mg tablets (either active herbs or placebo), taken twice per day for six months. Active tablets contained extracts from nineteen herbs. Fifty-eight patients were assessed, forty-four randomized to treatment, and forty completed therapy.

Side effects were modest and of a lower order of seriousness compared to drug therapy, although one patient was taken out of the trial due to palpitations, and two had their dose reduced because of temporary diarrhea and abdominal discomfort. The trial organizers concluded that the patients on the active herbs benefited from treatment, that the Chinese herbal approach warranted further development, and acknowledged that results were likely to be further improved by the use of individually customized prescription.

Of equal interest and note were the organizers' reasons for pressing ahead with this study in the face of opposition from vested interests and conservative elements within the medical establishment. Noting the limitations of interferon-based therapy, they commented:

> In Australia, it has been estimated that the cost of managing the patients with chronic hepatitis C infection will run into

Results of CH100 Trial		
	Treated Group	Placebo Group
Number tested	20	20
Age (years)	40.4	40.9
% male	59.1	59.1
Duration of HCV (months)	92	83
Alcohol g/d; past interferon	20	20
Past interferon	6	8
Initial ALT	120	102
Final ALT	82	102

billions of dollars by the year 2010. Many patients reviewing the literature on hepatitis C have decided that natural therapies may be a better way forward in the treatment of their own disease.... Recent publications have documented a protective effect of Chinese herbal preparations on the development of liver injury in rat models of liver injury or cirrhosis.... Studies demonstrate the presence of active components which may have the capacity to modulate liver disease in the clinical situation.

Thus Professor Batey acknowledges and affirms the reasoning and the thinking of many patients. Equally importantly he also refers to the very serious economic realities that make the application of chemotherapy on the necessary scale an expensive option. Professor Batey and his colleagues are to be congratulated for having the courage and professional integrity to open up this avenue of enquiry.

Call Cathay Herbal in Sydney, Australia, for further details: 61 2 9212 5151.

John Tindall's Protocols for Broad-Range Formulations for Hepatitis C

As a result of working intensively with hepatitis C patients for a number of years and close consultation with top Chinese herbal experts in the fields of liver disease and virology, Tindall has developed some broad-range tableted Chinese herbal formulae. While an individual consultation and prescription is still the best option, these preparations allow patients who wish to try Chinese herbs, but cannot get to a qualified specialized practitioner, the opportunity to do so.

Tindall has got around the problem of the diverse needs of patients by designing different products for the distinct profiles of HCV related disease he has observed. The closer the "fit" to one of the profiles listed below, the greater the chance of response. If you do not fit, avoid them. If in doubt, call the contact numbers listed below.

Patients trying these formulae should note the following lifestyle guidelines:

- Ideally, no drugs or alcohol should be consumed during this treatment. However, moderate occasional alcohol use with food (ideally wine) is unlikely to hinder the treatment.

- If you cannot give up cigarettes, try to cut down.

- Try to eliminate or at least reduce consumption of coffee, sugar, hot spicy food, and fried and fatty food.

- Try to adopt a relaxed approach to life; take time out if you are busy.

The Profiles

Some patients will fall outside these parameters and will need to obtain an individual prescription. Note that Chinese herbs usually take between two and fourteen days to have an effect. Where deep-seated symptoms are concerned—such as night sweats associated with cirrhosis—responsive patients have reported that up to six weeks may be required for neutralization. These formulae are primarily designed to be safe; potentially hazardous herbs have been omitted. They may be taken over the long term.

The herbs are designed in a modular format. Start by taking whichever of the first three (CATA, B, or C) best suit—you may have any of the indicators, but none of the contraindicators. As symptoms change, review the suitability of the formula. If they do not

Indications and Contraindications

Early Stage   CATA.001   **Peaceful River**

Indications:
Lassitude

Poor digestion, poor appetite, nausea, acid or bitter taste in the mouth

Bloating, gas, wind, abdominal cramps, stool loose or soft

Pain in the upper-right quadrant

Muscle ache, heavy feeling in the body

Intermittent feelings of alternate hot and cold

Mood swings

Tender liver

Raised ALT, AST, and viral load

Contraindications:
Pregnant or likely to become so

Colds and influenza

Fevers

Constipation, dry mouth and throat, migraines

Actions:
Regulates the Qi of the liver, spleen, and stomach

Clears damp heat

This formulation contains seventeen herbs including Dang Shen, Bai Zhu, and Hu Huang Lian.

work, then increase the dose (2 tablets, twice per day) or discontinue. If any discomfort is experienced, then reduce dose or discontinue. If you wish to try taking a stronger dose of "heat clearing" herbs, then add in "Eliminator" after the first three months; this has been designed to be taken in conjunction with the other formulations, but asymptomatic patients may try it on its own. None of these formulations have been subjected to placebo-controlled double-blind trials. They are, however, the basis of Tindall's herbal treatments, which have been well received by his patients.

Indications and Contraindications

Middle Stage   CATC.001   **Middle Way**

Indications:	Tired, disturbed sleep
	Liver pain, early fibrosis and inflammation
	Raised ALT, AST, and viral load
	Muscle ache
	Low mood, palpitations, irritable
	Thirst
	Painful periods
	Feeling of heat, frequent or persistent
	Incomplete stools or stools hard to pass
	Dark urine
	Dry skin, hair, and nails
	Tired eyes, headache
Contraindications:	Pregnant or likely to become so
	Fevers
	Diarrhea
	Migraines
Actions:	Tonifies the blood and Qi
	Cools the blood
	Eliminates damp heat and fire poison

This formulation contains sixteen herbs including Tai Ze Shen, Sheng Di, and Mu Dan Pi.

In addition Tindall has designed a fifth product called Adjunct, which is designed to be taken in conjunction with interferon or interferon-ribavirin adjunct therapy. Adjunct is formulated to offset the side effects of interferon-based drug therapy, particularly what TCM practitioners see as disrupted "kidney Qi," and also to enhance treatment. Again the formulation is based upon his clinical experience of treating HCV patients. A trial of Adjunct is currently being proposed in London.

Indications and Contraindications

Later Stage	CATB.001	Cool and Calm

Indications:
- Exhausted
- Night sweats
- Insomnia
- Vivid dreams
- Angry, depressed
- Thirst, dry mouth
- Sharp liver pain, fibrosis, inflammation, scarring and hardening
- Raised AST, ALT, and viral load
- Constipation
- Dry and itchy skin, split or brittle nails
- Stomach acid
- Joint ache
- Palpitations
- Hair falling out
- Dry and sore eyes, floaters, poor vision
- Headaches and migraine

Contraindications:
- Pregnant or likely to become so
- Fever, chest infection, gastroenteritis
- Diarrhea
- Cough and phlegm

Actions:
- Nourishes the Yin of the liver and kidneys
- Moves the Qi and the blood
- Clears stagnant fire poison

This formulation contains nineteen herbs including Sheng Di Huang, Bie Sha Shen, Mai Men Dang, and Dang Gui.

Indications and Contraindications

Supplement	CATD.001	Eliminator
Indication:	High viral load, ALT, and AST	
	On CATA, B, or C	
Contraindication:	Pregnant or likely to become so	
	Influenza, fever, and sweating	
	Not taking CATA, B, or C	
Actions:	Clears fire poison and toxin	

This formulation contains seven classic "heat clearing" and "fire toxin clearing" herbs including Bai Hua She She Cao.

In the U.K. these products are available from East West Herbs Shop, 3 Neals Yard, Covent Garden, London WC2H 9DP, phone: 44 (0)171 379 1312 or their office in Oxfordshire, phone 44 (0)1608 658862.

In the U.S. and Canada they are distributed by East West Herbs USA to practitioners only. Their Website is http://www.eastwest-herbs.com/.

These companies employ rigorous, extensive quality control procedures, comply with statutory regulations in the U.S. and EC, and are subject to regular inspection by government agencies. Price for one month's standard supply will be around £20 or $30.

"Do It Yourself" Chinese Herbal Tea for HCV

You can use this combination of seven Chinese herbs to make a tea that may help to support the liver. You need the following herbs:

- Fu Rong Hua. This is actually hibiscus, very good for the liver, having an opening and moving effect.
- Ban Lan Gen is an antiviral, used classically for hepatitis.
- Da Qing Ye. This is woad. It is the most commonly used antiviral for hepatitis in China.
- Yin Chen Hao is also antiviral but used for jaundice as well as hepatitis.

- Bai Hua She She Cao is a common herb that grows in Malaysia. It's actually an anticancer herb for the whole digestive system. It stops the liver becoming hard and breaks up tumors.

- Mei Gui Hua, miniature rose. This works on a physical and a mental level very well. On a physical level it keeps the energy of the liver moving and is good for digestion. The concept is that of a rose opening; it's like a small baby, it has bundles of energy, and it's wanting to burst open. It opens the liver and helps you to relax; it helps clear the mind of superfluous garbage. Regarded as useful for PMS and people who are liverish by nature.

- Jin Qian Cao is used for jaundice, like Yin Chen Hao. These two will make you urinate a lot, thus clearing heat through the urine.

To make the tea take 2 g of each herb. Add to 1 liter of water. Boil, and then gently simmer for about ten minutes. Let it cool down. Strain it and store the liquid. You then drink this over two days.

Classic Formulae

There are also a few classic broad-range formulae that have been used to treat hepatitis C; however you should consult a qualified herbalist before selecting one of these.

Sho-Saiko-To [Japanese Kampo name, also known as SSKT]/Xiao Chai Hu Tang [Traditional Chinese]. Also called Minor Bupleurum Combination, TJ-9, and SSKT, this formulation has seven ingredients (bupleurum root, pinellia tuber, scutellaria root, jujube fruit, ginger rhizome, ginseng root, and glycyrrhiza root) and is best known as a traditional treatment for malaria; it is also used in other "lesser Yang" disorders, which includes some types of chronic hepatitis, that "come and go." Researchers in Japan have focused on SSKT as a potential treatment for hepatitis C both on its own and in conjunction with drug therapy. Results have confirmed the presence of valuable medicinal properties, specifically the ability to prevent liver fibrosis[7] and boost interleukin production in the peripheral blood mononuclear cells of chronic hepatitis C patients.[8]

However, a certain amount of confusion and misinformation has arisen from this work. This is partly due to the inherent problems of applying one formulation across broad groups of people, particularly persons with a multifaceted condition such as hepatitis C. Other studies have shown that when combined with interferon therapy some patients developed serious lung disorders.[9] Early analysis suggested some kind of interaction was taking place; more recent reports have suggested that SSKT may induce such disorders on its own in elderly HCV patients with underlying lung disease.

It is thought that SSKT modifies immune response in such a way as to antagonize inflammation-related disease in lung tissue. Thus this formulation needs to be treated with a degree of caution and must be avoided by any patients with breathing or lung-related disorders, which may occasionally be linked to HCV. In TCM terms these adverse effects are explained by the fact that this formulation is "drying," a useful quality in typical "damp" manifestations of chronic liver disease, but hazardous to those more advanced patients who are already too "dry."

Inchin-Ko-To [Japanese Kampo name]/Yin Chen Hao Tang [Traditional Chinese]. This is another classic Chinese and Japanese formulation that would be used by herbalists in the treatment of some manifestations of liver disease. This formulation has been shown to protect liver cells from autoimmune-induced injury and death.[10] It is thought that much of the progressive injury to liver cells that takes place in chronic hepatitis C patients and results in fibrosis and oncogenesis is attributable to the increased presence of transforming growth factor $b1$. This substance is linked to the process of apoptosis—that is liver cell death—and is therefore seen as a danger sign. It has now been shown that this formulation inhibits this injury in both normal and precancerous liver cells. Further study suggests that the herb *Artimesia capillaris spica,* a key ingredient in this formulation and frequently used by expert herbalists to treat HCV, is responsible for this action. The other ingredients are fructus and *Rhei rhizoma.*

Xiao Yao Wan. This translates as "free and easy wanderer." It's a very common formula often prescribed for a range of conditions, notably PMS or general irritability. It can be used as a kind of pre-ventative measure to protect the liver. Memorably described by one patient as "like valium without the headfuck."

Miscellaneous Work on Chinese Herbs

Another interesting study examined the relative efficacy of a TCM formulation compared to three other powerful hepatic medicines in rats.[11] The other agents under study were hepatic stimulator sub-stance (HSS—an organ-specific, species-non-specific growth pro-moter thought to promote tissue regeneration); selenium + vitamin E (often self-prescribed by patients or used by some complementary practitioners—see chapter 18); and ciprofloxacin (an antibiotic known to help in recovery from ethanol invoked liver injury).

The report concluded that there was significant improvement in all treated groups compared to untreated controls. In relative terms the Chinese herbal treatment was found to be the most effective of the agents under study with respect to all of the parameters tested. In terms of histology none of the TCM- and ciprofloxacin-treated rats developed stage III cirrhosis; thirteen out of sixteen of the TCM group were graded 0 or 1, and eleven of the sixteen ciprofloxacin-treated group were 0 to 1. The HSS and selenium/vitamin E groups fared better than the untreated damaged rats, but were in signifi-cantly poorer state compared to the TCM and ciprofloxacin groups, with thirteen out of fifteen and twelve out of fifteen progressing to stage II or III cirrhosis, respectively.

Massage

General Purpose

Like acupuncture this moves the Qi and unblocks the meridians. It works according to the same principles as acupuncture but without the needles—fingers, palms, fists, elbows, and feet may all be used. The classical form of Chinese massage is called An Ma. When it was taken to Japan it became what is now called Shiatsu, which means finger pressure.

Massage may be used as an alternative to acupuncture in some circumstances. For instance, some patients cannot tolerate the idea of having needles stuck into them. However, massage will lack the precision of acupuncture. Massage is also more expensive than acupuncture because it requires the continuous, exclusive attention of a highly skilled practitioner—by contrast an acupuncturist can treat several patients simultaneously.

Typical Role in Treatment of HCV

Massage may be used to relax the patient. Many patients experience a lot of anxiety due to both the physical effects of the virus and the level of uncertainty its presence causes. Shiatsu massage is one of the most effective relaxing therapies available. Recent research into the health of human immune systems indicates that the ability to relax is linked to the effectiveness of the fight against infections. If the patient is tense and nervous (referred to as "fight flight" mode in the jargon), he or she will be at a disadvantage in the fight against HCV in their system.

Qi Gong

General Purpose

If you live in a big city and have been for a walk in the park recently, you may have seen people standing with their legs slightly bent at the knees and with their arms held out in front of them as though they were embracing an invisible giant balloon. Sometimes they stand in this position for an hour or more, and sometimes they move ever so slowly, apparently tracing invisible lines around their bodies with their finger tips. The chances are that these people are practicing Qi Gong (pronounced Chee Gung, also spelled Chi Kung). If they are moving about in a fluid but continuous manner, then they are probably practicing Tai Qi, which is a related discipline.

Some TCM practitioners are also Qi Gong masters, and they may recommend that patients try it. Qi Gong literally means "energy work." Since health is seen as a state of balanced energy, a system of exercises have been developed to enable practitioners to become more balanced and harmonized. Theoretically this allows the advanced practitioner to "treat himself" and means that he will not need medicines or acupuncture to correct illnesses, which can be seen as disharmonies in the Qi. If the Qi Gong student can bring about a balanced energy pattern in his body, he will by definition be perfectly healthy. In a sense it is the polar opposite of mainstream medicine, where the patient surrenders responsibility to a specialist who prescribes treatments to kill a virus—in our case HCV. In Qi Gong the approach is more like the following: "This is how healthy beings live, these are the energy patterns that correspond to health, look for this harmony and learn to live in accord with your own true nature. Then you will be as healthy as you can be."

Stephen T. Chang, a well-known practitioner from a long lineage of Qi Gong enthusiasts, has described the importance of Qi Gong as follows:

> Without proper consumption of nutrients, life will shorten. Without motion the body will atrophy. Without proper motion the body will weaken. It was with this last consideration in mind that the ancient Taoists created the Tao of Revitalization, the philosophy and method of thinking, breathing, and moving. The Tao of Revitalization is a system of many mental and physical movements, called Internal Exercises. Internal Exercises heal and energize the internal organs—the keys to youth, immunity against disease, and true health—through deceleration, smoothness, quietness, precision, naturalness, and an internal emphasis.[12]

The contemporary Qi Gong master Zhixing Wang has developed a form called Hua Gong, which can be translated as "transformation work." He describes the development of Qi Gong as follows:

> Qi Gong is an art for health, longevity, and spiritual cultivation that the Chinese people have been practicing for several thousand years. Archaeological findings show that it was already a common practice over five thousand years ago. It is believed to be the fundamental practice from which the old master thinkers such as Fu Xi (who invented Yi Jing, or *The Book of Change*) Lao Zi (who wrote *Dao De Jing,* which has been now widely translated into many languages), Confucius, Zhuang Zi, Lie Zi, etc. Traditionally, it is also the foundation for the

learning in Chinese herbal medicine, acupuncture, and Tua Na (massage and acupressure). Buddhist monks practiced it for wisdom and clarity. Taoist priests practiced it for longevity and immortality. Martial arts people practiced it for extraordinary fighting power. Over its long history, it has been the vehicle to attain wisdom, knowledge, and power. Its extraordinary healing effects have not only changed many people's life but also inspired many to think in a different way. Now there are over 60 million people in China and many more in other parts of the world practicing Qi Gong.

Qi refers to the state, quality, or energy (field) that is subtle and insubstantial. It has mainly two meanings when related with Qi Gong. First, it means the void energy field of the original state of being from which all matter evolved. It is the universal consciousness that is hidden in all existence. It is the force of creation that generates all living beings. Second, it refers to the subtle energy within the physical body that keeps the body alive and vital. It is the life force by which a living human being is differentiated from a corpse or a plant. Its vibration and circulation can be experienced through Qi Gong practice.

A good foundation practice is the palm healing sequence, which is demonstrated by Zhixing Wang on videotape and includes a "transmission." This, together with information on Qi Gong courses and retreats is available from Chinese Heritage in the U.K. (telephone 0171 229 7187) or Paul Markowitz in the U.S. (212-661-7399). Also try the TCM contacts.

Qi Gong is an option for all patients. It can be practiced by people who are ill or old, and may reward perseverance with improved physical and mental health. If you want to look for a teacher, bear in mind that there are many people now offering tuition in Qi Gong who are not sufficiently experienced themselves. The best teachers are not necessarily Asian, and be particularly cautious about parting with large sums of money—only very advanced practitioners with proven lineage can justify large fees, and they may not be that useful to beginners anyway.

So far as efficacy is concerned, there seems little doubt that practicing Qi Gong can benefit patients' mental and emotional health. Hep C patients can use Qi Gong to help address emotional problems and cultivate a degree of calmness. The importance of the link between mind and body in overall health, however, is still a controversial subject. There have been no studies into whether or not Qi Gong practice can clear HCV or even improve symptoms. What some practitioners claim is that Qi Gong can alter the course of an illness.[13] More work has been done on cancer and the results appear to be impressive; [14] Chinese hospitals organize Qi Gong for cancer patients and others with chronic ailments.

Typical Role in Treatment of HCV

Qi Gong is a long-term complete system of health promotion and maintenance. It is particularly good for cultivating a relaxed state of mind, which is thought to be important for healthy immune and liver function.

There are some exercises that are specifically aimed at people with liver problems. For instance, the "Swimming Dragon" is recommended to people with stagnant liver Qi or excess weight. Digestive Qi Gong is also important for HCV. One exercise you can try after eating or when experiencing indigestion is as follows:

Take off your shoes and kneel down, preferably on a carpeted floor or a piece of soft grassy ground. Sit on your heels, so that the soles of your feet are facing upwards, towards your buttocks. Lean backwards, placing your hands on the ground behind you. Tip your head right back, so you are looking behind you, and lift the knees off the ground. You may feel pain in the ankles. Hold for a few seconds to begin with. Repeat a few times. If it is useful, then practice regularly, holding the position for longer periods, up to five minutes. This exercise "opens the stomach and spleen channels."

Shen Qi

Shen Qi is an advanced but accessible practice. It is somewhat difficult to describe. The format superficially resembles a kind of Taoist AA meeting or discussion group. It could be categorized as a pure form of naturopathic energetic medicine, within which all forms of ill health are seen as energy blockages. By cultivating a strong Shen connection, manifestations of ill health will be ironed out or displaced. This system embraces mental health, particularly the role of the ego in obstructing access to the energy, and thereby optimum health function.

This modern-day practice has evolved out of Qi Gong. Master Ai Ping Wang has developed a system that utilizes the philosophy of the East—Buddhism—with the verbal interactive group process of the West. The intention is that this practice will help people to recognize their purpose in life, remove ego blocks that prevent the realization of natural abilities, cope with everyday challenges, and overcome ill health. Words are perceived as packages of energy that are given by the creator of the universe.

Key principles include taking a relaxed position by sitting comfortably, slightly opening the mouth, breathing slowly and deeply. The body can be regarded as an antenna that can receive universal energy. Internally reception is helped by not thinking, not caring, giving yourself permission to enjoy everything, not focusing.

Patients have reported that Shen Qi can be an enjoyable and powerful vehicle for change. If facilitated by a trained and experienced practitioner, initial benefits will include a powerful sense of relaxation and belonging.

Shen Qi Contacts

Zagreb, Croatia: 385 455 5350 (Ai Ping Wang)
Boulder, Colorado: (303) 545-6736 (Tom Thiele)
Phoenix, Arizona: (602) 266-3251 (Jane Brooks)
Buckfastleigh, Devon (U.K.): 44 (0)1364 642787
Yuan Centre, London (U.K.): Fax: 44 (0)171 916 7942

Finding a TCM Practitioner

It is most important to use only a qualified and experienced TCM practitioner with appropriate specialized knowledge.

The problem of finding a suitable practitioner is recurrent. Perhaps the best course is to seek a personal recommendation from another HCV patient, perhaps at a support group. Good practitioners will quickly build up an enthusiastic client base—the experience of patients suggests that hepatitis C is highly responsive to this approach.

Problems with Chinese Herbal Medicine and Ways of Avoiding Them

Since writing the first edition we have received a lot of mainly positive feedback on this approach. However, three problems have emerged:

Poor or Inappropriate Practitioners

At least one patient was being prescribed inappropriate herbs, presumably because some TCM practitioners do not appreciate the intricacies of hepatitis C (not uncommon in all branches of medicine).

HCV patients need specialized attention, preferably by practitioners with lengthy experience in the fields of hepatology, gastroenterology, and/or virology. The average Main Street practitioners offering treatment for eczema, asthma, and the like are less likely to be able to achieve significant results and to have access to quality-controlled and extensive herbal pharmacies.

Cost

Some patients have been charged large amounts of money for consultations and herbs. Check that the service fits your pocket. Some practitioners will offer reduced rates to those with financial difficulties, so you can try to negotiate.

Problems with Patent Remedies

Some patients taking patent Chinese herbal remedies for other problems, such as hair loss, unaware that they were contraindicated due to their HCV status, have exposed themselves to the risk of taking adulterated products from suppliers with inadequate quality control procedures. We have a reliable report of one patient developing jaundice as a result of using a patent remedy (He Shou Wu, for hair thinning and loss).

HCV patients are contraindicated from using standard formulations designed for other conditions—avoid all standard formulations unless they are specifically designed for HCV. HCV+ status effectively means that this factor has to be taken into account when herbs are formulated.

Contacts in the U.S.

National Certification Commission for Acupuncture and Oriental Medicine: (202) 232-1404, www.nccaom.org

American Academy of Medical Acupuncture (MDs and DOs): (800) 521-2262

Clinics and practitioners with good reports from patients include the following:

Zhang's Clinic
420 Lexington Avenue, Suite 631
New York, New York 10170
Telephone: (212) 573 9584
Website: http://zhang-clinic.com

Dr. M. Smith
Lincoln Clinic
New York
(718) 993-3100

Dr. Dan Bensky
Seattle
(206) 524-2724

Dr. Brian McKenna
call the Seattle number

Dr. David Eissen
Portland Oregon
(503) 239-0888

Dr. Magnolia Goh
New York
(718) 672-2011

Dr. Yujun Shao
New York
(212) 481-3388; Fax: (212) 679-3267

Quan Yin Healing Arts Center
1748 Market Street
San Francisco, CA
Has a long-standing reputation.
(415) 861-4964. Email: qyhac@aol.com

American College of Traditional Chinese Medicine
(415) 282-9603

National Acupuncture and Tetoxification Association
Phone/fax: (360) 260-8621.
Email: AcuDetox@AOL.com

East West Herbs
http://www.eastwestherbs.com/

Contacts in the U.K.

There is a **Register of Chinese Herbal Medicine** in the U.K. that maintains a list of trained practitioners. If possible, consult a practitioner with experience of treating patients with hepatitis C. Contact them by writing to P.O. Box 400, Wembley, Middlesex, HA 9 9NZ or telephone: 0171 224 0803

The Gateway Clinic has extensive experience of treating hepatitis C with TCM and also offers free Qi Gong classes. Telephone: 44 (0)171 346 5400

Sino-European Clinics have a good reputation for offering an effective and professional service to HCV patients. Call 44 (0)1225 483393 (Bath Chinese Medicine Centre and Network HQ) for details.

John Tindall can be contacted at 44 (0)181 690 9145. He also has information on the Yuan Centre, a new TCM-based clinic being set up in London. The new clinic will work closely with conventional medical experts and researchers and also aim to facilitate clinical trials.

National Acupuncture and Detoxification Association (U.K.): 0171 820 9892

TCM Experiences

Emma

I first visited the TCM center in January. I had discussed the idea with my specialist, but he seemed very wary about using herbal medicine. Despite this I decided to try it, largely because one of my friends worked at the center and were able to explain the way TCM works. At that time my ALT levels were nearly 300.

Two months after the start of treatment my ALT levels had dropped down to 121 and my specialist's attitude to TCM became more positive, although he was still clearly not exactly delirious about it. By this time I was feeling a lot more confident about myself; the depression and lethargy seemed to have been cleared by the herbs and acupuncture. I feel a lot better and a lot more hopeful about the future now.

Alessandria (Acupuncture Only)

Alessandria is a doctor of medicine. She was diagnosed as having chronic NANB hepatitis with cirrhosis in 1985. Doctors at the hospital she attended did not give her long to live—they told her that her condition was terminal. One of her friends, also a doctor, offered her some acupuncture; he had been studying the subject for a few years. Resigned to dying she decided to try it anyway.

After a few weeks she started to feel much better; energy and liver function seemed to be restored. After a few months she was able to go back to work. She still gets regular acupuncture, quite easy for her since she married the acupuncturist who treated her. She has since had a baby and shows no signs of imminent death.

Max

Shortly after my diagnosis someone told me that they had found that the treatment they had received at the Gateway had made them feel much better. When I discovered that the "treatment" involved having pins stuck into her and drinking odious teas based on cocktails of weird plants, I began to think that she was mad. However, she persisted in telling me how much better she felt and eventually persuaded me to book an appointment.

Despite my skepticism I went through with the treatment. A few days into my second herbal prescription, when I was still wondering whether the Gateway was run by lunatics for lunatics, I began to feel a hell of a lot better. My need for siestas disappeared, I found that I could eat without indigestion, my liver stopped hurting, and my outlook on life seemed to change for the better. I even decided to try a Qi Gong class, which seemed to be the height of insanity, consisting of a group of people waving their arms about and making strange noises.

I am now deeply appreciative of the Gateway and TCM. I realize that I did not know how ill I was until I began to feel better. I was only able to identify the hep C symptoms after they were relieved. Now I wonder how I ever got through the years that I was symptomatic. I find it really frightening that I didn't realize that there was anything wrong with me during that time.

I still go back for checkups and keep up the Qi Gong. Some symptoms can reappear, though they are not nearly as bad as they were. By and large I am in good shape today. I can even eat chips if I want. I don't know how it works, and I don't really care. Conventional doctors think that it is "psychological"; they are entitled to that view, but I think that they are mistaken. I was a complete skeptic. It works.

John

John S. contracted HCV in 1983. His ALT levels were always high, liver biopsies revealed fibrosis and chronic active inflammation, and he was very tired. Interferon treatments had no effect on his illness. In 1995, after two months of herbal treatments (at Zhang's clinic), his liver enzyme levels normalized and his fatigue and liver pain were gone. Recently Mr. S. underwent surgery to remove a gallstone. During surgery it was discovered that the inflammation and fibrosis were considerably reduced.

Spencer

Spencer S. works for a pharmaceutical company that produces interferon, so he went through three courses of interferon before trying Chinese medicine. Within two months of taking the herbs his liver enzymes were normalized for the first time in twelve years and his overall health greatly improved.

Susan

When Susan P. was first diagnosed with HCV in 1996, she refused interferon and sought advice from Dr. Andrew Weill, who suggested she try Chinese medicine. When she began acupuncture and Chinese herbs in 1998, her ALT and AST normalized for the first time.

Linda

In July of 1996 I was diagnosed with HCV, stage IV, with the beginnings of cirrhosis. My ALT was 85, and my AST was 68. A PCR taken in August, 1997, revealed a viral load of 18 million. By early February 1998 my ALT shot up to 386 and my AST was 213, despite a vegetarian diet, weekly autohemotherapy, ozone treatments, and a multitude of supplements. Frankly, I was desperate.

I had persistent arthritic pain in my joints, flu symptoms, brain fog, diarrhea, and digestion problems. A friend recommended Traditional Chinese Medicine and gave me the name and phone number of Dr. Zhang. On February 6, 1998, I began weekly acupuncture treatments and taking a variety of herbs throughout the day. By April 9, 1998, my ALT went down to 49, my AST went down to 44, and all the negative symptoms associated with HCV disappeared. Currently, I have more energy than I've had in years, and I'm optimistic about living a long, healthy life.

A Preliminary Report into the Efficacy of TCM in the Treatment of Hepatitis C

Twenty-four patients undergoing TCM for HCV were asked to complete a questionnaire. All patients were receiving herbs. Some were receiving acupuncture as well.

Subjective Identification of Symptoms and the Degree to Which TCM Relieved Them

Patients were invited to identify their symptoms and mark the degree to which they were helped by TCM.

Chronic continuous fatigue:

- Twenty-two patients said they had this symptom.
- Before TCM twelve described this as "severe," ten described it as "noticeable."
- After TCM seven said they were completely free; eleven said they were partially better; four said TCM had made no difference.

Sudden attacks of fatigue:

- Seventeen patients reported this symptom.
- Nine described this as "severe"; eight described it as "noticeable."
- After TCM four said they were completely free; thirteen said that improvement was "partial."

Indigestion/bowel problems:

- Nineteen patients reported this symptom.
- Fourteen described symptoms as "severe"; five as "noticeable."
- After TCM three said they were completely free; fourteen said they were partially improved; two said they were worse.

Aching joints:

- Seventeen patients reported this symptom.

- Thirteen described symptoms as "noticeable"; four as "severe."

- After TCM three said symptom was completely cured; eleven said "partially" improved; three said "no difference."

Depression/Malaise:

- All patients reported this symptom.

- Ten described it as "severe"; fourteen as "noticeable."

- Three said treatment had resulted in complete disappearance; nineteen said TCM had resulted in a "noticeable" improvement; two reported "no difference."

Objective Indicators and TCM

Few patients were able to respond to this section. None were able to respond as fully as I would have liked. No one was able to provide b-DNA or PCR results for HCV.

Six patients were able to provide ALT/AST results for before TCM and during/after. All results demonstrated improvement. There were no cases of deterioration.

Before		During/After	
AST	ALT	AST	ALT
73	87	48	55
140		40	
85	89	35	23
160	163		87
	288		53
177	192	58	51

Because ALT and AST levels fluctuate in HCV patients, these results are not conclusive. Greater numbers of patient responses are needed, and a wider range of tests need to be carried out. However, the initial conclusion is clear—Chinese herbs can seriously benefit patient liver enzyme levels.

Side Effects

Nineteen patients reported no side effects. One patient reported slight nausea, although she was undergoing interferon therapy as well.

There were no cases of toxicity. Readers who are interested in this should note that the Gateway Clinic, where a number of these surveys were completed, prescribes thousands of herbal formulae every year and has never had a case of toxicity reported.

General Observations

1. TCM is safe when administered professionally.

2. TCM makes most patients feel better in several respects.

3. TCM may improve clinical indicators; there are not enough responses here to prove that beyond doubt.

It is noticeable that patients who are cirrhotic tend to take longer to respond to TCM, or don't respond so well overall. Patients with other severe illnesses such as pancreatitis or cryoglobulinemia also demonstrate less clear-cut responses. Patients who have recently stopped interferon treatment also seem to take longer to respond.

Some of the patients who completed this survey had only been receiving treatment for four weeks or so, and may not have begun to respond. Chinese herbs generally take a few weeks to start to make a difference.

Having talked to patients who have used TCM clinics other than the Gateway, it is apparent that not all practitioners have the same approach to hepatitis C patients. Some appear to prescribe large amounts of tonic herbs, such as ginseng, which may make patients feel better in the short term, but will usually fail to achieve longer-term success or favorable changes in clinical indicators.

A Note about This Report

This is a preliminary report only. A full double-blind placebo-controlled study of the application of TCM to hepatitis C patients has now been designed. However, it will cost around £500,000 or $800,000, if comprehensive qualitative and quantitative tests are to be included.

Contacts are listed on pages 266–267.

Further Reading

Chinese Herbal Materia Medica. Dan Bensky, Eastland Press.
Chinese Medicine. Tom Williams, Element Books.
The Web That Has No Weaver. Ted Kaptchik.
Chinese Herbal Medicine—Formulae and Strategies. Bensky and Barolet.
Synopsis of Prescriptions of the Golden Champer. Zhang Zhongjing, World Press.
Acupuncture—A Comprehensive Text. Bensky.
Treatment of Disease with Acupuncture. James Tin Yau So.
Handbook of Chinese Herbs. Him-che Yeung, Institute of Chinese Medicine.
Handbook of Chinese Herbal Formulas. Him-che Yeung, Institute of Chinese Medicine.
Clinical Applications of Ayurvedic and Chinese Herbs. Kerry Bone, Phytotherapy Press, Queensland, Australia.

References

1. Adverse events involving certain Chinese herbal medicines and the response of the profession. Blackwell R. *Journal of Chinese Medicine,* No 50, Jan 1996.

2. Chronic hepatitis induced by Jin Bu Huan. Picciotto A et al. *Journal of Hepatology,* 28:165–167, 1998.

3. Effects of Oriental medicine on general condition and liver function following surgery. *17th International Conference of Internal Medicine,* Kyoto, Japan, 1984.

4. *Clinical Applications of Ayurvedic and Chinese Herbs.* Bone K. Phytotherapy Press, Queensland, Australia, 1996.

5. *Pharmacology and Applications of Chinese Materia Medica.* Vol 2, World Scientific, Singapore.

6. Preliminary report of a randomized, double-blind placebo-controlled trial of a Chinese herbal medicine preparation CH-100 in the treatment of chronic hepatitis C. Batey RG et al. *Journal of Gastroenterology and Hepatology,* 13:244–247, 1998.

7. Herbal medicine sho-saiko-to (TJ-9) prevents liver fibrosis and enzyme-altered lesions in rat liver cirrhosis induced by a choline-deficient L-amino acid defined diet. Sakaida I et al. *Journal of Hepatology,* 28:298–306, 1998.

8. Effects of Japanese herbal medicine "sho-saiko-to" (TJ-9) on in vitro interleukin-10 production by peripheral blood mononuclear cells of patients with chronic hepatitis C. Yamashiki M et al. *Journal of Clinical Laboratory Immunology,* 37:111–21, 1992.

9. Pneumonitis induced by the herbal medicine sho-saiko-to in Japan. Sato A et al. *Nippon Kyobu Shikkan Gakkai Zasshi—Japanese Journal of Thoracic Diseases,* 35(4):391–5, Apr 1997.

10. The herbal medicine inchin-ko-to inhibits liver cell apoptosis induced by transforming growth factor b1. Yamamoto M et al. *Hepatology,* 23(3), 1996.

11. Effects of hepatic stimulator substance, herbal medicine, selenium/vitamin E and ciprofloxacin on cirrhosis in the rat. Manna Z et al. *Gastroenterology,* 110:1150–1155, 1996.

12. *The Complete System of Self Healing.* Chang ST. Tao Publishing, 1994.

13. *Encounters with Qi.* Eisenberg D. Jonathan Cape, pp 208, 1986.

14. Guolin research report. Dr. Pao Ling. 2,873 terminal cancer patients practiced Qi Gong: 12% were cured, 47% improved, 41% no improvement.

16

Western Herbal Medicine, Medicinal Mushrooms, and Hepatitis C

Thanks are due to José Luiz M. Garcia, a qualified expert in agronomy, horticulture, plant biochemistry, and physiology, for research and editing of this chapter.

Introduction

THIS CHAPTER DESCRIBES herbal medicines that have either been used by HCV patients or appear to be potentially useful. In this context the word "Western" means "non-Chinese and non-Ayurvedic"; listed herbs include those of European, African, and American origin. Some of these herbs have Chinese or Ayurvedic counterparts, while others are unique to themselves. Many are extremely powerful and have been used to good effect for centuries, particularly for clear-cut problems such as jaundice. However, their application to the more subtle symptoms of HCV will require careful reflection.

Western herbal medicine lacks the sophisticated diagnostic system of TCM, which has its own logical structure developed over millennia. This means that medicinal herbs are often prescribed on an ad hoc basis. Some herbalists are now using TCM diagnostic techniques to prescribe Western herbs and are developing formulae that are becoming increasingly subtle. Conventional wisdom is that TCM herbs should never be mixed with Western herbal medicine. However, it is now possible to consult herbalists who will make use of both pharmacopoeias.

In general, herbal treatments are too complex to be meaningfully analyzed for their pharmacologically active ingredients. When one considers that many formulations use between ten and forty separate ingredients, that some of these are subjected to heating, drying, or other processing, that they are then concocted or subject to further varied preparation, it becomes obvious that the biochemistry of these formulations is too complex for definitive biochemical analysis. Traditional medicine systems often adopt a logical "energetic" system for categorizing these medicines, and these can work well in matching symptoms to complex prescriptions, particularly when backed up by a large inventory of empirical clinical experience. Other systems regard particular plants as carrying certain "messages," or as having the ability to convey a particular ancestral energy, or as embodying an aspect of universal energy. Primitive as these constructs may sound, they are generally better able to handle complex medicinal entities than the reductionist chemistry-based systems of the pharmaceutical model. It is also interesting to note that the most advanced biological molecular modeling techniques used to design protease inhibitors are once again talking in terms of "messages" and classifying both pathogens and treatments in terms of communication.

It is important not to take treatments without informing your doctor, regardless of which tradition he or she belongs to. Some herbalists are not as talented or experienced as others; certain herbs can cause problems in some individuals. No medicine is 100% safe. If you have faith in their judgment, you should be able to discuss all aspects of your treatment and agree on a course of therapeutic action. There are very few valid reasons for them objecting to you using herbs; medical contraindications are listed.

There is a long history of antagonism between advocates of herbal medicine on the one hand and pharmaceutical interests and the allopathic medical establishment on the other. For instance, German pharmaceutical interests insisted on the dismantling of the herbal medicine system in occupied France during the Second World War. It is thought that this was a purely commercial move. Their modern successors spend large amounts of money on "public relations" and even donate large sums to patient support networks that are sympathetic to their products. Some reckon that this debate goes back to the sixteenth century, the time of Paracelsus.

Some members of the conventional medical system are extremely hostile to the idea of herbal therapy and will attempt to persuade patients that it is at best useless and at worst dangerous. Various bodies with connections to the allopathic medical establishment regularly feed "scare stories" to the press concerning both Eastern and Western herbal medicine. Closer examination often reveals that these reports are misleading and merely part of an ongoing propaganda war, which has been being waged for centuries. Conversely there are those who believe that all modern patented drugs are inherently toxic, and that modern pharmaceutical medicine makes more people sick than well. Thus the debate proceeds; the important thing is for people living with hepatitis C not to get too agitated by such scare stories; if there is a relevant report, then it is important to read the text carefully and to check the source of the information—establish whether or not the assertions can be factually substantiated, or if the story has been taken out of context.

Methods of Taking Herbs

There are many ways of administering herbs. The following are the most likely methods to be prescribed for HCV patients.

Infusion simply means pouring boiling water over the herbs, waiting for ten minutes or so, straining off the liquid, and drinking it. Infusion is suitable for delicate leaf herbs.

Decoction is the process of simmering herbs for longer periods of time. Typically herbs should be put in a ceramic or stainless steel pot with a liter or so of filtered water, covered, and simmered for an hour. The resulting liquid should then be strained off and stored in a nonmetallic container. The process should be repeated twice, first with 0.75 liter of water for forty-five minutes, and then with 0.5 liter of water for thirty minutes. The decoction should be refrigerated. These quantities make enough for 8 standard cups of decocted herb tea. Doses should be slightly heated before use. They are usually best taken immediately prior to mealtimes. Decoction is suitable for robust herbs, such as roots and barks.

Gelatin capsules are often used to deliver herbs that are only required in small quantities or taste unpleasant. The herbs are pow-dered and tipped into the capsules. Vegicaps are vegetarian alterna-tives to the beef-based gelatin and are also easily digested.

Tinctures are concentrated extracts of herbs, usually suspended in alcohol, which may make them unsuitable for some HCV patients.

Most herbs or preparations thereof are best taken before meals.

Treatment Duration and Content

If Western herbal medicine is your primary chosen means of treat-ment, it is vital that you consult an experienced herbalist in order to obtain a long-term dynamic treatment strategy. Some herbs need only be taken for short periods, others over many months, and a few are best administered in bursts. A good herbalist will be able to mon-itor your progress and prescribe accordingly.

In general, a chronic condition such as HCV will require ongo-ing treatment. However, some of the symptoms may be cleared quite quickly, enabling the herbs to be adjusted to concentrate on the underlying condition. Usually herbalists will recommend breaks in the regime, typically one day a week or one month off after two months on.

Herbal Properties That May Be Pertinent to Hepatitis C Treatment

- Antacids are used to address overacid pH in stomach and intestines.
- Anthelmintic herbs aim to kill or eliminate parasites living in the gut.
- Antibiotics, in the herbal context, kill off bacteria and amoeba.
- Antipyretics are cooling herbs that prevent or reduce fevers.
- Antispasmodics stop muscle spasms and promote physical relax-ation.
- Antivirals kill or inhibit viruses.
- Astringents are substances that counter bleeding and swelling; they bind and constrict.

- Bitters increase the flow of gastric juices and promote hunger. Active herbs are often bitter, as the name suggests, and are useful to counteract wasting, often found in chronic liver disorders.

- Blood-purifying herbs or alteratives aim to remove toxins and neutralize acids in the blood. They are often powerful antivirals with immune-boosting properties.

- Carminatives help to relieve gas and pain in the bowels.

- Cholagogues promote the production and flow of bile; they do this by stimulating the gallbladder to contract and are important in addressing the liver/digestive aspects of HCV.

- Choleretics stimulate the secretion of bile by the liver as opposed to bile release by the gallbladder. Choleretics typically will decrease cholesterol levels since they reduce its synthesis by the liver and increase its excretion.

- Demulcents soothe and protect damaged tissue; often taken internally and used to address intestinal problems in HCV.

- Diaphoretics induce sweating, a means of toxin elimination and heat loss.

- Diuretic herbs promote the draining of excess bodily fluids via the kidneys in urine and are thus useful for fluid retention, common in cirrhotic patients. It is often argued that herbal diuretics are healthier than their pharmaceutical counterparts because they contain high doses of minerals that may otherwise be depleted.

- Emetics induce vomiting.

- Emmenagogues promote menstruation. Some liver herbs have this property and need to be used with care with female patients who may be pregnant.

- Laxatives promote bowel movement.

- Parasiticides destroy parasites in the digestive tract and skin.

- Rubefacients increase surface blood flow.

- Sialgogues stimulate flow of saliva and aid digestion.

- Stimulants increase the energy of the body, having a warming effect.

- Tonic herbs stimulate and support particular organs in their day-to-day functioning. They usually achieve this by providing large quantities of essential nutrients and enhancing the ability of these organs to assimilate these vital substances. Many of the herbs listed below are liver tonics although some apply to other organs as well. It is worth remembering that HCV does affect other parts of the body apart from the liver.

- Vulneraries encourage the healing of wounds by promoting cell growth.

Prescribing Herbs: Toxicity and Safety Issues

HCV+ status means that patients are more vulnerable to a range of undesirable side effects, modified action, or toxicity relating to the use of herbs. It is therefore very important to consult an experienced practitioner. Positive results are more likely if you do this in any case. It is unwise to self-prescribe, although some of these herbs, such as milk thistle seeds, are very hard to go wrong with. If you do decide to treat yourself, it is essential to check out contraindications before going ahead; this is particularly important if you are pregnant. Hepatitis C is associated with increased frequency of a range of conditions such as diabetes, which can have serious implications for the safety of herbal medicine. Patients should check with a herbalist. It is also strongly suggested that you use only one herb at a time if you are self-prescribing.

There are some herbs that are more likely to be unsuitable for HCV+ people. Examples include the following:

- Asfetida
- Comfrey root
- Germander *(Teucrium chamaedrys)*
- Gordolobo yerba tea
- Hops
- Kava kava (long-term, seek advice)

- Margosa oil
- Maté tea
- Mistletoe
- Pennyroyal
- Valerian
- Yohimbe

Germander has been reported to have caused outbreaks of hepatitis in France, where it was used as an adjunct in a slimming regime. Skullcap has also occasionally been found to have been adulterated with this herb.

This is not a comprehensive list, and contraindications will vary from one patient to another. Do take care and consult practitioners. Refer to toxicity references,[1] and the section "Safety, Toxicity, Quality Control, and Other Considerations" in chapter 15.

Prescribing herbs correctly requires skill and experience. Even experienced herbalists avoid prescribing herbs for themselves. It is therefore not a good idea for patients to go out and buy a selection of the herbs listed below and take them at will. Herbs can have unpredictable effects, particularly if taken in combination. It is important to consult a practitioner for formulae to suit you.

If you have a clear-cut medical condition, like Crohn's disease, and you haven't got access to a herbalist, then you may choose to try a single herb treatment; be aware that hepatitis C makes you more vulnerable to the possibility of unpredictable side effects. If you suspect that anything is wrong, then stop taking the herb immediately and seek medical advice. Many patients use herbs like milk thistle (silymarin) without consulting herbalists—this may be safe for short periods, but is inadvisable over the long term.

For a list of qualified medical herbalists in the U.K. write to: The National Institute of Medical Herbalists, 56 Longbrook Street, Exeter, Devon EX4 6AH. Enclose an A5 stamped addressed envelope.

In the U.S. contact the American Herbalists Guild, Box 1127W, Forestville, CA 95436.

A Selection of Herbs Commonly Used to Treat HCV and Related Conditions

Aloe Vera *[Aloeaceae]*
Liver, heart, spleen
Vulnerary, cholagogue, laxative
Important healer of skin and gut mucosa, by virtue of its enzyme-promoting properties. The gel can be consumed and has a detoxifying, antiviral, and immune-enhancing effect. The dried powder can also be taken—in this form it is a good laxative and liver decongestant.

Artemisia [Common Wormwood, Green Ginger; *Artemisia absinthium*]
Liver, gallbladder, digestive system
Bitter, anthelmintic, cholagogue, parasitic, anti-inflammatory
Used in acute hepatitis as a parasite killer, it may be more useful in chronic hepatitis for clearing the digestive tract of putrefactive bacteria and fungi. Also used as an organic pesticide and for malaria, it destroys the outer coat of many microorganisms. Taken by infusion or powder in capsules, in conjunction with plain rice or bean diet. Some herbalists recommend taking breaks from this herb if on long-term treatment. See the "Herbs" section of chapter 15 for more information.

Artichoke *[Cynara scolymus]*
Liver, gallbladder, kidneys
Cholagogue, diuretic, stimulates liver cell regeneration
Useful to address combination of liver and kidney disease common in HCV patients. It is often used in cases of diabetes mellitus and cirrhosis, both of which may be linked to HCV. Up to 4 g of dried leaves, stem, or root can be taken three times per day. Typical dry extract dosage would be 250 mg three times per day.

Astralagus [Huang Chi; *Astralagus membranaceus; Leguminosae*]
Spleen, kidneys, lungs, blood
Stimulant, immune stimulant, diuretic, tonic

This herb is commonly used in Chinese herbal medicine, where it is often used to prepare medicinal soups to increase energy and resistance to disease; it may be useful to patients who are feeling run down. The roots are used; they may be powdered and eaten directly, or simply added to herbal decoctions or soups. This herb is also a selenium accumulator. See the "Herbs" section of chapter 15.

Baical Skullcap [Huang Qin; *Radix scutellariae baicalensis*]
Gallbladder, large intestine, lung, stomach
Sedative, nervine, antispasmodic
Commonly used in Chinese medicine and also popular with Western herbalists. Prescribed to promote calmness, countering "liverish" behavior, and in helping withdrawal. See the "Herbs" section of chapter 15.

Barberry [Pipperidge Bush; *Berberis vulgaris*]
Liver, gallbladder, digestive system
Cholagogue, stimulating digestive and immune tonic
Useful in debilitated conditions associated with HCV. It stimulates blood supply to the spleen and activates phagocytosis.[2] Contraindicated if pregnant. The powdered bark is used, dried and powdered, three times per day.

Black Cohosh [Black Snake Root, Bugbane; *Cimicufuga racemosa*]
Liver, spleen, stomach
Astringent, emmenagogue, diaphoretic, diuretic
A native of North America, where it is used as an antidote to poisonous snake bites. Useful for female patients with irregular menses, those suffering from anxiety, and it may help to relieve arthritis in combination with angelica, prickly ash, and guiacum. It should be used in low concentrations, infused or decocted. Contraindicated if pregnant. Must only be used with professional guidance.

Black Root *[Leptandra virginica]*
Liver, spleen, gallbladder
Cholagogue, hepatic, laxative, diaphoretic, antispasmodic
A relaxing liver tonic with a range of applications in liver dis-

ease. It contains volatile oil with esters of cinnamic acid, ethoxycinnamic acid, and dimethoxycinnamic acid. Often used where there is liver-disease-associated constipation.

Blessed Thistle [Holy Thistle; *Cnicus benedictus*]
Liver, spleen, stomach
Liver tonic, alterative, bitter, homeostatic, appetite stimulant

A native of Southern Europe, where it has been cultivated for centuries. It is prescribed to relieve acute hepatitis, dyspepsia, fever, and jaundice. In high doses it is emetic (causes vomiting) and emmenagogue (promotes menstruation). It should be used in low concentrations, infused or decocted. It is best avoided by pregnant women or those who wish to become so. It is often combined with milk thistle.

Boldo *[Peumus boldus]*
Liver, gallbladder
Cholagogue, hepatic, diuretic

A traditional medicinal plant from Chile, boldo is commonly prescribed to treat gallbladder disease and in cases of liver toxicity. It has been shown to have hepatoprotective, choleretic, and anti-inflammatory effects in mice and rats.

The dried leaves are simply infused with boiling water. This herb is sometimes combined with fringe tree bark.

Bupleurum [Chai Hu, Thorough Wax; *Bupleurum chinense; Umbelliferae*]
Liver, gallbladder, pericardium
Antipyretic, alterative, analgesic

One of the best liver detoxifiers, and an important ingredient in many Chinese formulae for liver diseases. This is a strong herb and may cause nausea in some patients—it is best to consult a herbalist and to take small amounts to begin with. It seems to help to build up muscle tone, as well as being a powerful method of restoring normal liver function. Patients who have recently stopped drinking, taking drugs, or are coming off medication may find this herb particularly helpful. The root is used; it may be taken powdered (2–5 g) at a time, or decocted. See the "Herbs" section of chapter 15.

Burdock Root [Lappa, Fox's clote, Beggars Buttons; *Arctium lappa*]
Lungs, stomach, kidney, liver
Alterative, diuretic, diaphoretic, and nutritive

A native of Europe and common in Britain this herb is a relative of the thistle. It is a highly rated blood purifier and liver cleanser, considered to be in the same class as sarsaparilla. As well as providing nutrients valuable to the liver, it also benefits the kidneys. Japanese researchers believe that it has anticarcinogenic properties.[3] It is used to treat arthritis and rheumatism, as well as liver disease, and is very suitable for patients with these complications. It needs to be decocted. Practitioners usually stipulate starting with a low dose and building up slowly.

Californian Buckthorn [Sacred Bark, Chittem Bark; *Cascara sagrada, Rhamnus purshiane; Rhamnaceae*]
Colon, spleen, stomach, liver
Laxative, emmenagogue, nervine, emetic, and a bitter tonic

A native of North America, it is related to buckthorn species found in Europe but regarded as a more suitable variety for medicinal use. It is good for stimulating the entire digestive system and promoting the flow of bile; it benefits the spleen and the pancreas and is often used to treat constipation as well as liver congestion. The bark is the active part of the plant, and it should have been dried and aged for at least a year before use. The herb can be powdered and taken directly, mixed with honey, or infused (¼ teaspoon once per day is sufficient).

Cats Claw *[Uncaria tomentosa]*
Colon, immune system
Antioxidant, antimutagen, anti-inflammatory

Difficult to obtain loose, its properties are similar to the Chinese herb Bai Hua She She Cao. Solgar herbal range includes this herb. Not to be confused with *Uncaria guianensis*. Particularly suitable for patients with Crohn's disease, colitis, or irritable bowel syndrome.

European research suggests that it activates phagocytes, can reduce levels of precancerous indicators, and exerts an antileukemic action without adverse consequences for bone marrow.

Celandine (Greater) [Garden Celandine; *Chelidonium majus; Papaveraceae*]
Liver, colon
Alterative, diuretic, cholagogue, purgative, and antispasmodic

Common in Europe, this herb has a long history of medicinal application, notably for acute liver disease such as jaundice. It detoxifies the liver and is a blood purifier. It is also used as a cancer treatment (notably in Russia) and for bronchitis and asthma (notably in China). It contains a number of substances that are likely to help patients such as choline, saponins, and vitamin C. The juice of the leaves is sometimes used externally for eye problems, and the root is sometimes prescribed for toothache. The leaves contain the ingredients that will benefit HCV patients. They are infused or juiced to make a cordial.

Chaparral *[Larrea tridentata; Zygophyllaceae]*
Kidneys, lungs, liver
Alterative, antibiotic, anticarcinogenic, expectorant, diuretic

Regarded as one of the best herbal antivirals, it is a common ingredient in many herbalists' prescriptions for rheumatic pains, cancer, arthritis, flu, diarrhea, and urinary tract infections. It is also highly regarded as a deep detoxification agent by some practitioners, particularly for addressing residues from long-term drug use.

It is taken as an infusion three times per day. However, this herb may also aggravate hepatitis in some patients and should therefore only be used under close medical supervision.

Dandelion *[Taraxacum officinale; Compositae]*
Liver, spleen, stomach, kidney, bladder
Alterative, cholagogue, diuretic, stomachic, aperient, tonic

This is an inexpensive and useful herb. Root and leaves are commonly prescribed. The root contains many nutrients that help the liver, particularly in its blood purification processes. It also helps the spleen, pancreas, gallbladder, and kidneys, all of whose function can be reduced by HCV. It helps to boost digestion, assimilation, and elimination. It can help with blood sugar disorders. The root is often used to help the liver detoxify and may be more effective than silymarin for early treatment. Coffee, which is regarded as unhealthy for HCV patients, can be replaced by dandelion root coffee. The root should be decocted and may be taken up to six times per day.

The leaves can be infused to make a really effective diuretic. For patients suffering from fluid retention or poor elimination, this is a very useful herb. It is best drunk during the morning or early afternoon, since the diuretic effect would be disruptive if taken late at night, causing nocturnal urination, a symptom in some HCV patients.

Desmodium *[Desmodium ascendens; Papillonaceae]*
Liver
Hepatoprotective, antihepatotoxic, antiallergic, anti-inflammatory

This herb is found in the equatorial forests of Africa. The stems and leaves are used to treat jaundice and general weakness. It is thought to regenerate and protect hepatocytes and prevent lysis. It may help to prevent cirrhosis and normalize ALT.

Echinacea [Snakeroot, Purple Coneflower; *Echinacea angustifolia, E. purpurea*]
Lungs, stomach, liver
Immune tonic, antiinfective, stimulating alterative

Thought to stimulate the production of interferons and other substances associated with immune response, it might help to counter HCV at some level, although no research has been carried out. It is normally used to treat acute inflammation and/or infection, as a natural antibiotic. Mouthwash may help to alleviate oral symptoms of HCV. It is also used for cancer, and its efficacy in the treatment of HIV is being investigated. Some herbalists think that its effectiveness may decline if used persistently; if this is so, then it may not be so useful for long-term antiviral treatment of HCV. There are two species: *E. purpurea* is sometimes favored as an antiviral; *E. angustifolia* as an immune stimulant.

Echinacea is also thought to inhibit the activity of the enzyme hyaluronidase, serum levels of which are thought by Japanese researchers to be linked with fibrosis.

It is important to get this herb as fresh as possible; it can be infused or taken in dried, powdered form, every two hours or so for acute conditions and twice a day for chronic illnesses.

Elder Flowers [Sambucus nigra, S. canadensis; Caprifoliaceae]
Lungs, liver
Diaphoretic, alterative, stimulant

A useful, safe, and tasty herb for treating chronic flulike symptoms of HCV. Can be blended with hibiscus flowers, rosehip, and dandelion leaf (if a diuretic effect is desired) to make a really tasty antiflu infusion. Contains a lot of vitamin C.

Espinheira Santa [Maytenus ilicifolia]

Used in Brazil, where studies have supported claims of benefit to stomach ulcers and stomach cancer inhibition. Also used to soothe gastric discomfort.

Euphorbia [Phyllanthus; Euphorbiaceae subspecies amara and niruri]
Lungs, liver, kidneys, stomach
Astringent, diuretic, antiviral, stomachic, cholagogue, laxative, bitter tonic

Caution—can be toxic, although these reports may be confused by the fact that there are many different varieties and only the correct part of the plant should be consumed. Traditionally used in North Africa and Asia Minor for a number of conditions, this plant has been researched for use in clearing hepatitis A and B markers. The niruri variety has also been used to treat hepatitis C with good results in Brazil, according to one patient. In India the fresh roots are prescribed for jaundice. The leaves and resin are used externally—internal use is hazardous. A professional herbalist must be consulted prior to using this herb. See chapter 17 for further information on Phyllanthus (pages 324–325).

Fenugreek [Trigonella foenum-graecum; Leguminosae]
Colon, pancreas, stomach
Demulcent, digestive tonic, hypoglycemic, anti-inflammatory

Useful for patients with inflamed digestive tracts and or blood sugar problems. Simply take a teaspoonful of the seeds before meals washed down with a glass of water. Continue for two weeks on followed by a break of two weeks; repeat for as long as necessary. It may help to balance appetite.

Fringe Tree Root Bark *[Cortex radicus chionanthi; Chionanthus virginicus]*
Liver, gallbladder, stomach, spleen, pancreas
Bitter, astringent, diuretic, cold
Prescribed by herbalists for jaundice, cirrhosis, and fibrosis, this is a useful and safe plant. Properties are described as breaking up obstruction, promoting bowel movement, removing stagnancy, stimulating and dredging the liver and gallbladder, and clearing heat.

Indicators include pain in the flank or a sensation of fullness, fatigue, greyish dry stool, and constipation. These are quite common in hepatitis C patients. This herb may also help digestion and promote elimination through stool and urine, and have a cleansing effect.

Garlic *[Allium sativum; Liliaceae]*
Affects all systems
Alterative, stimulant, diaphoretic, expectorant, antispasmodic, antibiotic, nervine, carminative, vulnerary
Used to treat parasitic infections of the gut, lung problems, low blood pressure, infections, headaches, nervous disorders, heart disease, arteriosclerosis, colds, flu, high blood cholesterol, thrombosis. Also used externally to clear infections and promote healing. Some of these are part of the wider pattern of HCV symptoms. Patients with gut problems may benefit from garlic's ability to destroy malign pathogens in the gut, while not killing benign bacteria. It is best taken raw because cooking will destroy the active ingredients, especially the volatile oils. Contains germanium, an important mineral thought to stimulate immune response. It is often prescribed along with other alteratives and blood cleansers such as echinacea and dandelion root, in order to amplify the antiviral effect.

Gentian Root [Yellow Gentian; *Gentiana lutea; Gentianaceae*]
Colon, stomach, gallbladder
Bitter, digestive tonic, anti-inflammatory

Used to treat digestive problems, it may appeal to patients with stubborn gut problems and clinical conditions such as Crohn's disease and colitis. It stimulates bile production, aiding digestion of fats and soothes inflammation in the colon. The dried root and rhizome is taken three times per day. Some patients may be contraindicated—consult a practitioner before use.

Ginger Root *[Zingiber officinale; Zingiberaceae]* **and Galanga [Galangal, Chinese Ginger, Colic Root;** *Alpinia officinarium; Zingiberaceae]*
Stomach, colon, circulation system
Circulatory stimulant, vasodilator, diaphoretic, expectorant, pulmonary antiseptic
These herbs benefit the stomach, intestines, and the circulation and are also used to treat colds, flu, cramps, and nausea. Some dieticians suggest that ginger should be added to meat dishes in order to detoxify the flesh—it has now been established that this herb contains a potent digestive enzyme that is thought to act in a similar manner as papain, found in papaya. This herb is warming and may not mix very well with TCM treatment aimed at draining off heat and promoting cool, moist Yin energy. It can be eaten with food as a matter of course. If it is required for a particular acute symptom such as flu or sudden indigestion, it can be infused—use 1 oz or 28 g of ginger simmered for ten minutes in half a liter of water.

Gingko Leaf [Ginkgo Nut, Maidenhair Tree, Gingko Biloba; *Gingkoaceae]*
Circulation, brain, lungs, kidneys
Vasoactive
Claims made for the mental benefits of this herb have attracted a lot of attention. It is prescribed by herbalists for the treatment and prevention of Alzheimer's and senile dementia, and is primarily aimed at elderly people. However, some of its qualities may interest HCV patients. Those suffering from impaired concentration and other symptoms of cognitive dysfunction may benefit from gingko. It may also be beneficial to patients with other conditions related to poor peripheral circulation—Raynaud's syndrome affects a number of

HCV patients, and this may be helped. Gingko has to be taken for at least three months before benefits are felt. It can be taken as infused leaves; there are also a number of preparations on the market.

Caution: Gingko is a good example of a generally beneficial plant that might cause problems in hepatitis C patients. It is a strong inhibitor of platelets and has been associated with increased bleeding times and spontaneous hemorrhage, particularly in the brain. Additional risk factors for hemorrhage include some symptoms associated with hepatitis C—diabetes and hypertension. See toxicity references.[8]

Ginseng, American [Five Fingers; *Panax quinquefolium; Araliaceae*] and Ginseng, Siberian [Touch-Me-Not, Devil's Bush; *Eleutherococcus senticosus; Araliaceae*]
All body systems
Adaptogen, tonic—different types of ginseng benefit different systems, stamina booster, vasoactive

A part of the Chinese pharmacopoeia for millennia, the properties of this group of herbs are now widely accepted in the West. Both types of ginseng are classified as adaptogens, which means that they may be able to help the body to adapt in whatever way is necessary to deal with whatever stress it is currently facing. For instance, if HCV is creating particular problems in the liver for one patient, but is causing greater dysfunction in the digestive system in another, ginseng might be able to help both patients to respond effectively to the differing pattern of disease.

These adaptogenic qualities may be linked to the presence of a hormonelike substance in these plants.

The American variety is the most expensive and probably the most suitable for HCV patients; it is regarded as a Yin tonic and would be used to build up inner strength and organ tone. It would be used to strengthen debilitated patients and might be expected to benefit the digestive system in particular. It stimulates the production of digestive enzymes and helps to normalize the appetite.

Siberian ginseng is less expensive and is now included in many immune tonic formulae. It increases resistance and is a vasodilator. In both cases the root is used either powdered, decocted, or infused by simmering for at least ten minutes.

Note: Patients should note that the most widely available ginseng, Asian or Korean (Latin name *Panax ginseng*), is regarded as being generally unsuitable for HCV patients with classic symptoms of heat and inflammation on account of its warming, Yang stimulant properties. It may well exacerbate such symptoms.

Golden Seal [Puccoon Root, Yellowroot; *Hydrastis canadensis; Ranunculaceae*]
Colon, liver, stomach, heart
Alterative, anti-inflammatory, bitter tonic, aperient, homoeostatic, astringent

This herb is often prescribed for gastric disorders associated with hepatitis. It is a powerful antibiotic—it cleans the gut walls. However, it may kill benign bacteria as well as pathogens. It can also be used externally. It is contraindicated in pregnancy. It tastes extremely bitter and is quite expensive. It can be infused or taken powdered, ¼ teaspoon at a time. This plant is under threat of extinction due to overexploitation; therefore try to use only plants grown under sustainable techniques.

Licorice [Gan T'sao; *Glycyrrhiza glabra; Leguminosae*]
All systems, especially the liver
Expectorant, alterative, demulcent, laxative

The root is commonly used to balance herbal formulae and to treat flu, gastric ulcers, liver disease, and chronic fatigue syndrome due to its ability to improve cortisol utilization. It is contraindicated for patients with fluid retention. It is sometimes used to treat patients who have recently undergone steroid therapy; it may help to boost glycogen storage in the liver, and hence increase stamina. Bilirubin levels may rise. May be taken dried or powdered, or decocted.

This plant has attracted much attention in Japan and among the HIV community on account of antiviral properties. It forms the basis of the medicine SNMC, featured in chapter 14, page 216, which appears to slow advanced liver disease progression.

Milk Thistle Seeds [St-Mary's-Thistle; *Silybum marianum, Carduus marianus; Compositae*]

Liver, spleen

Hepatoprotective, bitter tonic, demulcent, antidepressant

Many patients are aware of this herb and its properties. It contains some of the most potent liver-protective substances known as well as exerting a powerful antioxidant effect. The main active ingredient is silymarin, which is a mixture of the flavanoids silibinin, isosilibin, silidianin, and silicristine. These substances block the formation of leukotrenes, which damage liver cells, stimulate cell synthesis, and protect against hepatotoxins such as carbon tetrachloride. It is also thought to help to prevent glutathione deficiency in liver cells. It is known to positively influence the course of chronic hepatitis, even where patients already have cirrhosis.[4]

It has been used successfully to treat patients suffering from acute mushroom poisoning. It has been shown to prevent liver failure when subjects are exposed to otherwise fatal substances. Along with NAC, lipoic acid, and vitamin C, it has been used in high doses to try to affect liver regeneration; lower doses are commonly used to try to arrest liver disease progression. It also reduces fat deposits in the liver. It can be purchased in the form of silymarin. Legalon is a well-known brand of milk thistle extract. If preparing at home, note that the seeds need to be broken down with pestle and mortar or a blunt instrument before they can be decocted. (1–4 g of dried seeds or equivalent to be taken three times per day). A few patients have complained of skin rashes developing after prolonged use.

There is a useful review of milk thistle in *The American Journal of Gastroenterology,* Flora K, 93(2):139–143, 1998. This report summarizes liver studies that have shown protection against genomic injury, increased protein synthesis, decrease of tumor promoters, stabilization of mast cells, and increased iron chelation. Additional references for the use of silymarin are listed at the end of this chapter.[5]

Oregon Grape Root *[Mahonia aquifolium, M. repens; Berberidaceae]*

Liver, gallbladder

Cholagogue, alterative, anti-inflammatory

This is a popular herb for treating both chronic hepatitis and associated conditions such as arthritis and bowel problems. It is also used to treat cancer, along with other powerful alteratives such as red clover, echinacea, chaparral, pau d'arco, cascara, ginseng, and astralagus. For hepatitis it is often combined with dandelion root. It is regarded as a cooling herb. It may be infused, decocted or taken powdered (0.5–2 g, three times per day).

Pau D'Arco [Tabebuia, Lapacho, Ipe Roxo; *Tabebuia avellanedae; Bignoniaceae*]
Blood, liver, lungs
Alterative, antifungal, hypotensive, antidiabetic, bitter tonic, digestive, antibacterial, anticarcinogenic, immune-stimulant, anti-inflammatory

Hailed as a "wonder herb," this plant is from South America. It has attracted a lot of attention, particularly from those seeking cancer treatments. Apart from this HCV patients may value its immune-boosting and digestive tonic qualities. It may also be used to treat autoimmune diseases. The shredded inner bark is the active ingredient. Infused tea should be drunk 3–4 times per day.

Peony Root [Shao Yao; *Paeonia lactiflora; Ranunculaceae*]
Liver, blood, uterus, skin
Alterative, hepatic tonic, antispasmodic

This is a popular liver tonic and blood purifier. It is often prescribed for women on account of its beneficial influence on PMS. Although it is most popular in TCM, it is grown in the U.K. on an island called Steep Holmes in the Severn estuary. The root can be decocted or dried and powdered. See the "Herbs" section in chapter 15.

Picao Preto *[Bidens pilosus]*
Used to treat hepatitis in Brazil.

Pokeweed Root *[Phytolacca Americana; Phytolaccaeae]*
Lung, spleen, kidneys
Alterative, antirheumatic, anti-inflammatory, emetic, cathartic

Controversial herb on account of claims and counterclaims about its efficacy in cancer detection and treatment—some believe that it stimulates production of a number of immune-related substances that counter tumors and correct cancerous growth; others say that it can cause serious illness.

It is traditionally used to treat inflammatory autoimmune conditions such as rheumatoid arthritis. Some people do have adverse reactions to this herb—it should only be taken on the advice of an experienced herbalist and should be started in small doses.

Psyllium Seeds *[Plantago ovata, P. psyllium; Plantaginaceae]*
Colon, spleen, stomach
Lubricating laxative, anti-inflammatory, demulcent, healing

Prescribed for dry constipation, inflammation in the colon, and intestinal putrefaction, they may appeal to patients with this pattern of symptoms. The husks must be included in the decoction. Take 1 teaspoon each evening or use one of the many preparations on the market.

Sarsaparilla *[Sarsaparilla officinalis, Smilax officinalis; Liliaceae]*
Liver, stomach, kidneys
Alterative, heat clearing, anti-inflammatory, antipruritic, diaphoretic, tonic

Used to treat eruptive skin disorders, hepatitis and gout, it has been shown to contain substances known as saponins that bind with endotoxins, allowing them to be eliminated. It is regarded as a useful but gentle liver cleanser (1–4 g of dried root is taken three times per day).

Slippery Elm [Red Elm; *Ulmus rubra; Ulmaceae]*
Lungs and stomach
Nutritive demulcent, expectorant, vulnerary

Often prescribed for patients with bowel inflammation, ulcers, diarrhea, and constipation. It is used to make a gruel, along with honey and ginseng, that is given to severely debilitated patients, particularly those who are suffering from nausea. The inner bark is the active part of the plant; it is infused.

St. John's Wort [*Hypericum perforatum; Hypericaceae*]
Immune system, kidneys
Antiviral, antiretroviral, antidepressant, diuretic, antineoplastic

This herb is of particular interest on account of its antiviral and antidepressant qualities.

Scientifically shown to demonstrate broad-range activity against enveloped viruses. It is thought to interfere with the assembly of viral components by infected cells, therefore inhibiting the development of mature virions. In the case of HCV it is thought to interfere with virus uncoating during cell invasion.

Work in Germany (led by Dr. Anne Steinbeck-Klose) and in Israel (led by Dr. Gad Lavie) has investigated HCV antiviral action of a concentrated extract from St. John's wort called hypericum. Sixteen out of nineteen hypericum-treated patients were found to have achieved significant reductions in circulating HCV RNA after twenty-two months of study. Three converted to PCR negative and remained that way for four- to six-month follow-up.[6] Dosage was equivalent to an average of 0.05 mg per kg of body weight. There were no side effects, although these have been observed at much higher doses (photosensitivity and mental conditions).

Antidepressant qualities and action are controversial. However, it should be noted that hypericum has overtaken Prozac as the best selling antidepressant in Germany. Hepatitis C patients with depression seeking to minimize exposure to possible hepatic disease cofactors found in many antidepressants might wish to consider this approach. It has been suggested that the antidepressant effect is achieved through MAO inhibition. If this is the case, then patients with signs of liver toxicity should avoid it until this has been resolved.

It also reduces fluid retention and has some remarkable photo-reactive qualities that may be of use in cancer diagnosis and treatment by laser.

Suma [Para Toda, Brazilian Ginseng; *Pfaffia paniculata; Amaranthaceae*]
Spleen, pancreas, lung
Energy tonic, demulcent, nutrient, adaptogen

Para todo means "for everything" in Brazil, where this plant is highly regarded. Michael Tierra, author of *The Way of Herbs,* is very enthusiastic about the benefits of this South American herb for patients with chronic fatigue or low energy. Since this is a primary symptom of HCV, it may prove useful. It is difficult to obtain in Europe. (3–6 g of the root should be taken three times per day until symptoms subside or disappear.) It is rich in germanium, a rare mineral, thought to be medicinally valuable by Japanese researchers.

Wild Yam [Colicroot, Rheumatism Root; *Dioscorea villosa; Dioscoreaceae*]

Liver, gallbladder, kidneys, spleen-pancreas
Antispasmodic, anti-inflammatory, cholagogue, diaphoretic, expectorant

Often used to make medicinal soups along with other robust herbs such as astralagus, it is prescribed to patients with chronic hepatitis and associated flatulence, intestinal cramps, rheumatoid arthritis, and gallstones. It is often combined with oregon grape root. The root is decocted or dried and powdered.

Yellow Dock [Curly Dock; *Rumex crispus; Polygonaceae*]

Liver, colon
Cholagogue, alterative, mild laxative, blood tonic

One of the more powerful Western liver herbs, it is often included in strategy for treatment of chronic liver disease. Properties ascribed to this herb include decongesting the liver, reducing inflammation, cleaning the blood, and increasing bile flow. It is often combined with burdock and sarsaparilla. The root should be thoroughly decocted.

A Note about Availability

Most of the above herbs will be available from quality herbalists. However, some of the South American species are difficult to locate. If you have difficulties, call Naturatech in Sao Paulo, Brazil: telephone 55 (0)11 228 0955; fax 55 (0)11 229 1463.

Medicinal Mushrooms

There are a number of mushrooms and fungi with notable medicinal properties that may be of use in treating conditions linked to hepatitis C. Classical knowledge and modern medicinal research yields information that may inform their application; because these plants and extracts thereof can be very powerful, relevant practitioners should be consulted prior to usage. Some mushrooms, such as Fu Ling, the useful diuretic, are covered elsewhere in the book.

Maitake *[Grifola frondosa]*
Thought to be anticarcinogenic and immunomodulating.

Maitake is available in tablets, powder, and sometimes in its natural form; it may be used as a culinary ingredient.

Some cases of allergic reaction have been reported.

Reishi *[Ganoderma lucidum]*
Traditionally used to treat liver disorders, hypertension, and arthritis in the traditional medicine systems of Asia.

Thought to have antiallergic, anti-inflammatory, antibacterial, and antioxidant effects. Increased appetite has also been noted.

Reishi can be used as a culinary ingredient and is also available in tablet and syrup form.

Shiitake Mushroom *[Lentinus edodes]*
Active ingredient is thought to be lentinan, a polysaccharide, which is widely available in health food shops.

This is an immunomodulating anticancer agent that has been widely researched. Found to increase production of various cytokines (the chemical messengers associated with intracellular immune response) and killer cells in many studies, particularly in Japan. (For example, "Recent progress in immunopharmacology and therapeutic effect of polysaccharides." Kawasaki. *Develop. Biol. Standard,* 77:191–197.)

This is also a rather tasty mushroom that, if organically grown and cooked gently, may retain some of these medicinal qualities, and thus be a good general addition to the culinary shopping list.

Turkey Tail *[Tremetes versicolor]*

Also known as *Boletus versicolor, Polyporus versicolor,* and *Coriolus versicolor;* karawatake is the Japanese name, and it is known as Yun-Zhi in China.

The principal property of interest is immunomodulating anticancer action, which has been researched in Japan. The second, and less well researched property, is possible antiviral activity.

Principal active ingredient is thought to be PSK, or krestin, a water-soluble, protein-bound polysaccharide. PSK has been subjected to multiple clinical trials on cancer patients in Japan. A good summary of these trials appears in "Cancer Immunotherapy" published by *Life Sciences,* August 5, 1977. In general it was found to generate few side effects and to have clinical benefits to a number of patients who had not responded to conventional therapy. However, liver cancer response was poor.

It has been found to induce an increased production of interferons, stimulate macrophages, and induce potent antimicrobial activity against a range of microorganisms including *Staphylococcus aureus* and *Candida albicans.* See the book *Medicinal Mushrooms* in the "Further Reading" section for details.

This mushroom and its extracts may be of use in the preemptive treatment of possible cancer, a component in antiviral therapy, and as a general immune tonic.

Formulations

Some Western herbalists have now gained considerable experience in treating hepatitis C patients. They stress the importance of consulting a practitioner; however, Peter du Ruyter was prepared to recommend two general formulations for hep C.

For a general-purpose "liver tea," obtain a packet each of

Dandelion root (unroasted)

Rosemary leaves (dry)

Licorice root (omit this herb is you have severe high blood pressure)

Gotu Kola (sometimes called hydrocotyl)

Calendula flowers

Take 1 tablespoon each and put in a nonaluminum teapot. Add 4 cups of boiling water, replace lid, cover, and leave for six to eight hours. Drink 1 cup twice daily, warmed up. Tea is safe to take long term, four to six months at a time.

Or, for a general-purpose herbal formulation *(not to be taken while also on the above tea regimen)*: go to a herbalist and have the following made up into a tincture:

Baical skullcap	15%
Astralagus	15%
Bupleurum	5%
Silybum	15%
Schisandra	20%
Licorice	15%
Echinacea	15%

Take 3 ml three times per day before meals, diluted in some water. Build up the dose slowly.

Also, if liver function is abnormal, go to a chemist or herbalist and ask them for Picrorrhiza tablets (see chapter 17 for details on this herb). Take ½ tablet twice daily before meals, until all functions are normal. Then continue for two months at ½ tablet daily.

Ses Salmond has written about her experience of treating hepatitis C.[7] She offers detailed analysis of both disease pattern and clinical strategy including the following list of key therapeutic aims:

- Boost the immune system
- Prevent necrosis
- Support regeneration
- Promote bile flow, waste elimination, and detoxification
- Address addictions

She comments:

> The use of botanicals in the treatment of viral hepatitis offers tissue support, the prevention of necrosis of liver cells, and alternative pathways of metabolism to circumvent inflammation....

A clinical observation that I have made is that the prescription of herbal antioxidants has a marked effect in lowering liver enzymes and improving liver function.

Mindy relates her experience of herbal medicine:

My walk with the dragon started in March of 1997, when I tried to donate blood and the little beast showed himself. Mine was an all-too-familiar story: evidently I contracted the hep C virus from a blood transfusion during surgery, thirteen years prior. I saw a gastroenterologist, who recommended a biopsy and then treatment with interferon. In the meantime, a friend begged me to go to our local health food store, which aggressively treats all types of illnesses with good one-on-one support.

I went to the health food store rather reluctantly. Up until that time, my idea of eating healthy meant that I ordered a small order of French fries from McDonald's instead of a large. Was I ever in for a change! The professionals at the health food store recommended a diet for me. It consists of all organic foods and is limited to whole-grain products, raw or steamed vegetables, and small amounts of protein. I eat very little dairy products and no sugar, as viruses feed off of sugar. This includes fruit, as fruit turns into sugar in your bloodstream as it is processed by the body. In addition, I use a product called "Green Vibrance," which is mixed with water and contains all kinds of natural herbs. I take quite a few supplements, including milk thistle, Liv-a-Tox (cleanses the liver), vitamins, ACES (vitamins A, C, E, and selenium), B vitamins, carotenoid, folic acid, and more.

After ten months, my liver enzymes were fluctuating between normal to just a few measurements over normal. I had lost twenty-five pounds, looked better, and felt better. The diet is a permanent lifestyle change.

However, my viral load continued to climb—from 2 million to over 4 million in that ten-month period of time. I went back to the health food professionals for advice, and they started me on what they described as an "aggressive herbal treatment," targeted to eliminate the virus. In just eight weeks, the viral load dropped from over 4 million to just over 500,000. I will be tested again in two months to see if it has continued to decrease. I do not have a spleen, so the reduction in the viral load is even more remarkable.

The herbal treatment is made up of herbs produced by Gaia Herbs, Inc. Each herb comes in a small dropper bottle, and I mix up a batch according to the following recipe. Dosage is one dropper (¼ teaspoon four times a day). Side effects include extreme fatigue; I know that is also a symptom of the hep C, but the herbs seem to make it worse. The herbs need to be mixed and stored in an amber bottle, as exposure to light lessons their potency. The formula is as follows:

5 parts milk thistle

5 parts turmeric

3 parts schizandra

2 parts licorice

2 parts eclipta

2 parts phyllanthus

4 parts reishi/bupleurum

4 parts camp coleus forskohlii

4 parts lomatium

4 parts echinacea

My disclaimer: I didn't for one minute think this would work. But the store that is helping me offered to provide all of the above at no charge, just on an experimental basis. Who knows? This may be a temporary improvement. They worked very carefully on an individual basis with me, so the treatment might be slightly different for someone else.

I believe the most important factor in all of this was prayer. Constant. Makes all the difference in the world.

Todoxin

Another herbal antiviral that might be explored is the compound Todoxin, which has been used effectively in the treatment of HIV.[8]

A powerful herbal immunomodulator with over forty ingredients that are subject to a secret process, it is provided on a patient study participation basis to HIV patients. Some HCV patients have also now been recruited to the trial—interim PCR test results suggest that a significant antiviral response is taking place. This would certainly suggest itself as an option to HIV coinfected patients. The average ALT and AST of a tested population with 45% HCV coinfection showed a marked average decline to within the normal range during Todoxin therapy.

Details on Todoxin are available from the Society for the Study of Complementary Medicine in the U.K. Call 44 (0)171 436 0821. Call the same number for details of access to the study in America.

Hepatico

This is a four-herb combination used as a traditional remedy for hepatitis in Georgia, former USSR. It is currently undergoing a 100-patient trial in Canada, where it is being tested for impact on liver function in HCV patients.

Further Reading

Back to Eden. Jethro Kloss.
Herbs of Grace. Forida Davidson.
Planetary Herbology. Michael Tierra.
School of Natural Healing. Dr. J. Christopher.
The Herbal Handbook, A User's Guide to Medical Herbalism. David Hoffman. Healing Arts Press, Rochester, Vermont, 1988.
The New Holistic Herbal. David Hoffman. Element Books.
Green Pharmacy, The History and Evolution of Western Herbal Medicine. Barbara Griggs. Healing Arts Press.
The Information Sourcebook of Herbal Medicine. Edited by David Hoffman. The Crossing Press.
Complementary Medicine: New Approaches to Good Practice. British Medical Association. Oxford University Press.
Natural Health, Natural Medicine—A Comprehensive Manual for Wellness and Self-Care. Andrew Weil, MD. Houghton Mifflin Company, Boston.

Eastern/Central Medicinal Plants. Peterson Field Guides. Steven Foster, James A. Duke. Houghton Mifflin Company.

The Complete Medicinal Herbal. Penelope Ody. Dorling Kindersley.

Spontaneous Healing. Andrew Weil, M.D. Knopf, New York.

The Honest Herbal. Varro Tyler. Haworth Press, Binghamton, NY.

Herbs of Choice. Varro Tyler. Haworth Press.

The Energetics of Western Herbs, Volumes I and II. Artemis Press [Reference].

Medicinal Mushrooms. Christopher Hobbs. Botanica Press.

References

1. Toxicity references: note that each of these papers has subreferences. Also refer to the "Safety, Toxicity, Quality Control, and Other Considerations" section in chapter 15 and professional herbal reference material.

Traditional remedies and food supplements—a five-year toxicological study (1991–1995). Shaw et al. *Drug Safety,* Adis International, 17(5): 342–356, Nov 1997.

Risks or remedies? Safety aspects of herbal remedies in the U.K. Shaw D. *Journal of the Royal Society of Medicine,* 91:294–296, June 1998.

Subarachnoid hemorrhage associated with Gingko biloba. Vale S. *The Lancet,* Vol 352, July 4, 1998.

2. Sack RB et al. *Infect Immune,* 35:471–5, 1982.

Murray M. *The 21st Century Herbal Vitaline,* 1988.

3. A desmutagenic factor isolated from burdock. Kazuyoshi M et al. *Mutation Research,* 129:25–31, 1984.

4. Immerman. V13 *ACA Journal of Chiropractice,* Apr 1979.

5. Silymarin references:

Immunomodulatory and hepatoprotective effects of in vivo treatment with free radical scavengers. Lang I et al. *Ital J Gastroenterol,* 22:283–7, 1990.

Liver-protective action of silymarin therapy in chronic alcoholic liver diseases. Feher J et al. *Orv Hetil* (Hungary), 130:2723–2727, 1989.

Effect of silymarin on chemical, functional, and morphological alterations of the liver. A double-blind controlled study. Salmi HA et al. *Scand J Gastroenterol,* 17:517–521, 1982.

Results of a double blind study on the effect of silymarin in the treatment of acute viral hepatitis, carried out at two medical centers. Magliulo E et al. *Med Klin* (Germany), 73:1060–1065, 1978.

Effect of silimarin (Legalon) therapy on the antioxidant defense mechanism and lipid peroxidation in alcoholic liver disease (double blind protocol. Muzes G et al. *Orv Hetil* (Hungary), 131:863–866, 1990.

Randomized controlled trial of silymarin treatment in patients with cirrhosis of the liver. Ferenci P et al. *J Hepatol* (Netherlands), 9:105–113, 1989.

6. Effective reduction of HCV RNA blood levels following therapy of chronic hepatitis C patients with hypericin containing preparations from hypericum perforatum. Steinbeck-Klose AM et al. Unpublished. Correspondence contact Dr. Gad Lavie, Blood Transfusion Centre, Sheba Medical Centre, Tel-Hashomer, 52621, Israel. Telephone 972 3 5302178 for reprint requests.

7. Herbs and hepatitis C. Salmond S. *International Journal of Alternative and Complementary Medicine,* pp 24–26, Sept 1997, and subsequent issue.

8. The prolonged virological and clinical efficacy of todoxin in the treatment of HIV-1 infection. Jovanovic T et al. *Raum and Zeit* (Austria), 82–96, 1996

17

·

Ayurvedic Medicine and Hepatitis C

AYURVEDA MEANS "knowledge of life." This vast and ancient system has its origins in the Indus civilization of northwestern India. It is concerned with both health maintenance and disease treatment and is the oldest intact medical system in the world. Some of the texts, or Vedas, which lay out the philosophical and practical bases for the Ayurvedic approach to the diagnosis, treatment, and prevention of disease are over 5,000 years old. Most medical treatments available today have their roots in Ayurveda.

A number of the concepts that inform the Traditional Chinese Medicine system, such as the classification of conditions and treatments according to energetic qualities and the idea of the existence of invisible meridians of energy, have their origin in systems of thought native to India. The spread of Buddhism from its northern Indian origins to China via Tibet is usually regarded as being the historical key to the transmission of these ideas. Although Ayurveda embraces a number of metaphysical concepts, it is emphatically not a religion itself; Indian doctors who are Buddhists, Hindus, Jains, Muslims, or belong to many of the other faiths native to India will use Ayurvedic knowledge and principles to advise and treat their patients. However, there is a pronounced spiritual dimension to Ayurvedic practice; as in TCM both diagnosis and treatment can have a meditative dimension.

Practitioners may also talk of attaining optimum health as a duty, even a karmic imperative, and have been known to commence treatment by lecturing their patients along these lines. Thus there is a strong element of personal responsibility. Much of the role of the doctor will be to assist the patient to establish what agrees with them and what does not. Treatments are aimed not so much at curing diseases directly, but at assisting the body to engage its innate capacity to heal itself. This is directly comparable to TCM, homeopathy, and naturopathy; the latter approach in particular draws heavily upon Ayurveda.

Ayurveda is directly relevant to hepatitis C because of the present and historical prevalence of liver disease in India and the consequently large body of experience gained. Interested patients may be able to tap into this, although good and experienced practitioners are particularly hard to find in the West. The application of this "knowledge of life" requires lengthy training and experience. Because the system is so wide ranging, most practitioners specialize in particular aspects of both disease and treatment.

The main components of Ayurveda are herbal medicine, yoga, dietary therapy, detoxification (panchakarma), meditation/prayer, and lifestyle adjustment. There are many subcategories such as color and/or music therapy, the use of minerals and metals, crystal or gemstone affinity, astrology, and surgery. In all cases the application of these bodies of knowledge is individually prescribed. Each person is seen as a unique fragment of universal consciousness. Thus this is a "patient-centered" approach requiring individual consultation. While TCM has been partially systematized, as demonstrated by the growing incorporation of standard Chinese herbal formulations and acupuncture points into mainstream medicine around the world, Ayurveda is still a largely individualized and alternative system.

In the words of Shyam Singha, a renowned practitioner, "If there are 6 billion people on the planet, there will be 6 billion different solutions; whatever is required to unblock an individual will be unique. It may be a diet, herbal medicine, even sounds or colors."

Thus a fixed-name disease such as hepatitis C may be a secondary issue in the diagnostic process. An Ayurvedic doctor will first categorize the patient according to dominant body energy, or *dosha*. These doshas consist of

- **Vata:** associated with air and space, tend to be thin, light sleepers, anxious.

- **Pitta:** associated with fire and water, often medium build, intelligent, aggressive.

- **Kapha:** associated with water and earth, often heavy build, calm, likes sleeping.

Everyone will have a balance of these three energies; disease will be associated with imbalance. Ayurveda also has a clear concept of mental energies, or Gunas, of which there are three types, Sattva, Rajas, and Tamas. Patterns of behavior can be clearly diagnosed in this system. For instance, a patient who is told by their doctor to abstain from eating a particular food, understands the reasoning for the advice, agrees with the advice, and accepts it, but is completely incapable of abstaining from the proscribed food might be said to be suffering from a particular deficiency in one of the mental elements. As with the imbalances in the physical elements, there will be classically prescribed treatments for these conditions.

Patients will be subjected to an eightfold examination consisting of pulse reading, tongue analysis, voice analysis, skin examination, eye assessment, general appearance review, urine analysis, and stool analysis.

Having said this, there are some principles and specific practices originating in Ayurveda that are likely to be of general value. Because the system is so vast, what follows are snippets. If this approach seems appropriate, try to track down a suitable practitioner; some contacts are listed at the end of this chapter.

Diet, Dietary Therapy, and Liver Disease from the Ayurvedic Perspective

Ayurvedic medicine has an extensive set of instructions regarding the "right" way to eat; according to classic texts the correct foods need to be taken in the correct quantities at the right time at the right temperature in order to meet the body's seven needs. These needs are "required" plasma, blood tissue, muscle, fat tissue, bone tissue, and reproductive tissue. Only when all of these needs have been met can energy be spared for the Ojas, the seventh level of need, associated with health, aura, and positive supreme energy.

In the case of hepatitis C patients, the prescription of a "correct" diet would usually be accompanied by the prescription of medicine to treat liver disease. In the words of Dr. Arpana Bapat, an Ayurvedic specialist in chronic fatigue syndrome and pulse diagnosis:

> If the liver is not functioning correctly, the energy transformation will not be efficient and toxification will be more likely. Therefore the liver problem is the immediate priority. I would look at general body detoxification (panchakarma) followed by the prescription of herbal medicine. (See below for panchakarma.)

Dietary advice and general lifestyle counselling is given to patients with chronic liver disease. In classical Ayurvedic terms the liver is responsible for blood formation, along with the bone marrow and the spleen. Therefore blood-forming foods might be emphasized, along with herbs such as dandelion root. More importantly fatigue would be seen as a sign of blockage and stress; therefore counselling might aim to identify the cause of the negative cycle and help the patient to escape. Unexpressed emotion would be a prime candidate for linkage to chronic fatigue or liver disease.

If liver disease was chronic, immune system dysfunction might be suspected; diagnosis might be supported by stool analysis, particularly for the presence of candidiasis, a classic sign of poor immune function in Ayurveda.

Dietary rules have been adapted to modern Western needs by Shyam Singha, an Ayurvedic practitioner who specializes in dietary therapy (i.e., food and dietary adjustment is seen as a powerful method of treatment in and by itself) and has treated a number of HCV patients in the Netherlands and Italy. Some general principles are as follows:

- Avoid microwaved food; it is "dead."

- Chew food very well.

- Avoid distractions while eating and allow plenty of time for digestion.

- Favor alkaline-forming foods, as in the Hay diet.

- Eat only when hungry.

- Choose foods intuitively; don't become obsessive.

- Reduce cold drinks in favor of hot or warm ones.

- Try to have your main meal in the middle of the day.

- Avoid any foods that cause reactions; gluten and dairy products are prime candidates.

- Try to reduce exposure to herbicides, pesticides, additives, and refined and processed foods of all types; reduce meat intake because concentrations of toxins are higher further up the food chain. Eat organic if possible.

Singha sometimes suggests radical diets to his patients. This goes well beyond general dietary guidelines and should be regarded as a distinct form of therapy. In this approach the kinds of effects usually only associated with the use of medicines—such as herbs or drugs—are achieved through the adoption of precise regimens.

With regard to hep C specifically Singha is reluctant to give general advice. However, he would tend to start by addressing the immune system. If the liver was in reasonable shape, he might suggest the grilled orange monofast, a Singha classic, often recommended to HIV patients as well.

Blood-Purifying Diet: Consume nothing but grilled oranges and hot water for one week. To grill oranges, simply cut in half and place under the grill until a brown crust appears. Cook four at a time, four times per day. Scoop out the flesh, along with loose pith, with a spoon.

After seven days, continue for a further ninety days with four grilled oranges for breakfast. At other meals eat 70% raw food, 30% cooked. Avoid red meat, sugar, wheat, and milk completely. Drink 4 cups of dandelion coffee and 2 cups of nettle tea per day. Eat plenty of plums, kiwi fruit, red onion, cos or romaine lettuce, and broccoli.

Combine with taking leisurely walks, plenty of sleep, and relaxation. Friction baths and Dead Sea or Epsom salt baths are helpful.

This is thought to be helpful because oranges are strongly alkaline forming and, when grilled, particularly rich in bioflavanoids. (Note that oranges can cause adverse reactions in liver disease; this is an immune-enhancing strategy that assumes that the liver can take the strain. Consult a practitioner and avoid if unsure.) Further dietary advice with a view to protecting immune function consists of

- Avoid all foods containing gluten.
- Avoid all other antagonists or allergens.
- Avoid all processed foods (e.g., butter is better than margarine).
- Avoid microwaved foods.

The occasional colon and liver detox, cleansing diet such as a grape monofast and regular breathing exercises are all highly recommended to support immune function. Regular laughing is also regarded as being an extremely powerful immune tonic by Singha, who often arranges laughing therapy, wherein participants are asked to pair up and tickle their partner for ten minutes continuously.

For the **general health of the liver,** Singha recommends the following fresh juice recipe. (Note that all juices should ideally be freshly squeezed. Any nonorganic fruits with skins, such as grapes, need to be soaked in a salt solution for an hour to extract pesticides or herbicides; this is necessary because most such toxins are water insoluble.)

Take 1 tablespoon of dandelion flowers with roots (from a herbalist) and boil in 500 ml of water until 125 ml remains. Add 375 ml of equal amounts of the following juices (approximately 95 ml each):

- Carrot
- Raw beet
- Parsley
- Radishes (with leaves)

Drink 1.5 liters of the juice per day. Avoid fatty foods and alcohol.

Singha also has a specific prescription for an **"angry liver,"** which may be of interest to some of us. Make 375 ml from equal amounts of the following juices:

- Cooking apple

- Celery
- Carrot

Then prepare a mixture by boiling 2 tablespoons of dried dandelion leaves and root (from a herbalist) with a pinch each of powdered clove, salt, and cinnamon, in 500 ml of water until 125 ml is left. Add the mixture to the juice. Drink while chewing 25 g of fresh parsley—on an empty stomach, once or twice a day.

For **candidiasis,** which is seen as a symptom of serious immune dysfunction in Ayurveda, he recommends: For seven days eat four rotten overripe black bananas (mashed and with a pinch of pepper) with 500 g of live bioyogurt every four hours. Nothing else, except hot water between "meals."

For the next twenty-one days have two rotten overripe mashed black bananas with 250 g of live bioyogurt and some added pepper. Eat nothing else for two hours afterwards. Eat only cooked vegetables during the day. Drink hot water and herb tea. Avoid other drinks, particularly stimulants such as tea, Coca Cola, and coffee.

For the next two months eat two rotten bananas with 250 g of live bioyogurt with added black pepper for breakfast. Wait for two hours before eating other food. For all other meals eat 70% cooked food and 30% raw.

During the whole three months strictly avoid

- Milk, sugar, wheat, and red meat
- Yeast in any shape or form—fermented products such as alcohol, cheeses, yeast spreads such as marmite; read labels carefully. For instance, vitamin supplements may contain brewer's yeast.

Singha has a wide range of radical dietary treatments for a number of hepatitis C-related disorders, such as arthritis (potato skin monofast!), depression, fatigue, kidney disorders, colon disease, indigestion, and eye problems, which are listed and explained in his remarkable book (see the "Further Reading" section at the end of this chapter).

Amaroli—Urine Therapy

Urine therapy has the double advantage of being free of charge and universally accessible! Judging by the sales of recent books on the subject, it is also becoming popular both in North America and Western Europe. If you wish to pursue this option, you might wish to read it up in more depth—books are suggested below. You may also wish to discuss this with your doctor, although words along the lines of "I am thinking of drinking my own urine; I understand it may be highly therapeutic" have been known to trigger extreme reactions among the conventional medical profession.

Urine therapy is a serious and deeply rooted medicinal practice. It involves the drinking of urine, or its external application, usually one's own. It has been recognized for its medicinal value by many different peoples—for example, the Lapps, European alchemists, and some contemporary American doctors. However, India is home base for this very interesting therapy. A 5,000-year-old Ayurvedic text called Shivambu Kalpa Vidhi ("The Drinking of Urine in Order to Rejuvenate") describes its indications, applications, and efficacy. The practice is still very popular there; senior citizens regularly attribute their longevity to this practice, and there are even annual festivals for enthusiasts.

Urine therapy is safe, although it may precipitate a detoxification reaction or healing crisis. Urine is actually filtered blood, a product of the kidneys. There are no reports of any adverse effects, despite an instinctive apprehension about such "recycling" of an apparent waste product. Pharmaceutical companies are major buyers of urine; it is used in skin care, contraceptive, and anticoagulation products.

Technique

Simply take a sample from the midstream of your urine, usually first thing in the morning. Start off by drinking only a few drops. Build up to an eggcup sized dose over a period of two weeks. Continue indefinitely or use as required.

For external use simply apply urine to broken skin or a wound that needs to heal. Urine can also be used in massage or even in facial compresses; enthusiasts will extol the benefits to skin tone.

HCV patients with optical problems may be advised to massage urine into the area around the eyes before going to bed. Consult an Ayurvedic practitioner before trying this.

Contraindications

- People who are taking drugs or chemotherapy should avoid urine therapy.

- People with edema (swelling) of the ankles, high blood pressure, or proteinuria (abnormal protein in urine) should consult their doctors.

- Avoid if suffering from urinary tract infections.

Dietary Recommendations While Using Amaroli

Try to reduce acid-inducing foods (see the "Food Combining and the Hay Diet" section in chapter 22). Avoid or reduce meat. Reduce salt and refined, processed, and hormone- or additive-containing foods. Try to eliminate alcohol, coffee, tobacco, and junk food.

Indications and Actions

There have been no double-blind placebo-controlled studies of urine therapy. Given the inherently noncommercial nature of this approach, there are never likely to be any. However, there is such a long standing, commercially disinterested, and widely based enthusiasm for this form of therapy that some sort of benefit is almost certainly occurring.

How and why urine therapy may deliver results is not precisely known. There are various theories. The most obvious one centers around the medicinal value of the substances found to be present in urine. These include creatine, serotonin, a range of amino acids, albumin, protein antibodies, urokinase, protease, thiamine, vitamins B_2, B_6 and B_{12}, nicotinic acid, ascorbic acid, a wide range of hormones, DHEA, prostaglandin, and interleukin-1.

Other theories center on possible homeopathic action or examine the possibility of some kind of biofeedback mechanism which creates a homeostatic balancing effect. The possibility of a psychological or psychosomatic action is also put across strongly by some doctors, who may focus on the boost obtained by consuming one's own medicine!

Urine therapy is often promoted as a generally healthy, life-enhancing practice and, as such, requires no specific indicators. However, some Ayurvedic practitioners have found it to be specifically helpful in treating liver disorders such as hepatitis C; urine therapy may be beneficial due to the opportunity it presents for reabsorption and reuse of nutrients. It has been suggested that faulty liver function or biliary duct inflammation may lead to bile flow obstruction and consequent seeping into the blood. Urine therapy may offer the opportunity to reabsorb bile into the digestive tract. Thus bile and other liver enzymes can be reused.

For fatigue, allergies, and rheumatic and skin disorders, the reabsorption of some hormones may provide a necessary correction. In particular the hormone melatonin may have a calming and anticarcinogenic effect.

The ingestion of urea may have a number of benefits. It is thought that urea is converted into glutamine, and a Dr. Danopoulos has suggested that it may be helpful in treating liver cancer

People with immunodeficient conditions (such as AIDS) or with susceptibility to developing immunodeficiency (such as HIV) may be advised to try amaroli by Ayurvedic doctors. Amaroli appears to be quite popular in this community at present. There are many anecdotal reports of improvements in HIV and AIDS patients who have tried this (see the "Further Reading" section below).

Panchakarma

This is an important element in Ayurvedic medicine that may be recommended to hep C patients, particularly those with clear signs of liver toxicity or lymphatic disease. It embraces five classic purification techniques, though we would probably use the word "detoxification." These therapies are best delivered in a clinical environment; it is advisable to book into a specialist Ayurvedic center if you wish to pursue this option. Panchakarma consists of

- **Emesis:** Deliberate use of herbs or agents designed to induce vomiting. Often used to help treat long-term poor dietary habits or toxin accumulation.

- **Purgation:** Use of laxatives and other medicines and techniques that encourage bowel evacuation. Often used to treat "hot" diseases, such as hep C-related fever.

- **Enema:** Use of enemas to clean the bowel; this therapy is quite likely to be recommended to hep C patients because the bowel is linked to the liver in Ayurvedic medicine. Bowel cleansing would be thought to "help" the liver, by alleviating the detoxification load. Note that this therapy and its rather hip relatives such as colonic irrigation have their roots in Ayurveda. In this context they are used as one element in an overall treatment strategy.

- **Nasal drops or snuff:** Medicated oils, powders, or ground herbs may be taken through the nose. Usually only prescribed for ear, nose, throat conditions.

- **Bloodletting:** Phlebotomy. This has a known value in the treatment of hep C, reducing liver iron cell concentrations and consequently lowering chances of liver disease progression. In Ayurveda metal instruments or leeches may be employed for the purpose. Medicinal pastes may be applied to the bleeding point to enhance the effect. Again this is likely to be recommended on account of its classical indication by inflamed liver and spleen.

All of these treatments may be preceded by certain preparatory therapies such as

- **Aromatherapeutic massage** and/or **essential oil treatment.** These very pleasant therapeutic tools are designed to soften the body, making it more responsive to the main treatment.

- **Sweating therapy** is also prescribed as a panchakarma precursor and may include the application of poultices. Again there are strong links to modern therapies involving the application of hot and cold presses.

Ayurvedic Herbal Medicine

There are many extremely powerful and interesting medicinal agents in the Ayurvedic materia medica; it is not confined to herbs, also containing minerals (particularly prevalent in the related field of Tibetan medicine) and metals. Western herbalists and biotechnology companies are eagerly pouring over some of these substances, particularly the herbs listed below.

In general Ayurvedic medicine places less emphasis on the art of herbal prescription than TCM. Therefore it will be hard to find a practitioner with the necessary skills to provide individualized and complex formulations tailored to meet individual needs. There is a greater emphasis on the use of standard formulations. As with Chinese herbal medicine, practitioners are not interested in the biochemistry of these agents so much as the energetics or biorhythmic properties. Again it is this system of classification that underpins the science of synergistic formulation, which in turn delivers the power.

Caution

Patients or practitioners wishing to explore this approach should be aware of two currently serious drawbacks:

1. Although a lot of work has been done in India on the impact of these herbs on liver disease and hepatitis in general, there is very little data on hepatitis C. While some TCM practitioners have now done extensive work adapting and adjusting formulations to meet the distinct needs of HCV patients, very little work has been done in Ayurveda to date.

2. The quality control of Ayurvedic herbs can be haphazard. There are no Ayurvedic herbal companies operating to the level of reputable TCM companies such as East West and Spring Wind, who run manufacturing facilities in the West that are subject to regular and random scrutiny by statutory agencies. While some Ayurvedic herbal companies do have extensive quality control procedures, these are not subject to scrutiny in the U.S. or EU. There have been a number of recent reports

in the Indian press highlighting the shortcomings of some of the herbal operations currently in that country; criticisms range from adulteration to the failure to prepare herbs according to traditional Ayurvedic guidelines.

Therefore patients or practitioners wishing to access the power of some of these agents need to take steps to verify the species of the herbs or the quality control procedures of suppliers. It will also be necessary to think carefully about the distinct needs of HCV; most of these formulations appear to have been tried out mainly on hep A and hep B patients. As explained earlier, the dynamics of these viruses are distinct from those of hep C.

A note about safety—don't even think about combining any of these formulations or herbs with any other concurrent herbal medicine. Always consult a practitioner prior to using these formulations.

Some Formulations

Liv-52 is a well-known Ayurvedic formulation for liver disease. It contains the following (classic Ayurvedic plant name in brackets):

- *Capparis spinosa* [Kabra]: hepatic stimulant and appetite inducer; hepatoprotective, diuretic, aperient; supports glycogen storage.
- *Cichorium intybus* [Kasni]: hepatic stimulant, tonic, and diuretic; checks vomiting and diarrhea; supports glycogen storage.
- *Solanum nigrum* [Makoi]: hydragogue, often used to try to reduce anasarca and ascites; diuretic; moderate hepatoprotective and laxative.
- *Cassia occidentalis* [Kasondi]: tonic, diuretic, stomachic, and choleretic; may act against nausea.
- *Terminalia arjuna* [Arjuna]: cardiac tonic.
- *Achillea millefolium* [Gandana]: stimulating tonic and carminative.
- *Tamarix gallica* [Jhau]: hepatic stimulant and digestive. Mildly hepatoprotective and glycogen storage supporting.
- *Mandur bhasma*: not a plant but a preparation of ferric oxide

"triturated in the juices of innumerable powerful hepatic stimulants and cholagogues. It is a powerful haematinic tonic and is valuable in the treatment of haemolytic jaundice and microcytic anaemias."[1]

- *Eclipta alba* [Bringharaj]: anti-inflammatory and tonic; may relieve hepatic and spleenic enlargement.

- *Phyllanthus amarus* [Jar-amia]: stomachic and diuretic; antiviral found to have anti-HBV activity—see below and references.[2]

- *Boerhaavia diffusa* [Sant]: antibilious, anti-inflammatory, carminative, diuretic, aperient, and tonic; often used to treat jaundice and ascites.

- *Tinospora cordifolia* [Giloe]: stomachic; stimulates bile secretion; reduces fever and improves appetite.

- *Berberis aristata* [Daruhaldi]: widely used in the treatment of jaundice.

- *Raphanus sativus* [Muli]: stomachic, laxative, tonic, and carminative; tonifies the spleen.

- *Phyllanthus emblica* [Amla]: tonic, laxative, and carminative.

- *Plumbago zeylanica* [Chitrak]: astringent to the bowels, anti-inflammatory, tonic, and aperient.

- *Embelia ribes* [Baberang]: appetite stimulant, carminative, and laxative, often used in ascites.

- *Terminalia chebula* [Hirda]: tonic, stomachic, and carminative; often used in ascites and nausea.

- *Fumaria officinalis* [Pit-papara]: improves appetite and has tonic qualities.

Liv-52 clearly contains many tonics, particularly those used to treat manifestations of late-stage liver disease, such as ascites. Therefore it may be of interest to doctors treating patients in this category. Thus this formulation may be of use as a temporary treatment— perhaps three to nine months—for patients with pronounced liver disease who are also cold or unreactive.

The concentration of tonic agents might make it unsuitable for long-term use. Again it is important to stress that the impact of Liv-52 on HCV-related liver cirrhosis is unknown; adverse effects cannot be ruled out.

Liv-52 has been tested on chronic viral hepatitis, although this may be predominantly HBV and HDV, as mentioned above. Findings of one double-blind placebo-controlled study concluded:

> Following Liv-52 treatment, significant clinical improvement was observed along with improvement in biochemical parameters in both infective hepatitis and chronic active hepatitis.[3]

Perhaps the most likely role for Liv-52 would be as a component in the treatment of cirrhosis. Impact upon cirrhosis has been subject to several double-blind placebo-controlled studies in India. Examples of findings and conclusions include

> The Liv-52 treated cases showed markedly superior clinical improvements which were borne out by biochemical liver function tests and histopathological assessment after six months of therapy.[4]

> The results of hepatic function tests and needle biopsy specimens demonstrated definite improvement in hepatocellular function and structure with Liv-52. For this prolonged treatment for at least nine months was necessary.[5]

It is also worth noting that some Western hepatologists are suspicious of the standards used by Indian doctors in these trials. Reciprocally some Indian doctors accuse the Western doctors of being in the pockets of pharmaceutical companies, who, in turn, are supporting unfair and restrictive trade practices that block access to products such as Liv-52. For more information on Liv-52, obtain the monograph in the references.[1]

Another formulation that may be of interest to patients with rheumatoid arthritis is called Maha Yograj Guggul. This product has a very good reputation for addressing RA and may be at least as effective as any of the patent medicines currently approved for use in the West. Again this is a complex compound that should not be taken by a hepatitis C patient without expert advice.

There are many other formulations, both classical and modern, that may be of interest to hepatitis C patients and their practitioners. A company called Envin Bioceuticals, which does operate extensive quality control procedures in India, produces a number of formulations available in capsules or syrup.

Optiliv is primarily designed as a hepatoprotective medicine. This contains *Andrographis paniculata, Aphanamaxis rohituka, Picrorhiza kurroa, Azadirachta indica, Eclipta alba,* and *Boerhaavia diffusa.*

EuMil (AKA Stresseeze) is designed as an antistress, antioxidant, and adaptogen, also protecting organs including the liver from lipid peroxidation in animal studies.[6] This contains *Ocimum sanctum* and *Withania somnifera* and has been shown to have effective free radical scavenging properties.[7]

Proimmu is designed to enhance immune function and contains the following herbs: *Ocimum sanctum, Withanium somnifera, Tinospora cordifola,* and *Emblica officinale.*

While more work needs to be done to demonstrate safety and effectiveness in HCV patients, it is clear that many of these herbs possess properties that are likely to be of great value.

Andrographis paniculata has attracted interest from biotech companies looking for HIV antivirals and is well known in Chinese herbal medicine (Chuan Xin Lian). A number of Indian studies have demonstrated beneficial impact on both key processes such as digestion and aspects of body structure such as liver cell integrity.[8]

Phyllanthus amara and *Phyllanthus niruri* have attracted great interest and have also been the focus of much poorly informed comment. In part confusion has arisen due to inherent problems associated with trying to analyze traditional medicines from a Western "scientific" perspective; it seems that the antiviral properties of *Phyllanthus amarus* vary according to where it grows, the time of year it is harvested, how it is processed, and, to some extent, which other herbs it is prescribed with.

The *Lancet* study listed below found that 59% of treated subjects cleared a key marker for hepatitis B compared to only 4% in a control group. Subsequent studies failed to confirm this finding, but also used plants not from India. No one has yet studied phyllanthus for clearance of HCV markers.

Phyllanthus has also been observed to have mild hepatoprotective properties, to inhibit HIV replication in vitro, and also be able to lower blood glucose.[9] Active antiviral agent has been tentatively identified as repandusinic acid A. Kerry Bone, a well-known phytotherapeutic authority, has concluded: "Phyllanthus sourced from India may have a role in viral liver diseases, but it should be used in combination with other treatments."

Picrorhiza kurroa is well known for its benefits to liver function in both Ayurveda and TCM (Hu Huang Lian), where it is a classic heat clearing agent. Used by Western herbalists such as Peter de Ruyter to normalize liver function, it comes in a tablet form known as Picroliv. It has been the subject of many studies in India.[10] This is thought by some to be the most powerful hepatoprotective plant of them all; it has also been observed to exert a strong choleretic and cholagogue effect, to be antioxidant, to reduce bronchial allergic reaction, to be anti-inflammatory, to enhance phagocytosis, T and B cells, and, possibly, to act against certain parasites.[9]

Ocimum sanctum has been shown to enhance certain important immune functions in animal experiments.[11]

Withania somnifera appears to be another extremely useful plant for both immune-enhancing and antipathogenic effects. This plant might be suitable for use to offset bone-marrow-related side effects of drug therapy as well as for general medicinal value. Many studies have been done on animals.[12] It has been observed to have adaptogenic, tonic, anti-inflammatory and antitumor effects.[9]

Osbeckia octandra is another Ayurvedic herb that has attracted attention as a hepatoprotective agent. This plant is commonly used in the deep south of India and Sri Lanka. An animal study conducted at King's College in London found clear biochemical benefits related to this herb and concluded that "the results support the use of Osbeckia as a hepatoprotective agent."[13]

Yoga

This is a vast subject. In general, patients need to distinguish between schools that stress physical work such as Hatha Yoga, and the more esoteric schools such as Kundalini. For physical work on both treatment and disease prevention, Hatha Yoga will be the most obvious option. Practitioners who have been taught by the famous master Iyengar will be a good basic choice.

Yoga may be of particular benefit to joint problems and help to maintain flexibility. Postures and exercises can be suggested to address almost any physical, mental, or emotional condition by a good practitioner. For instance, the immune system or the liver can be helped by particular postures. Always tell the teacher that you have hep C.

Refer to the "Qi Gong" section in chapter 15 for more information on various aspects of this type of approach to treatment.

Contacts, Practitioners, and Other Information

For further information on Ayurvedic medicinal plants and formulations, quality control issues, and applicability to hep C, contact **Indian Herbs Research and Supply Co**, P.O. Box 5, Sharda Nagar, Saharanpur 247 001, U.P., India. Fax 91 132 726288.

The Herbal Database is a computer based information resource in London, England. Call McAlpine, Thorpe, and Warrier Ltd at 44 (0)171 370 2255 for access details.

For practitioner contacts you could try the following:

U.S.

American Association of Ayurvedic Medicine
P.O. Box 598
South Lancaster MA 01561

American Institute of Vedic Studies
P.O. Box 8357
Santa Fe NM 87504

The Ayurvedic Institute: (505) 291-9698

The Ayurvedic Institute of Wellness Center
1131 Menual N.E. Suite
Albuquerque NM 87112

Chopra Centre for Wellbeing: (619) 551-7119

U.K.

Suryoda (Shyam Singha's center)
The Old Rectory
High Street
Gislingham, Suffolk, IP23 8JG
Telephone: 44 (0)1379 783527

The Hale Clinic
7 Park Crescent
London W1N 3HE
Telephone: 44 (0)171 631 0156
(This center offers a range of therapies, has an excellent health product shop called The Nutricenter and a bookshop.)

Further Reading

Ayurveda. Gopi Warrier and Deepika Gunawant, MD. Element Books, 1997.
The Secrets of Natural Health. Shyam Singha. Element Books, 1997.

Reading List for Urine Therapy

The Golden Fountain: The Complete Guide to Urine Therapy. Coen van der Kroon. Amethyst Books, 1997.
Urine Therapy—It May Save Your Life. Dr. Beatrice Bartnett. Water of Life Institute, Hollywood, Florida, 1989. Also call for information: (505) 258-3046.
Your Own Perfect Medicine: The Incredible Proven Natural Miracle Cure That Medical Science Has Never Revealed! Martha M Christy. Future Med Inc, Scottsdale, Arizona, 1994.
Die Heilkraft der Eigenharn-Therapie. Ingeborg Allmann. Verlag Dr. Karl Hohn KG, Biberach, Germany.
Urine Therapy: Self Healing through Intrinsic Medicine. Dr. John F O'Quinn. Life Science Institute, Fort Pierce, Florida, 1982.

References

1. Liv.52 A Monograph. Published by The Himalaya Drug Co. Shivsagar E, Dr. Annie Besant Road, Bombay, 400 018.

2. *Lancet,* 764, Oct 1, 1988.

3. Liv.52 in infective hepatitis and chronic active hepatitis. Mandal JN and Roy BK. *Probe,* 4, 217, 1983.

4. Clinical, biochemical and histopathological observations with Liv.52 in cirrhosis. Singh KK et al. *Antiseptic,* 7, 393, 1979.

5. Placebo controlled study of Liv.52 in cirrhosis. Mukherjee AB et al. *J Ind Med Prof,* 17, 7853, 1971.

6. Protective effect of zeetress on lipid peroxidation in different organs of rats subjected to immobilization stress. Chatterjee S. *Indian J. Vet Med,* 15(1):14–17, 1995.

7. Hydroxyl radical scavenging effect of stresseeze. Tripathi VK and Ghosal S. *Indian J. Indg Med,* 10(2), Mar 1994.

8. Andrographolide increased the rate of mitosis of hepatocytes..., Srivasta S. *Indian Journal of Pharmacology,* 28:45, 1996.

9. *Clinical Applications of Ayurvedic and Chinese Herbs.* Kerry Bone. Phytotherapy Press, Queensland, Australia, 1997.

10. It was reported that the biological activity of Picroliv might be due to the enhancement of protein and nucleic acid synthesis. Singh V et al. *Indian J Exp Biol,* 30:68, 1992.

11. O. sanctum leaves increased the number of T-Lymphocytes as well as total leucocyte count in rats. Ghodwhani et al. *J. Ethnopharmacol,* 24:193, 1988.

12. W. somnifera root extracts showed immunoprotective effects in gamma irradiated and cytotoxic drug treated animals. It restored the number of total leucocytes, bone-marrow cellularity, NK-cell activity, hemoglobin concentration and red blood cell count in immunocompromised animals.

Praveen Kumar et al. *Amala Res Bull,* 14:69, 1994.

Kuttan G. *Indian Exp Biol,* 34:854, 1996.

Praveen Kumar et al. *Amala Res Bull,* 15:77, 1995.

Praveen Kumar et al. *Indian J Exp Biol,* 34:848, 1996.

Ziauddin et al. *J Ethnopharmacol,* 50:69, 1996.

13. Protective effects of Osbeckia octandra against galactosamine and tertbutyl hydroperoxide induced hepatocyte damage. Thabrew MI et al. *J Ethnopharmacol,* 49(2):69–76, Dec 1, 1995.

18

Vitamins, Minerals, and Amino Acids

WHILE IT MAY BE TRUE that a good diet provides adequate supplies of vitamins and minerals for most healthy people, HCV patients are likely to have deficiencies. There is also a growing body of evidence that suggests that environmental factors, such as poor air quality, or lifestyle factors, such as smoking, give rise to a need for additional vitamin intake even in the general healthy population. Despite longstanding skepticism toward the value of vitamin supplements on the part of the conventional medical establishment, there is currently a shift towards acceptance of the need for patients with chronic illnesses such as HCV to take supplements to address proven likely deficiencies.

One problem is that individual assessment of needs is expensive. Some private practitioners offer blood tests for vitamin, mineral, and amino acid profiles and hair analysis, but these are very expensive and need to be taken regularly in order to ensure that supplementation is having the desired effect. This branch of medicine is still developing and is highly specialized.

A general approach based on the likelihood of deficiency, experimentation, and common sense is more practical for most people. A number of patients interviewed for this book have reported benefits from taking high-quality multivitamin supplements. Some of these products have over 100 ingredients; it is not practically possible to assess which of these is having a positive effect. It is unwise to take multivitamins continuously because some of their ingredients may be harmful to HCV patients if taken over a prolonged period. There is also a theory that vitamin levels in the body are self-balancing—this means that taking supplements achieves only a temporary boost. Thus it is best to take vitamins in short courses rather than continuously. Patients on restricted diets may have a greater need for supplements. There are also some vitamins and minerals that can cause problems for HCV patients, particularly those with significant liver damage.

Vitamins That Should Be Avoided or Taken with Caution

Vitamin A can damage the liver. Beta carotene is a vitamin A precursor. It is biochemically similar to alcohol. It is safer to avoid A supplements; some specialists suggest that the "emulsion" form of vitamin A is safer. In any case no more than 25,000 IU should be taken daily. Symptoms of excess include loss of appetite, dry skin, hair loss, headaches, and nausea. Multivitamins containing high doses of A should be taken for short periods only. This vitamin is usually included in immune-boosting supplements; HCV patients may be better off using other antioxidants, such as C, E, NAC, and so on, and getting A from foods such as carrots.

Vitamin D is the most potentially toxic of all the vitamins and should be treated even more cautiously than vitamin A. Symptoms of excess include those for A plus constant thirst, irritability, and depression.

Iron supplements need to be treated with caution. Patients with cirrhosis and HCC have been found to have increased concentrations of stainable iron deposits in liver cells. Premenopausal women are less susceptible to this condition than other patients because of blood loss via menstruation. It is not known whether this is a cause or a consequence of the development of liver cancer, but it is thought that increased concentrations of iron correlate with the likelihood of liver cell mutation.

Because of this it is wiser not to take multivitamins containing these ingredients for long periods and to avoid food supplements, such as cod liver oil, that contain high concentrations of vitamins A and D.

Melatonin, a controversial product, should be avoided by patients with autoimmune diseases. There are also unresolved safety concerns about this product, which is now a popular treatment for jet lag.

Useful Vitamins and Minerals

B complex vitamins are often prescribed for liver problems. They support the cytochrome P450 system, which governs the liver's detoxification processes.

Thiamin, B_1, is useful to the spleen and nervous system and is often deficient in liver disease patients.

Pantothenic acid, sometimes referred to as B_5, is theoretically very good for rheumatoid arthritis (RA) and fatigue; it also supports adrenal function and plays an important role in supporting certain liver functions detailed in page 378.

B_6, pyridoxine, deficiency impairs immune function. B vitamin supplements often turn urine bright yellow—this is perfectly normal. Excessive amounts cause headaches.

B_{12} is normally found in the liver. There is an injectable, long-lasting B_{12} complex called "Neo Cytamen" produced by a company called Evans. This is a deep red liquid that comes in ampoules. Some patients have reported that this is an effective "pick-me-up," particularly good if you are run down. It acts against pernicious anemia, tiredness, poor appetite, and mental dysfunction.

Biotin supports T cell function and is thought to help eczema, exhaustion, and fat metabolism.

Vitamin C is useful and widely regarded as being nontoxic. Best taken in a "buffered" pH neutral form with bioflavonoids, it supports all aspects of the immune system and is thought by many to be anticarcinogenic.

It's best to take magnesium ascorbate or calcium ascorbate, rather than ascorbic acid, because these forms are more easily assimilated. Chelated forms are better absorbed. Preparations with bioflavanoids are thought to be more effective. It is also a good idea to gradually adjust vitamin C intake to avoid possible "rebound" effects. Some practitioners will favor the use of time-release forms of vitamin C.

Some doctors, notably Linus Pauling and Robert Cathcart, have advocated vitamin C as a powerful therapy in itself, as well as being an essential nutrient for good health (megadoses of vitamin C had previously been used to treat seriously ill cancer patients with variable results). Cathcart has suggested that megadoses of vitamin C could have powerful antiviral qualities that might be sufficient to help HIV patients. "Bowel tolerance" dosage means that the patient takes as much vitamin C as he or she can before developing diarrhea; the dose is repeated several times a day over a period of weeks. He has suggested that the higher the tolerance, the greater the need. However, in order to achieve an antiviral effect, it is also necessary to take other nutrients, such as zinc, manganese, selenium, and vitamins A, B, and E. No one I know of has tried this for HCV yet. It is also advocated by nutritionists aiming for an elimination effect.

Another reason to take vitamin C is to support the body's collagen production. Collagen is the protein that makes up much of the body's connective tissue and constitutes the basement membrane of the glomeruli in the kidneys, which can be diseased in HCV patients.

High doses of vitamin C may result in increased iron uptake from the bowel, and may therefore be hazardous for patients with high levels of iron in liver cells. As with other immune "boosting" supplements it is worth noting that a healthy immune function is not necessarily a hyperactive one; this is particularly true for patients susceptible to autoimmune conditions.

As with other supplements it would seem that cautious and careful experimentation is the most sensible policy.

Calcium is essential to the phagocytosis process and for bone strength.

Calcium magnesium caprylate is known to kill intestinal fungi, such as *Candida albicans,* while not inhibiting the good bacteria.

Choline, also known as lipotropic factor, is useful to the liver and helps mental function. Found in lecithin.

Cobalt also helps white blood cells.

Coenzyme Q12 supplements may help to boost cellular energy; lower levels are found in diseased tissue and older people.

Vitamin E, also known as tocopherol is a powerful antioxidant, particularly useful to combat fatigue, support the immune system, and improve skin tone. It is thought to boost cell-mediated immunity. Vitamin E deficiency is linked to cirrhosis and poor metabolism of fats.

Its role as a reducer of oxidative stress and the potential significance of this to patients with HCV has attracted the attention of researchers in the Department of Medicine at the University of California. They claim to have clear evidence that it prevents molecular changes that are associated with the development of cirrhosis. They summarized the results of one study as follows:

> This study provides insights into the molecular mechanisms of fibrogenesis as well as potential therapeutic approaches for patients with chronic hepatitis C.

A recent German study of the impact of high-dose IV vitamin E (2 × 400 IU alpha-tocopherol/day) on hepatitis C patients undergoing interferon therapy clearly established that liver enzymes were significantly improved by concurrent supplementation.[1] The authors suggested that it should be offered more widely as supportive therapy.

Folic acid is an important vitamin whose levels may be reduced if liver function is impaired. It is essential to the production of red blood cells, protein metabolism, and the use of amino acids and sugars. It may be a particularly good supplement during drug therapy and if consuming alcohol. It is closely interlinked with vitamin B_{12} and PABA; if taking a lot of vitamin C, it is advisable to also increase folic acid. The latest research into Alzheimer's disease suggests that folic acid supplementation just might reduce the likelihood of developing this condition. It is found in leafy vegetables such as kale and spinach.

Germanium sesquioxide (not germanium oxide) is a controversial mineral believed by some to have powerful therapeutic properties. Japanese researchers have advocated its use in HIV. Findings include immune modulation, homeostasis (i.e., balancing of the body functions), and analgesia. Banned in the U.K. after a misleading anti-health-fraud campaign, it is present in garlic and Siberian ginseng.

Glucosamine is needed to make glycoproteins that protect the gut wall. Believed to help lactic bacteria in the gut and to block the proliferation of harmful species.

Inositol helps to support liver function and metabolizes fats.

Iodine may be useful because HCV patients are prone to thyroid problems. Kelp is a good source.

Vitamin K deficiency is associated with liver disease. Live yogurt is a good source. Poor blood clotting is a symptom of deficiency.

L-glutamine is advocated by some nutritionists to heal ulceration and help with "leaky gut" syndrome.

Magnesium levels may be depressed if digestion is poor.

Manganese helps white blood cells ingest and destroy toxins. Supplements may help to address muscle weakness, a symptom of HCV.

MSM (methyl-sulfanyl methane) is a natural form of organic sulfur thought to benefit cell development. MSM has been used by vets for many years, often to treat joint problems in horses. It is thought to have been helpful by some patients.

Niacin will help to promote a healthy digestive system.

Potassium works with sodium to regulate the body's water balance. If you are taking diuretics to address fluid retention problems, then this might be useful. Good diuretics such as Fu Ling and dandelion leaf contain potassium.

Selenium is an extremely important mineral that plays a role in a number of processes that are important to the body's ability to manage viral infections, such as HCV.

- It works with glutathione and is vital in the maintenance of normal immune function.

- It inhibits the oxidation of lipids (see "Fats" section in chapter 22), which will be particularly important in the management of fats by the liver.

- It has a specific role in the prevention of tumor development.

- It is strongly epidemiologically linked to the ability to combat viruses. Populations with deficiencies suffer from high levels of particular diseases.

- Selenium may support impaired thyroid function (hypothyroidism), which is quite common in HCV patients, particularly those undergoing interferon therapy)

- It has been found to protect the liver in cases of alcoholic cirrhosis.

Its presence in foods varies widely due to soil differences. Some parts of the U.K. and the U.S. have low levels in soil; chemical farming may be a cause of further lower levels in food. Thus the likelihood of needing supplements will vary. Signs of deficiency include dry skin, dandruff, cataracts, and fatigue. Organic garlic is a good source. Supplements can be combined with vitamin E, zinc, and NAC or glutathione for maximum impact. Excessive levels lead to a sense of lassitude, which may be confused with "brain fog," hair loss, and indigestion.

Ethan Taylor, a molecular biologist, has done a lot of work on selenium; visit his Website at www.rx.uga.edu for further information.

Superoxide dismutase is a powerful cellular antioxidant.

Zinc has an important role in the regulation of the immune system and the management of a large number of body processes. It can help to counteract irregular menses. Deficiency may be associated with liver disease.

In addition there are some preparations that are suitable for patients. These include "Reduced Glutathione" and "Hep 194" produced by Biocare.

Food Supplements and Miscellaneous Substances

Alpha-lipoic acid is an important and versatile antioxidant that enhances the functions of vitamins C and E and glutathione and may therefore be supportive of liver function.

Bromelain is a protein-digesting extract of pineapple; it may counteract food allergy and intolerance.

Chlorella is a unicellular microalga. Much hyped by the natural health care community, it is regarded as an excellent low-calorie source of numerous micronutrients. It is a rich source of vitamins, minerals, and amino and fatty acids. It may be particularly useful to vegetarians because it contains some nutrients, such as vitamin B_{12}, that may be deficient in this diet. It does contain a range of substances that are thought to be good for the immune system, the blood, and the liver, being particularly rich in detoxification agents. It is a good single source of nutrients. Chlorella varies in quality and price.

Colloidal minerals come in liquid form. The word "colloidal" refers to the presentation of the minerals in a form that is easily absorbed by the gut and utilized by the body. Most preparations are derived from ancient plant matter deposits. If you believe in the "overfed but undernourished" analysis of contemporary diet or want to address possible mineral deficiency, then this supplement may be a good option.

Colloidal silver has been touted as a natural antibiotic with activity against viruses as well as fungi and bacteria, which can be safely consumed indefinitely. The sales pitch is that this substance disables the oxygen metabolism of all single-celled pathogens. Long-term use can cause argyria, an unpleasant and dangerous condition characterized by silver salt deposits in internal organs, eyes, and skin. Consult a reputable practitioner prior to use.

Essential fatty acids: See chapter 22, pages 391–393.

Grapefruit seed extract is currently regarded as a good natural treatment for candidiasis by Dr. Leo Galland, a practitioner specializing in intestinal diseases. It is also regarded as being safe.

Kelp is a great cheap source of minerals, including iodine. However, it contains a lot of sodium and should be avoided by patients on a low-salt diet.

Kombuchka tea mushroom has been used by some patients in London. It looks like a prop from a David Cronenburg film—a large fleshy pale mushroom. It is floated on a blend of ordinary tea and sugar in a bowl, which it somehow processes into a drink with a number of supposed medical qualities.

Patients' reactions are varied. It is traditionally used by middle-aged and elderly people in Central and Eastern Asia. It may benefit older patients more than the younger group of patients who tried it. Some safety issues have still not been resolved.

Caution: Hepatotoxicity has been reported. This mushroom acts like a sponge, and this may be explained by the absorption of toxins from other sources. Airborne pollutants may become concentrated in this preparation.

Lecithin is a type of phospholipid that helps to protect liver cells and may prevent "fatty liver."

Linseed oil is a good source of essential fatty acids and anti-inflammatory agents. It may be useful to patients with colon problems and those at risk of thrombosis.

Liver extracts from animals, typically pigs or cattle, are sometimes recommended by dietary practitioners

Para-aminobenzoic acid (PABA) is an important antioxidant and constituent of folic acid, a deficiency of which may cause depression, fatigue, and indigestion.

Papain is a protein-digesting extract of papaya fruit that helps digestion.

Probiotics and **ecobiotics** are terms used to describe products containing active intestinal flora. They come as powders or in capsule form, and are literally living bacteria such as *Lactobacillus acidophilus, Bifidobacterium bifidum,* and *Lactobacillus thermophilus* plus, in some cases, nutrients that support these organisms. The object is to restore a healthy balance of bacteria within the gut. Practitioners such as Leon Chaitow specifically link a healthy balance of intestinal flora with better absorption of foods, reduced liver toxicity (linked to "leaky gut" syndrome), and a reduced risk of autoimmune disease (such as rheumatoid arthritis). In conjunction with dietary therapy probiotics can help to cure conditions such as Crohn's disease and candidiasis that affect many HCV patients.

Pycnogenol is an extract of pine bark and is thought to be a powerful and easily utilized antioxidant that also supports tissue repair and may inhibit histamine production, which is linked to inflammation. However, lowered levels of histamine may correlate to poor response to interferon-based therapy,[2] so avoid if on this treatment. Like grape seed extract, pycnogenol is classed as an oligomeric proanthocyanidin.

Shark cartilage is thought to contain substances that inhibit the development of new blood vessels. It has been touted as an anticancer agent and is used as a general supplement by some patients. It has also been suggested that it may help arthritis and other inflammatory conditions. It is rich in calcium and phosphorous. Read labels carefully as some products contain other ingredients; shark cartilage should be white.

Spirulina, sea or **lake plankton** are very rich in nutrients. However, these are often grown in uncontrolled conditions, which may be the reason for a few patients having reported adverse reactions.

Tibetan yogurt culture, also known as **kefir,** has been used by a number of patients. This is a "do it yourself" medicinal yogurt culture from Tibet. One simply pours milk over it and drains it off twenty-four hours later; it is then drunk, usually last thing at night. Detailed instructions come with it; it is passed from person to person informally and is free. It doubles in size every twenty days or so. It resembles soggy cauliflower heads. It is used to treat hepatitis, liver cancer, and as a general health tonic in Tibet and has been around in Europe for some time. Some patients who have tried it have found it to be useful; others report no benefits. Most note that it results in healthy weight gain and a sense of relaxation. It is claimed that it boosts the immune system; helps the heart, liver, pancreas, and spleen; cleanses the digestive system; heals inflammation; cures kidney problems; prevents cancer; and acts as an antidepressant!!! (Note that these aren't my claims—just those that come with the instructions.) It is unsuitable for people with a milk allergy.

Tissue salt CALC SUL 6X is recommended by Peter de Ruyter; dissolve 1 tab, three times per day.

Wheatgrass is another very rich source of vitamins, minerals, and trace elements. Wheatgrass or its juice is sometimes prescribed in radical dietary therapy, particularly for cancer.

Amino Acid Therapy and Hepatitis C

Amino acids are the building blocks of protein—without protein life cannot be sustained. The liver plays a vital role in assimilating amino acids; poor function can adversely affect overall levels, although the cause of deficiency may be more complex in HCV patients.

Amino acid therapy is a new branch of medicine, and it is founded on the belief that some individuals or sections of the population have imbalanced amino acid profiles that are associated with ill health. The aim of therapy is the correction of these imbalances. Some amino acid deficiencies are thought to have very serious consequences. It appears that HCV patients constitute a group with a serious pattern of deficiency; therefore, in the eyes of therapists, they are likely to achieve significant improvements in their immediate health or prognosis if the imbalance can be corrected.

N-Acetyl Cysteine (NAC)

NAC is a popular supplement that is frequently used by people with hepatitis C. Some patients report definite subjective benefit, and it is generally regarded as a safe supplement with a greater prospect of benefit coupled with minimal chances of adverse effect. However, the situation with regard to clinical need and efficacy of action is still obscure. Here are some findings and speculations about NAC.

During the course of researching this book I came across some interesting material that appears to demonstrate that interferon therapy has significantly improved biochemical results when combined with NAC.[3] The small study that caught my attention was carried out at the Department of Internal Medicine at the University of Navarra, Pamplona, in Spain. NAC (600 mg) was administered daily to fourteen patients who had not responded to interferon despite taking it for four months. This combination of therapy for a further five to six months resulted in complete normalization of ALT levels in 41% of these previously unresponsive patients—a result that clearly bucks the trend. All patients demonstrated a steady reduction in ALT levels. The results were published in August 1993.

The author concluded that "NAC enhances the response to interferon in chronic hepatitis C. Controlled studies are needed to ascertain whether antioxidant therapy might act in synergy with interferon in chronic viral hepatitis."

There are two properties of NAC that are of interest with regard to hepatitis C:

- It is hepatoprotective.
- It has been shown to counter glutathione deficiency and is an antioxidant.

These properties may be interlinked. NAC is a "glutathione precursor." This means that when NAC is assimilated by human beings it is metabolized and converted into glutathione. Thus the ingestion or injection of NAC leads to higher levels of glutathione.

Glutathione is a "nonessential amino acid" with powerful therapeutic properties. It is described chemically as a tripeptide comprising the amino acids cysteine, glutamic acid, and glycine. It is the major intracellular damage limiting agent. As such it plays a leading role in the process of detoxification. It is essential for life and helps cells to produce energy. These properties are reflected in its typical use as an antidote to paracetamol poisoning, which may cause liver failure if untreated.

Glutathione may also be an immunomodulator—in other words, it may activate killer lymphocytes. This could be very important for HCV patients. As we have seen in the first part of this book, HCV is an extremely subtle and changeable virus that appears to be able to elude immune system detection and response. It is for this reason that it has been used in HIV treatments and is popular with that community of patients

Glutathione levels within cells are associated with healthy immune responses. Hence NAC may confer its hepatoprotective properties by raising levels of glutathione within liver cells. Deficiency is somewhat difficult to quantify, there being a number of different levels one could measure. In the case of HCV patients, levels of glutathione within liver cells would be a key indicator. These have not yet been adequately measured. The situation is further complicated by the fact that glutathione levels may be influenced by environmental and lifestyle factors as well as viral infection.

Whether or not HCV patients are consistently deficient in glutathione, and therefore generally indicated for supplementation, is a question that has yet to be satisfactorily answered. The research carried out in Pamplona established that HCV patients in the trial had reduced levels of glutathione in plasma compared to unaffected controls. Another well-known hepatology consultant has confirmed to me that many HCV patients have "severely depressed" levels of glutathione. However, the picture is still not entirely clear; one recent Swiss study showed that plasma levels were acceptable in a small population of HCV patients.

The question of deficiency within liver cells is critical because it plays a vital role in supporting the liver's detoxification and self-defense processes. Its presence is associated with the reduction of hyperoxides, which cause damage to cells and genetic structures. Conversely if glutathione levels are severely depressed, the liver's ability to protect itself from damage and to eliminate toxins is reduced;

thus HCV patients, already subject to liver damage, would be less able to deal with the ongoing stress and more vulnerable to serious hepatic injury.

Research into NAC

NAC has been explored as an antiviral therapy in its own right for HIV patients, who have been found to be deficient in levels of glutathione in blood cells. An important general finding was that NAC was generally well tolerated and regarded as a nontoxic form of treatment. Absence of side effects will be appealing to those who wish to avoid these side effects or for whom interferon is contraindicated.

The Stanford NAC Study, a report that was published in March 1997 [*Proceedings of the National Academy of Sciences, USA.* Herzenberg et al. 94(5):1967–1972] is the most important study of NAC to date. The key findings were that a low level of glutathione was strongly associated with diminished survival in AIDS and that oral NAC improved levels of glutathione within blood cells. Earlier findings indicating limited effectiveness were discredited and found to be based in methodologically flawed study design.

Furthermore it was discovered that the survival difference was large, with 60–80% of the high-glutathione, NAC-taking group surviving for longer than three years and less than 20% of the low-glutathione group surviving this long.

Research by Clotat [Effects on surrogate markers of IV NAC in AIDS patients. Eighth International AIDS Conference, Amsterdam, abstract PoB 3013, 1992] is interesting. Using 3,000 mg of NAC diluted in 500 ml of 5% glucose infusion administered over one hour during fifteen days, he appeared to achieve an antiviral effect.

Ho has found that NAC has a powerful antiviral effect on HIV in vitro [Glutathione and NAC suppression of HIV replication in human monocyte/macrophages in vitro. Ho WZ et al. *AIDS Res and Human Retrovir,* 8:1249–1253, 1992].

Its value as an antioxidant and free radical scavenger is further confirmed by the findings of Italian researchers experimenting on some unfortunate mice:

NAC significantly improved survival during the six days following sepsis induction and caused lower liver toxicity. These results suggest that NAC works as a direct antioxidant and scavenger of free radicals generated from other sources.[4]

NAC may be of particular interest to those concerned about the carcinogenic properties of HCV. (All cirrhotic patients take note.) Leon Chaitow in his book *Amino Acids in Therapy* reports that trials into the use of glutathione as a cancer regression agent have demonstrated clear cut results. In rats exposed to the chemical aflatoxin B (see page 370–371), which would usually produce 100% liver cancer development, 80% were still alive and well after two years where they were also administered glutathione. [*Science*, 179; 588–591, 1973].

Dutch cancer researchers reach similar conclusions:

> This implies that carcinogenic compounds can initiate tumor growth only in amounts saturating detoxification mechanisms. In this context it is well known that glutathione plays a crucial role in the detoxification of xenobiotics (poisons). NAC, an aminothiol and precursor of intracellular cysteine and glutathione, has been shown to possess important preventative properties.[5]

Since HCV patients with significant liver damage are vulnerable to liver cancer, it seems to be possible that benefit would be obtained by taking NAC or other glutathione-boosting agents on a regular basis.

NAC may also be of particular benefit to patients who drink alcohol; according to Leon Chaitow:

> Alcohol-produced damage of the liver is thought to be prevented in several ways by glutathione. In the first place there is the actual reduction of hydroperoxides, prior to their attacking saturated lipids, as well as the conversion of lipid hydroperoxides into harmless hydroxy compounds.[6]

For further information about the role of amino acids in detoxification, refer to pages 378–379.

Dosage and a Note of Caution

- The recommended dose is 500–600 mg 3 times per day with food, preferably taken with vitamin C; some recommend taking selenium and zinc with NAC as well.

- NAC may aggravate stomach ulcers

- It should be taken with food, not before it, according to Mark Lands, a well-known nutritionist.

- If the liver is severely damaged or toxic, consult a specialist practitioner. If in any doubt, take glutathione instead. This is because under these circumstances the liver may be unable to convert NAC into glutathione. Instead the unconverted NAC may inhibit a substance called NF kappa B, which in turn would reduce levels of T cells, a highly undesirable effect.[7]

- Diabetics on insulin should consult their doctor before taking cysteine supplements.

- Metabolism of NAC may "use up" minerals, particularly zinc and copper; therefore mineral supplementation may be advisable if taking NAC.

- Recent research suggests that bovine thymic extracts can also boost levels of glutathione.

Other Amino Acids That May Be Useful to HCV Patients

Lysine is thought to play a role in viral control. Fatigue, indigestion, dizziness, and anemia may be signs of deficiency. It has been shown to be very helpful to people with the herpes virus.

Methionine is a powerful detoxification agent and will help to clear heavy metals from the liver. It is included in many liver nutrient packages. It works with cysteine and selenium to combat free radicals and is particularly useful in combating the adverse effects of alcohol. Deficiency of methionine has been linked to fatty liver conditions and low levels of choline. S-adenosyl methionine is also reported to be good for repairing the liver and increasing intracellular glutathione levels.

Tryptophan can help symptoms of liver inflammation, insomnia, depression, and obesity. It is linked to serotonin levels in the brain and is contained in many carbohydrate foods. Some reckon that the poor dietary habits noted in some people suffering from depression may be linked to a craving for serotonin-boosting foods. It is thought to be potentially dangerous in high doses and is not available on its own, but can be obtained through general amino acid supplements.

A new product called L-5-hydroxytryptophan is now available; it is reported to be useful in the treatment of sleeplessness and depression related to low levels of serotonin in the brain. Also called 5-HTP, it is derived from a small African bean, *Griffonia simplicifolia*. Avoid if it is mixed with valerian.

Proline is linked to the health of connective tissue and joints, and therefore may be useful to patients with rheumatoid arthritis.

Taurine helps gallbladder function and maintains the ability to digest fats.

Glutamine and **glutamic acid** is regarded as a "brain fuel" and may help with concentration problems. It may help patients with blood sugar irregularities—hypoglycemia—and is also thought to protect against the effects of alcohol.

Glycine helps in liver detoxification and reduction of free radicals.

Amino acid supplements are best consumed following meals, particularly nonprotein foods. Another way of taking amino acids is to consume supplements such as **chlorella,** which are packed with both essential and nonessential amino acids, vitamins, and minerals. Because these products are foods in themselves, they can be eaten on their own and digested without the risk of competition from other foods. There are anecdotal reports that hepatitis C patients with patterns of liver-spleen deficiency (symptoms such as indigestion and loose stool) derive particular benefit from consuming chlorella.

Patient's Experience of Supplements: José

I'm approaching two months of selenium therapy and feeling better all the time; I'm taking about 800 mcg per day. I know a lady in Texas, Sue, who has been taking it for over six months.

She has reported increased energy levels and all of her levels—viral load, liver enzymes—are low. . . . The most remarkable effect for me was the clearing of psoriasis in less than two months (I had psoriasis for more than seven years) and the normalization of T3 hormone, thereby getting rid of a number of symptoms including hypoglycemia. The arthritis has also improved.

Note that both José and Sue were also taking vitamins E and B_6 and NAC.

Contacts

In the U.S. **Direct AIDS Alternative Information Resources** has been suggested as a good source of food supplements (see Resources for further U.S. contacts).

In the U.K. some of these products can be difficult to find. Some contacts are as follows:

For colloidal minerals, call **Lydia** at 0181 678 9589.

For chlorella, try **Emerald Life** at 0181 674 2722.

For NAC, try **East West Herbs** at 0171 379 1312.

For a comprehensive selection of vitamins, call **The Nutricentre** (in the Hale Clinic) at 0171 436 5122.

Further Reading

Prescription for Nutritional Healing. James Balch and Phyllis Balch. Avery Publishing Group, 1993.

References

1. Vitamin E improves the aminotransferase status of patients suffering from viral hepatitis C: a randomized, double-blind, placebo-controlled study. von Herbay A et al. *Free Radic Res,* 27(6):599–605, Dec 1997.

2. Histamine and the response to IFN-alpha in chronic hepatitis C. Hellstrand K et al. *J Interferon Cytokine Res,* 18(1):21–22, Jan 1998.

3. NAC enhances the response to interferon alpha in chronic hepatitis C: a pilot study. *Journal of Interferon Research,* 13(4):279–82, 1993.

4. Effect of NAC on sepsis in mice. *European Journal of Pharmacology*, 292(3–4):341–4, Mar 1995.

5. NAC for lung cancer prevention. van Zandwijk et al. *Chest*, 107 (5):1437–44, May 1995.

6. *Amino Acids in Therapy*. Chaitow L. Thorsons, p 90, 1985.

7. Antioxidants inhibit stimulation of HIV transcription. Staal FJ. *AIDS Research and Human Retroviruses*, (4):299–306.

19

Homeopathy and Hepatitis C

HOMEOPATHY IS AN IMPORTANT and widely accessible alternative medical system. Unlike Traditional Chinese Medicine it does not work well in conjunction with conventional "allopathic" medicine. In the introduction to the book *Homeopathy: The Potent Force of the Minimum Dose* by Keith Scott (Thorsons), it is described as "... treating diseases with remedies which are capable of producing symptoms similar to the disease in question." Allopathic medicine usually treats disease with remedies that produce effects opposite to, or different from, those of the disease. Therefore the two principles are in direct contrast to each other and do not mix well.

The term "homeopathy" is derived from two ancient Greek words: *homois* meaning similar and *pathos* meaning suffering. The maxim often used by homeopathic practitioners is *"Cembalo similibus curentur"* which is Latin for "Let likes be treated by likes." In the foreword to the same book Dr. George Lewith summarizes homeopathic principles and practice as follows:

> Biological systems respond in a very marked way to small changes in their environment. Homeopathy has capitalized on this simple principle by using such small changes to activate and harness the body's own healing potential. Homeopathy's strength is its evident effectiveness. Its weakness is a lack of scientific evidence to support its mechanism of action, and a dearth of clear statistical data evaluating its efficacy.

Gareth James of the HEAL Trust has extensive experience in the treatment of HIV, HBV, and HCV patients. Like a number of other alternative medicine practitioners he challenges the somewhat military language used to describe the dis-ease process. Instead of regarding HCV as an invading alien, something which we "have," he views hepatitis C as a process. He feels that the language is important, particularly because he notices that many of his patients have become scared by verbal constructs employed by their doctors (viruses as invaders, pharmaceutical drugs as armory, T-cells as defenders, etc). James thinks that this fear may contribute to stress, which is extremely undesirable and a probable cofactor in disease progression. He thinks that it is both more accurate and more helpful to focus on the patient, emphasizing that symptoms are individual reactions to the presence of a pathogen, and that these reactions can be modified. He describes the homeopathic approach as follows:

> This model views the body as the finely tuned end product of millions of years of evolution and credits the constitution with intelligence and knowledge far exceeding our own modish scientific trends and fashions. It considers symptoms—which by definition imply a prior cause—to be an intelligent statement indicating where that individual has become diseased or "stuck." Homeopathy defines health as the ability to constantly adjust to changes within ourselves and our environment. Chronic disease is defined as the inability to adjust to such changes and thus symptoms are considered to be expressions of resistance to change....
>
> In this model microbes are actively employed by the constitution in an attempt to re-adjust and recover. So, rather than viewing microbes as the cause of disease, homeopathy suggests that microbes only "effect" symptoms when the organism is already diseased at some level, so rather than prescribe a drug to contradict the intentions of the system, it would give a remedy to assist and resolve the process.
>
> In this sense we prompt a change in reality. If chronic illness indicates resistance to change, and acute illness is an attempt to get better, with microbes being part and parcel of this phe-

nomenon, then they cease to be the enemy. The need to stamp the intruders out with chemical warfare is lost, and all the military metaphors fall away, becoming redundant misconceptions.

Homeopathic remedies usually consist of small white pills containing minute traces of a substance reckoned by the practitioner to be suited to the individual nature of the patient. These remedies are prescribed individually. The practitioner will usually spend at least half an hour with a new patient running through all kinds of questions about personality, background, likes, dislikes, affinities, and aversions. Once the patient has been classified according to his or her responses, the homeopathic materia medica can be consulted, which will usually suggest an appropriate remedy, selected for its symptom-producing potential. The practitioner will determine the correct potentiation of the remedy—the lower the trace of the substance, the more powerful the effect—based on his or her experience. In this respect the hepatitis C patient will be treated in exactly the same way as anyone else.

Homeopathy is thought to work as an energy level therapy, like acupuncture. However, homeopathy aims to create a particular energetic resonance by reaction, while acupuncture seeks to adjust energy flow within the patient. Practitioners will adjust treatment on a dynamic basis, attempting to be sensitive to every aspect of the patient's condition. For instance, a patient presenting with post-diagnostic shock might be prescribed a remedy based on Arsenicum album, which is known to cause shock and anxiety, the intention being to induce calm and balance.

Longer-term treatment may be related to three standard homeopathic classes of condition: *Inflammation; Liver and inflammation; Liver, chronic.*

Chelidonium and Carduus-mar are often employed as general organ support treatments. Specific liver-related remedies often include Lycopodium, Mercury, Natrum sulph, and Nitric ac. Where drug or other toxic liver condition is suspected as well as hep C, Nux vomica and Phosphorus may be prescribed.

Some homeopaths prescribe nosodes to hep C patients. Nosodes are remedies that are usually made from tissue infected with the pathogen that is being treated. Again they are potentized, meaning that there is only the faintest energetic trace in the medicine. There is no question of any live genetic material being present in a nosode.

Some HCV patients have received nosodes derived from the thymus gland as well as ones made from liver tissue. This indicates that some homeopaths are now cognizant of hepatitis C pathology and may adapt treatment to target key organs. They are usually prescribed to patients who have not yet developed serious symptoms. This is the only respect in which treatment for hepatitis C patients differs from that of other patients. These treatments aim to provoke a more active immune response.

There are a number of new homeopathic products in the market that appear to be designed to meet the needs of HCV patients. There are some "homeopathic interferon" products and, in Italy, even an HCV antiviral preparation from a company named Vanda called "HCV Anti-Virus."

Another product that employs the homeopathic principle is DNCB, which stands for dinitrochlorobenzene. (DNCB has been used by HIV patients for a number of years; some HIV patients believe that this medicine has helped them enormously and have pointed to log drops in their viral load to substantiate their claims.) The crystalline substance is dissolved in various strengths of acetone, which are then applied to a small patch of skin. The purpose is to provoke a significant immune response—the skin becoming red and itchy is interpreted as a good sign. The idea is that the DNCB is picked up by immune cells that migrate to nearby lymph nodes, in turn provoking a proliferation of CD4 T-helper cells, which then initiate a cell-mediated immune response. Other elements of the immune system are activated in the attempt to rid the body of the DNCB antigen; it is theorized that in the process other infected cells are also dealt with.

The key point made by supporters of this approach is that pathogens such as HCV usually exist within cells, including immune cells themselves, such as lymphocytes. Thus, in a situation where immune cells themselves can act as reservoirs, the only effective approach is logically confined to enhancing intracellular antiviral activity. This line of thought leads back to the homeopathic view of chronic infection by a pathogen as an immunological disorder as opposed to a virological disorder.

Homeopathic treatments tend to be more suitable for patients who are drug and alcohol free and eat healthy diets. Patients who are "clean living" report that remedies can have a powerful impact, particularly on the immune system, where they may precipitate autoimmune symptoms.

Homeopathy can be regarded as a long-term health management strategy that may or may not help to prevent the onset of severe symptoms. Patients' experience of the impact of homeopathy on hepatitis C is very difficult to assess. Most have used homeopathy for general health management for years prior to diagnosis. There are some anecdotal reports of homeopathic patients testing sero negative after treatment.

Contacts

DNCB information can be obtained from the **DNCB Treatment Group** in San Francisco (telephone: 415-954-8896) or the **HEAL Trust** in London (telephone: 0181 265 3989).

20

Miscellaneous Treatments for Hepatitis C

Aromatherapy and Essential Oils

Aromatherapy can offer general symptomatic relief. One specific treatment likely to be suggested to patients is the aromatherapeutic lymphatic drainage massage. This is consistently reported to be a very pleasurable experience regardless of clinical impact. It is likely that the sense of relaxation it is reported to induce will be beneficial to the immune system. Patients with lymphatic-system-related symptoms may be particularly attracted to this approach. If lymphoma has already developed, this approach must be strictly avoided.

The prescription of essential oils, either in massage, added to baths, or heated to create particular aromas (vaporized), is closely linked to herbal medicine. An experienced practitioner should be consulted as some of these oils exert powerful effects. Oils specifically indicated for liver congestion include carrot seed, celery seed, helichrysum, linden, rose, camomile, lavender, frankincense, calendula, Spanish sage, turmeric, and lemon verbena. Juniper and rosemary are recommended for cirrhosis.

A specific treatment for liver inflammation consists of alternating hot and cold compresses on the liver area. Compresses are prepared by filling a bowl with very hot water, to which an essential oil is then added. A towel is then dipped into the water and applied to the liver area in alternation with an ice-cold water-immersed towel.

Castor oil is also used for direct liver compresses by some practitioners.

Several patients have reported that they find clary sage, ylang ylang, and lavender particularly helpful for stress relief and PMS.

Colonics

This approach to treatment is secondary. It includes enema, the use of lower bowel cleansing herbal regimes, and colonic irrigation. Conditions such as irritable bowel syndrome, bowel diseases such as Crohn's, and liver toxicity may be helped by this approach. In addition some patients have reported that the common symptoms of "brain fog" and frequent headaches may be significantly eased by colonics. This is interesting because the colon is linked to the brain in TCM. Laxatives are used to treat encephalopathy in Western medicine.

Practitioners of colonics link the presence of bowel problems such as "leaky gut" syndrome and coeliac disease to impaired liver function. They reason that if the bowel can be cleansed and the gut wall helped to heal, then fewer toxins will leak from the gut into the blood, whence they are transported to the liver.

In general there is a distinction between retention enemas, which should be retained for about fifteen minutes and are thought to support liver cleansing, and cleansing enemas, which are retained for only a few minutes and are used for colon health. Coffee retention enemas are reported to have a powerful impact and can also eliminate excess iron. Some people prefer using chamomile instead of coffee because it is "gentler."

When preparing enemas, use unprocessed ingredients (e.g., coffee beans, not granulated instant coffee) and distilled water. Prepare as a hot tea, filter, and allow to cool. Health stores and pharmacies sometimes stock kits.

Dry Brushing

Dry brushing is recommended by some practitioners for lymphatic health maintenance. The technique usually involves first taking a bath with Epsom salts. After getting out of the bath the technique is to brush the body from all extremities in turn toward the heart.

Osteopathy and Cranial Osteopathy

Osteopathy and cranial osteopathy have been reported to be helpful. Both of these therapies warrant further investigation.

Ozone Therapy

This approach has been consistently reported to have a positive impact upon symptoms. However, posttherapy relapse is also reported to be very common. Some practitioners are now offering patients a treatment wherein their blood is directly oxygenated and reinjected; this is supposed to have an antiviral effect. Such a treatment is unlikely to reach many HCV reservoirs.

21

Hepatitis C and Naturopathy:
The "No Treatment" Option

IT IS CLEAR THAT a significant number of people diagnosed as having hepatitis C choose not to have treatment. For some this will be a result of taking the view that it is not a serious illness, an impression that was widely promoted in the early '90s. For others it will be the result of a conscious decision. Armed with the facts about hepatitis C, it is perfectly reasonable to decide not to take treatment or to defer the decision. There is much to be gained by simply making the lifestyle changes outlined in the next part of the book. The following lines of thinking are quite common.

Approach 1: Waiting for Better Treatments
to Emerge or Further Clarification of the Efficacy
of Those That Are Currently Available

Given the fact that many HCV treatments are still in the early stages of development, it is reasonable to decide to wait until the picture becomes clearer. This option is obviously more attractive to patients who are not yet experiencing severe symptoms or who feel that they are unlikely to develop them.

The current picture is one of disappointing success rates coupled with significant side effects in conventional medicine. It is reasonable to expect that better drugs will appear in the future. While Traditional Chinese Medicine can be shown to have benefited a proportion of patients, its long-term impact on the course of illness is still unclear, availability is uneven, and it can require hard work on the part of patients. Some Western herbs are good for the treatment of particular ailments, but their application to HCV as a whole has not yet been properly thought through. Homeopathy is very difficult to assess. Other complementary and alternative treatments are beginning to tentatively address hepatitis C, but they are still in the early stages of understanding what it is that they are treating.

Approach 2: Having Other Priorities

Because hepatitis C is primarily a chronic illness, patients with another pressing health problem often choose to address that first. For instance, patients with severe drug or alcohol problems quite rightly regard these as being a more immediate threat to their well-being than HCV. In other words hepatitis C is not necessarily a patient's primary health concern. Much depends upon one's individual situation.

Naturopathy

Naturopathy could be described as a tradition of health care that excludes intervention of any kind. The body is regarded as a self-regulating mechanism whose health is best maintained by a good diet and appropriate exercise. It is defined as "a system of preserving health by means of a simple diet, regular exercise and the avoidance of drugs or anything that seems artificial" *(The Penguin Medical Encyclopedia)*. The closest it comes to treatment is the adoption of restrictive diets, particular forms of exercise such as the adoption of certain yoga positions, and the practice of fasting. Diet and exercise are covered in the relevant chapters.

Fasting

Caution: Some hepatologists are extremely antagonistic to the idea of fasting; some believe that the liver may deteriorate as a result of deprivation of nutrients for a day or more. They are particularly concerned about the effect of a lack of protein. Their advice to HCV patients is usually "Don't even consider it." Others note that fasting is common practice in some countries with very high rates of HCV prevalence—Egypt for instance—and are quite open-minded.

Some HCV patients who are committed to natural health care undertake regular fasts and obviously feel that they are beneficial. If you are considering trying fasting, it is important to obtain the advice of a reputable practitioner and to start with a short one, say twenty-four hours or thirty-six hours maximum. Fasting is best avoided if you have a history of eating disorders or serious liver disease.

Naturopathy is particularly associated with the Ayurvedic traditional health system of India, where the practice of fasting is reckoned to have physical, mental, and spiritual benefits. Fasting actually has nothing to do with diet—it is seen as a method of treatment. Long fasts are sometimes undertaken, but they are closely supervised.

David Curtin, a prominent homeopath practicing at the Hale Clinic in London, reckons that most people can safely do a forty-eight-hour water-only fast. Some people cannot tolerate this, and they need to take fruit and vegetable juices. Others can fast for five days, although Curtin says that he would usually introduce juices and grapes after the first forty-eight hours. Asked what the benefits of fasting to patients were, he answered as follows:

> It rests the bowels and the whole digestive system including the liver and the pancreas. Often a good thing to do in conjunction with that is to use enemas. Colonic irrigation is even better. Coffee enemas can also be useful for detoxifying the liver. I'm sure that fasting has benefits for the immune system as well although precisely why I couldn't tell you. There is certainly some connection between the liver and the immune system. Also the immune system has to work when you eat because you are introducing substances into the body; the immune system has to make a decision about whether the substance is foreign and whether it needs to be attacked or not.

Michael Tierra, author of *The Way of Herbs* (Pocket Books, 1990), lists the following reasons for undertaking a fast:

- A way of becoming more sensitive to the body
- For a curative effect, especially with chronic ailments
- To lose excess weight or excess water
- To clean out accumulated wastes
- To free the blockages of energy flow in the body
- For longevity
- As a way of developing calmness, control and willpower

He goes on to discuss the concept of the "healing crisis":

> It is not uncommon with effective therapy that one seems to get worse before getting better. When the body is engaged in the elimination of toxins accumulated over the years, one may experience aches, pains, and symptoms of diseases, from the most recent to those of childhood. This is because the toxins are being liberated from their storage places and are now actively affecting the body with full force. This is the healing crisis.

A well-established fasting regime is as follows: Start the day with a glass of prune juice. Top up with small glasses of organic apple juice diluted 50:50 with purified water throughout the day. Use camomile enemas twice a day, more often if headaches become severe. Maintain the regime for up to four days. If this is your first fast, then stop after thirty-six hours. Break the fast with stewed apple sprinkled with cinnamon. The next couple of meals should consist of steamed vegetables, but avoid sulfur-rich varieties such as cabbage and broccoli. Incorporate carbohydrates and proteins last.

Headaches are common, particularly through the afternoon and evening of the first day. Apparently these are caused by the toxins that are being drained out of the body. The diluted organic apple juice is to maintain blood sugar and is reckoned to be good for detoxifying heavy metals, a particular problem for people living in cities.

Different practitioners will have varied regimes. For instance, many will recommend coffee enemas because these are supposed to be good for liver detoxification. (Incidentally, enema kits are available at some pharmacies.) Juicing is also recommended to hepatitis C patients by many natural health practitioners. A blend of organic carrot, beet, and lemon juices is a common liver detox recipe. However, carrot juice contains a lot of beta carotene, which is metabolized into vitamin A and may be bad for some patients (see chapter 18.)

Peter de Ruyter advises the "utmost caution" for liver disease patients contemplating fasting; he provides some guidelines and cautions:

1. Avoid "hard fasts" (just water); such regimes can result in a massive release of stored toxins into the bloodstream, which can overload an already struggling liver. Symptoms such as headaches can be easily confused with those of a "healing crisis."

2. Restrict the fast to one or two days at a time, particularly to begin with. Cleansing could also be promoted by adopting a diet of only rice, filtered spring water, plus freshly made diluted vegetable juices.

3. The best juices would be lettuce, broccoli, bell pepper, bok choy, celery, as well as small amounts of carrots. My personal view is not to mix fruit and vegetable juices together as there is some indication that this further stresses the digestive system.

'Juicing" may be a powerful and appropriate approach for some patients; refer to chapter 17, pages 314–315, for some recipes.

Liver-Cleansing Regimes Developed and Described by Dr. Stone

Cold-pressed olive oil with lemon is a cleanser for the liver. Cooked and fried oils are harmful.

Daily Breakfast

(No food to be taken with this morning cleanse.)

Mix 3–4 tablespoons of pure, cold-pressed almond, olive, or sesame seed oil, with 6–8 tablespoons (twice the amount) of fresh squeezed lemon juice (fresh ginger juice may be added to taste). Add fresh grapefruit, orange, or tangerine juice to taste. Liquefy with 3–6 cloves of garlic. Drink and follow with herbal tea containing licorice, anise, fennel, and fenugreek (simmered) and add peppermint and violet leaves.

If you are constipated: Add more licorice root and fresh garlic.

If you have diarrhea: Omit licorice, ginger, and the liver flush, but substitute cinnamon bark in the tea. Also try eating ground cinnamon with baked apples or dates and raisins or cinnamon cooked with rice or barley.

Also, chew citrus seeds, keeping in the mouth for at least fifteen minutes to gain the benefit of enzymes, vitamins, and minerals. The bitter essence is helpful to the liver and also helps to relieve the garlic odor, along with parsley or whole cloves.

A Patient's Experience of Fasting: Camillo

Camillo has been through the mill of conventional HCV treatment— an early participant in interferon trials, he had a particularly rough ride and did not have a sustained response. He has since used "natural" medicine and has become expert in its adaptation to hepatitis C. He fasts regularly for up to four days. This is his experience.

> The first afternoon and evening is the worst because of the headaches—the more toxins you have stored up, the more severe they are. My mental and emotional state is really up and down; you know, for the first and second days, I can become quite manic. On the third day I usually start to feel really good and can function quite well. On the fourth day I get quite high, sometimes hallucinating.
>
> I feel that I have definitely benefited from fasting. Before I used to feel really tired and sometimes had to spend days in bed. Along with using herbs and a balanced diet it has contributed towards me feeling much better.

Part

4

Lifestyle Issues

22

Diet, Alcohol, Drugs, and Environment

Diet and Digestion

DIET IS A VITAL but controversial issue. Divergent recommendations are handed out by various authorities on the subject, frequently resulting in a sense of confusion and despondency.

This chapter will outline the types of advice patients are likely to encounter and an explanation of the reasoning or lack of it that underlies the prescription. If any particular approach seems to make sense to you, then try it. Since there is no definitive hepatitis C diet, patients will often need to experiment to find one that suits.

Of all the facets of hepatitis C, diet is the one that really cuts through to the core of peoples' belief systems. It's a subject that goes right to the center of what any given culture believes to be good and wholesome, and its views on health and medicine usually conform to these beliefs regardless of the effects on the population. Experts often appear unwilling to condemn an aspect of diet that is linked to cultural identity, regardless of the impact on the health of their subjects.

Thus people who want to take diet seriously may have to wade through the superfluous cultural bias of nutritional recommendations before they can get to the core of what is likely to yield benefit and what is likely to cause damage.

It is important that both patients and dieticians appreciate that chronic hepatitis C is a dynamic condition associated with a number of divergent clinical profiles. Therefore there is no such thing as a "Hepatitis C Diet," and anyone who claims that there is, is clearly not conversant with the facts. A patient with normal liver enzymes and a good appetite will have very different requirements than one who is underweight and has cirrhosis of the liver.

There is a basic distinction between general dietary guidelines and the distinct field of radical dietary therapy, which may consist of lengthy monofasts or other such demanding regimes. It is essential not to adopt a radical dietary strategy without consulting your doctor or having a very clear awareness of your overall health status. Most HCV patients who do adopt strict diets have been working on themselves for some time previously and have gradually adopted the regimen. Such patients have a clear perception of what does and does not agree with them as individuals; they have usually gained this understanding through a process of experimentation.

Unhealthy diets rich in refined carbohydrates and sugars are common in newly diagnosed patients. It seems likely that a taste for these foods may be a response to feeling tired and depressed, and might represent an intuitive attempt to boost energy levels. For instance, many patients experience sudden "attacks" of fatigue and the ability to obtain a degree of relief by immediately eating confectionery, bananas, or drinking caffeine-based drinks laced with sugar. Long-term problems such as fluctuating body weight are classic indicators of liver disease. There are also a number of people who have adopted extremely strict health diets prior to their diagnosis, knowing that something was wrong, but being unable to identify the problem.

What follows is a summary of the dietary advice suggested by various medical and health practitioners together with patients' experiences of following these suggestions.

Traditional Dietary Advice

There are a dwindling number of dieticians who fall into this category. Basically they will not recommend any particular diet to hepatitis C patients beyond the balanced fare suggested to everyone else unless there is advanced liver disease. This approach evolved during the first half of the twentieth century against a background of widespread malnutrition or poorly balanced diets common throughout

Europe and North America at that time. Accompanied by technical advances in the fields of biochemistry and molecular biology, a "scientific" approach to nutrition was formulated. Processed food was still rare, additives were used sparingly, and food production methods were less intensive than they are today. The emphasis of this approach was to avoid deficiencies in the diet by ensuring that patients consumed all of the ingredients identified as being "essential" in sufficient quantities.

Little attention was paid to the question of whether or not ill health might be caused by excesses of certain foods. The increasing consumption of substances like sugar and salt was rarely acknowledged as a potential risk to health. Only a few dieticians became alarmed as the food and drink industry began to incorporate additives and agents into their products. Indeed increasing proportions of these "food scientists" were employed either directly or indirectly by such interest groups. Changes in the environment, such as urban air pollution, which affected vast numbers of people, were not considered to have any implications for human dietary requirements.

The "big eating" school of thought is exemplified by the Royal Free Hospital's dietary handout to liver patients, which offers the following advice.

> **Calories.** The liver plays an important role in energy metabolism, so if an individual with a liver condition does not eat enough calories, they will be more at risk from poor nutrition than someone whose liver is functioning well. Research has shown that in chronic liver injury there is less glycogen (short-term storage material) in the liver, that glycogen breakdown is reduced (the energy cannot be used so easily), and that there is an increased breakdown of protein and fat to provide energy (a process that actually wastes energy)....
>
> Make sure you are eating enough. If eating is becoming difficult try the following: Eat more of the foods you like; eat a variety of foods; eat frequently, three meals a day plus snacks; "little and often" may help; minimize restrictions; don't fill up on low calorie foods; tuck in, especially on better days; try supplement drinks (ask advice); don't despair—every mouthful helps, so keep eating....

Protein. Protein is necessary for many vital functions in the body. The liver has a unique role in protein metabolism and if it is not working properly this may be impaired. Some proteins, like albumin, prothrombin, and transferrin, are made only in the liver from amino acids derived from dietary protein. Cutting back on protein will result in insufficient of these building blocks being available to the liver for protein production. It has been shown that inadequate dietary protein causes hepatic necrosis and fibrosis in experimental animals....

It is important not to cut back on the amount of protein eaten and to try to eat a protein rich meal twice, if not three or four times a day.... Never reduce the protein in the diet or start a low protein diet unless you are following medical advice....

Vitamins and Minerals. We do not need to be too concerned about vitamins and minerals if we are eating well.... This does not mean that they are not extremely important in the diet and there may be some occasions when it is necessary to take extra vitamins and minerals as supplements....

Restrictions. It is the symptoms of liver disease [not the causes] that may be helped if certain foods are avoided or limited.... It makes sense therefore that if an individual does not have a particular symptom they will get no benefit from following a restricted diet. And so they should eat as normally as possible....

The thrust of this advice is therefore to carry on with a "normal" diet until an identified pattern of symptoms manifests that would necessitate restrictions. No mention is made of sugars, salts, fats, additives, medicinal drugs, processed foods, pesticide residues, and so on. Salt reduction is only prescribed after fluid retention has become obvious, low-protein diets are only recommended after encephalopathy has been diagnosed, and a reduction in fat intake is only suggested after steatorrhoea (inadequate bile production related to poor fat absorption) has become serious.

This is in stark contrast to natural medicine systems, such as TCM, where hepatitis progression is seen as a process whose potential characteristics are to be anticipated and treated before they appear. Symptoms are seen as being of more importance in these systems and are believed to amplify the power of the progression pattern; in this way cause and symptom are not seen as being entirely separate. Therefore a reduction in fat consumption, the use of cholagogues (bile stimulating), such as Oregon grape vine, and diuretics (flush out excess fluids), such as dandelion leaf, are all considered at an early stage in order to head off disease progression. By doing this practitioners seek to halt and then reverse the progression.

Thus the standard dietary advice given to HCV patients without advanced symptoms of liver disease typically consists of the following:

- Eat plenty of protein in the form of meat, eggs, cheese, or fish. Avoid a vegetarian diet.
- Balance this with vegetables, carbohydrates, and fruit.
- Fried foods and fatty foods are OK, but don't eat them all the time.
- Coffee and sugar are alright if taken in "sensible" amounts.
- There is no need to avoid processed foods or particular additives.

When patients mention alternative diets, they are often told that there is no evidence to support the recommendations. Patients are not told that this is usually because such research has not been carried out in the first place. Typical of the standard advice proffered to patients is contained in a patient information booklet produced by Roche:

> A normal healthy diet is perfectly appropriate for most people with hepatitis C. If you develop cirrhosis, your doctor may advise you to take a low salt diet to reduce fluid accumulation.[1]

Hepatologists are particularly concerned about cirrhotic patients who are underweight. Dr. David Patch had the following to say on the subject of nutrition and patients with advanced liver disease:

> Liver patients often have difficulty in keeping their weight up. One very important factor in building them up before a transplant is getting them to take enough calories. People tend to

lose weight in hospital anyway and hospital food doesn't usually tempt them to eat more. That's why we encourage them to take supplements and may resort to putting feeding tubes down into their stomachs. Of course a lot of patients complain about it, but it may be the only way to get down the 2,000/3,000 calories the patient needs.[2]

One exception to the general reluctance to advise restriction is shellfish. Because shellfish can sometimes harbor hepatitis A, which is known to be additionally hazardous, even potentially fatal to people with hepatitis C, some doctors and nutritionists do now advise patients to avoid them. What do biologists really think?

I recently went to a wedding where I got into a conversation with a molecular biologist working as a researcher for a major pharmaceutical company. He'd had quite a bit to drink. He had the following to say about organic food and pesticides:

> Look, mate, there's just billions of really nasty looking little mutant microbes out there. I spend all day looking at the little bastards down my microscope. Some of these f***ers are really vicious, man. I mean we make antibiotics out of these things and we screen out 9,999 out of 10,000 because they are absolutely deadly or we don't know what would happen if they got loose in the body. So I'd go for the sprayed fruit and vegetables every time. You eat organic and you really don't know what you're getting, I mean those tomatoes with the cobwebs on them, I wouldn't touch them. These guys who go on about organic food really don't know what they're talking about. . . .

The "eat your chemically controlled meat and two sprayed veg" school of thought is clearly alive and well!

A Note about Aflatoxins

Although many nutritionists appear to be unaware of the severe risks posed by aflatoxins in the diet, particularly to people who already have liver disease, this problem is well known to epidemiologists. Figures from China are unambiguous: aflatoxins are a definite dietary cofactor in the development of liver cancer.

Residents of this area are at high risk for development of hepatocellular carcinoma, in part due to consumption of aflatoxin-contaminated foods.[3]

Aflatoxins are carcinogenic chemicals formed by fungi. They are found in a number of crops, though they are noted as being a particular problem in peanuts.

Until screening and removal is 100%, patients might be well advised to avoid all foods that might potentially contain any traces of aflatoxin. This includes all peanuts. Foods with low levels seem to be perfectly safe to the general population, but may present a small risk as cofactors to HCV in triggering the development of liver cancer.

The Digestive System and Health

Digestive problems are very common in people with hep C. Since poor digestion means that foods will not be properly assimilated, many people conclude that the first objective in compromised patients is to strengthen this process; what is the point of discussing diet if foods are not being properly assimilated? Thus it is entirely rational to commence dietary therapy by optimizing the efficiency of the digestive system first.

Holistic health systems always stress the importance of the link between healthy digestion and good liver function and regard this symptom as being inextricably linked to faulty liver function. Treatment of liver disease often commences with treatment of the digestive system. This is exemplified by the approach adopted by experienced practitioners of Chinese herbal medicine. Treatment will often commence with a range of herbs designed to kick-start both appetite and digestive energy; for instance the formulations "Peaceful River," "Middle Way," and "Cool and Calm," (see pages 253–255) contain plants classically prescribed to those with weak digestion.

Many medical practitioners see both the development of illness and the restoration of health as long-term processes, with the state of the digestive system being a key factor and good function regarded as a prerequisite for recovery. Some dietary practitioners, such as the cornflakes breakfast cereal inventor John Harvey Kellogg, become obsessive about bowel health. Some contemporary experts have equally emphatic "gastrocentric" views of health dynamics. For instance, Brian Wright, author of *Cycles of Disease and Health,*[4] describes the processes of disease progression and recovery in terms of the health of the digestive system as follows:

1. Disease Progression

Poor food ⟶ lack of nutrients ⟶ food toxins ⟶ antibiotics ⟶ stress ⟶ drugs ⟶ poor digestion ⟶ allergy ⟶ putrefactive intestine ⟶ candidiasis ⟶ parasites ⟶ dysbiosis ⟶ leaky gut ⟶ intoxicated liver ⟶ overwhelmed elimination ⟶ DISEASE

It is notable that Wright suggests that a poor diet and lifestyle along with faulty digestion may lead to the development of a toxic liver state even without the presence of a pathogen like HCV. If a "leaky gut" state is also present, then unsuitable toxins will be transported to the liver for breakdown. Some of these, particularly those related to heavy meat protein, can be dangerous—it is postulated that partly digested meat proteins in the gut attract pathogenic organisms that produce toxic putrefaction. This may also trigger immune reaction and allergy.

The autoimmune problems that plague HCV patients may therefore also be triggered or antagonized by digestive problems. Gluten is often identified as a food allergen correlated to inflammation of the intestinal tract. It may also be linked to the development of lymphatic cancer, particularly in conjunction with celiac disease, a form of "leaky bowel":

> The increased incidence of lymphoma in celiac sprue (CS) is well documented, and the risk of developing this malignancy is 40–100 fold greater than in the general population. The author believes that gluten may also be at the root of lymphomas in asymptomatic and latent celiac sprue, as well.[5]

The much-discussed candidiasis phenomenon may also feature. The health of the cytochrome P450 enzyme system in the liver is seen as being crucial. Because HCV patients are also likely to have sustained some damage due to infection, this may be particularly relevant. Wright goes on to explain:

> Toxins leaking through the gut are carried to the liver where the cytochrome p450 enzyme system oxidizes and breaks down toxins, conjugation combines the toxin with another molecule, usually making it water soluble and less destructive, and antioxidants neutralize the corrosive effects of oxidation.

According to this model at this point the whole body can be seriously compromised by being overwhelmed by such toxins or by not receiving the nutrients it needs; when this stage is reached toxins that are normally eliminated accumulate in dangerous concentrations. A pattern of disease similar to that experienced by some HCV patients can then emerge. The kidneys, colon, bile duct, lungs, and mucus membranes become clogged and their efficiency deteriorates. The skin may develop rashes, eczema, or psoriasis. Urine smells strongly and diarrhea may be persistent. Aches and pains will occur throughout the body, and autoimmune diseases may develop as the immune system struggles to respond. Other degenerative diseases may manifest, organs may fail, and the patient is at risk of developing cancer, which can be seen as a last-ditch attempt by the body to protect itself.

2. Health Restoration

Improving elimination ⟶ detoxifying and healing the liver ⟶ colon cleansing ⟶ healing leaky gut ⟶ clearing candidiasis and other parasites ⟶ clearing allergy and fasting ⟶ complete digestion ⟶ no stress ⟶ no drugs ⟶ optimum nutrition ⟶ HEALTH

Elimination is seen as being of primary importance in the treatment of HCV by many natural health practitioners. If the body can be supported in efficiently getting rid of toxins and waste products. then damage to the organs will be minimized and the immune system will be less likely to start malfunctioning.

They suggest drinking plenty of pure water—distilled is better than mineral. Next the skin, the kidneys, and the lungs can be helped perhaps by prescribing some of the following—vitamin C, niacin, dandelion leaf, ginger, burdock root and sarsaparilla. Then the liver can be detoxified by using herbs like milk thistle seeds (silymarin), burdock root, dandelion root, and yellow dock. Vitamins and amino acids are also seen as powerful helpers in this process, particularly N-acetyl cysteine. These are discussed later in this chapter and on pages 338–344.

Next the health of the colon can be addressed. The following substances may be of use here: linseed, psyllium husks, slippery elm, fennel seed, fenugreek seed, L-glutamine, aloe vera, cat's claw, glucosamine, and butyric acid. Beneficial bacteria can be introduced by eating plenty of live yogurt or probiotics containing the benign acidophilus, bulgaricus, or salivarius species. These beneficial bacteria manufacture vital B vitamins and counter the proliferation of pathogenic bacteria. Some claim that they can alleviate autoimmune diseases like rheumatoid arthritis.[6]

Some malign intestinal parasites, such as the notorious fungal stage *Candida albicans,* may require stronger treatment. (A white coating on the tongue is a common symptom of candidiasis.) This may consist of grapefruit seed extract, which has achieved promising research results,[7] artimesia, pulsatilla chinensis, barberry, prunus mume, ginger, zanthoxylum, rhizoma coptidis, calcium magnesium caprylate, Pau D'Arco, thyme, rosemary, lemon balm, garlic, and vitamin C. This condition may also require long-term and strict dietary adjustments; the complete elimination of sugar, sucrose, yeast, and refined foods of all types for up to two years is recommended by many authorities on this condition, such as Leon Chaitow.

Identifying and avoiding allergens is another important step; allergens are substances that cause sensitivity reactions in certain individuals. There are varying degrees of reaction—a true allergy is characterized by severe and immediate reactions usually characterized by vomiting, bloating, diarrhea, or constipation. The weaker term "food intolerance" is now used to embrace longer-term and less dramatic reactions; because these reactions typically resemble some of the symptoms of chronic hep C—aching joints, indigestion and irritable bowel syndrome, fatigue, frequent headaches, depression, mouth ulcers—it may be a good idea for patients seeking to improve their quality of life to establish whether or not they have any specific sensitivity.

Two common dietary antagonists are wheat and dairy products. Gluten, which is contained in barley, oats, and rye, as well as wheat, is a commonly identified allergen. A number of patients have adopted diets free of one or both of these ingredients. Because these products are so common in standard diets, it can be quite difficult to identify all culprit foods, particularly those containing gluten. For instance, many cereals, a high proportion of processed foods, and many condiments, such as most types of soy sauce, contain gluten, as well as bread and pasta. With care it is possible to adjust. For instance, there are wheat- and gluten-free cereals available, and some classic wheat-based products are now made from substitutes such as spelt, a related but distinct species.

The development of such reactions may be subtly linked to chronic liver disease (refer to the work of Linda Lazarides later in this chapter). Tests that enable the identification of these substances are now widely available. When digestive health is definitely improving. the adoption of restricted or carefully tailored diets may be an excellent method of further enhancing digestive function (see below for some suggestions). If indigestion persists, then patients may consider using the following supplements:

- Betaine HCl—a source of stomach acid, helping to digest protein and minerals
- Protease—a group of enzymes that digest protein, helping to make amino acids
- Lactase—enzyme for the digestion of the milk sugar lactose
- Lipase—helps to break down fats
- Amylase—helps to break down starches and sugars
- Cellulase—helps to break down cellulose fiber
- Papain—an extract of papaya that digests proteins and starches
- Bromelain—an extract of pineapple that can reduce effects of food allergy
- American ginseng—tones the stomach, pancreas, and intestine

- Fenugreek—supports the pancreas, controls appetite, and balances blood sugar cycle
- Gentian root—anti-inflammatory, stimulates bile flow, and improves fat digestion

Liver Function and Specific Dietary Advice

The leading British nutritionist and director of the Society for the Promotion of Nutritional Therapy, Linda Lazarides, recently wrote a highly informative feature on the subject of the liver and diet [The liver of the matter. Lazarides, L. *Continuum*, 5(1), Autumn 1997]. Key points are as follows:

The vital functions of the liver can be separated into two distinct phases: detoxification (phase I) and biotransformation (phase II). Diagnosis and prescription of dietary adjustments, supplementation, or foods to avoid may be determined by assessing the overactivity or underactivity of these two phases and the relative balance between the two.

Detoxification embraces the processes of oxidation, reduction, and hydrolysis, which are catalyzed by the group of liver enzymes known as the cytochrome p450 oxidases. Thus toxins and metabolites absorbed by the digestive tract are presented to the liver for conversion into "intermediate substances"—alcohols, free radicals, and aldehydes, such as chloral hydrate (a well known "knock out" agent). If function is poor, these "intermediate substances" hang around for too long and are absorbed into general blood circulation. Other intermediate substances resemble endogenous benzodiazepines, which may also give rise to powerful sedative effects; thus the chronic fatigue experienced by so many HCV patients may have a clear biochemical link to faulty liver detoxification, or phase I activity.

The key dietary point is that these intermediate substances are far more toxic than the original toxins and that their harmful effect can only be controlled by an ample supply of antioxidant nutrients and enzymes and/or a reduction in intake of or exposure to these factors. The greater the volume of toxins consumed, the more p450 enzymes are induced in the liver, the greater the likelihood of "toxic overload." Substances identified by Lazarides as *inducing* p450 enzymes and therefore to be avoided or reduced by HCV patients with liver toxicity are as follows:

- Caffeine
- Alcohol
- Dioxin (found in some herbicides) and other pollutants
- Exhaust fumes
- High-protein diet
- Oranges and tangerines
- Organophosphorus pesticides
- Paint fumes
- Steroid hormones
- Acetaminophen/paracetamol and many other drugs
- Diazepam tranquilizers and sleeping pills
- The contraceptive pill
- Cortisone
- Dish-washing liquid residue (contains solvents and detergents— always rinse thoroughly when dish-washing).

Substances that can *inhibit* the action of p450 enzymes and therefore lead to a greater probability of aldehydes building up include the following, which may also be noted by patients:

- Carbon tetrachloride
- Carbon monoxide
- Barbiturates
- Quercetin
- Grapefruit—contains naringenin

Lazarides identifies the following as key symptoms of inhibited p450 enzyme function and the buildup of aldehydes:

- Brain fog
- M.E. and chronic fatigue syndrome

- Increased sensitivity or allergic reaction to previously tolerated substances
- Alcohol intolerance
- Vasculitis

Thus Lazarides provides a rational explanation for some of the symptoms that many patients find hardest to understand and get others to accept. Perhaps this is a key to the understanding of "brain fog." Maybe the allergic reactions reported by some hep C patients might be traced back to inhibited p450 enzyme function.

Candida albicans overgrowth in the intestines may also cause an unmanageable buildup of excess aldehydes. Because this notorious condition, known as candidiasis, appears to be common in HCV patients, particularly women, this is another avenue worth exploring if these symptoms present. Another cause of the buildup of aldehydes may be an increase in formaldehyde gas in the environment (often given off by new carpets or other furnishings).

Substances known as amines, which are found in chocolate, cheese, and adrenaline, are also oxidized by the p450 enzyme system. Symptoms of amine buildup may include hypertension and chemical sensitivity reactions.

Biotransformation, or phase II liver function, is composed of various conjugation processes. Essentially conjugation involves the joining of a metabolite or toxin with another molecule to make them water-soluble so that they may be excreted. Types of conjugation, their dependence on the presence of particular amino acids, and symptoms of inadequate function include the following:

Acetylation requires a good supply of pantothenic acid. Symptoms of poor function include the slow clearance of drugs and chemical sensitivity.

Acylation embraces a number of conjugation processes. The amino acids glycine, glutamine, and taurine are required for the conjugation of bile acids produced by the liver. These are potentially toxic, particularly if they build in the digestive tract and block the assimilation of fats and vitamins. Buildup is also associated with impaired cholesterol metabolism. This process is also pH sensitive, and some nutritionists may "alkinize" overacidic patients by prescribing sodium and potassium bicarbonate to facilitate these reactions. The amino acid glutathione is necessary for the conjugation of xenobiotics (foreign biochemical entities), such as aromatic disulphides, napthalene, anthracene, and phenanthacin. Glutathione deficiency found in many patients will inhibit these processes. Another disruptive factor is the presence of heavy metals in the liver, which prevent or slow down the recycling of glutathione, again leading to a toxic buildup of xenobiotics.

Sulfation embraces the conjugation of a number of toxins that require the presence of sulfate for detoxification. Some people, notably Parkinsonism and Alzheimer's patients, have an impaired ability to produce sulfate from the amino acid cysteine. A buildup of these toxins can cause damage to nervous tissue over the long term according to a Dr. Steventon of Birmingham University in the U.K. Impaired sulfation may therefore be linked to some of the nervous problems experienced by some patients such as peripheral neuropathy.

Methylation embraces the conjugation and detoxification of substances such as amines, thiols, and adrenaline that are then excreted through the lungs. Methionine is the amino acid whose presence is necessary for this process. A classic symptom of poor methylation is chemical sensitivity. Magnesium or methionine can be prescribed to patients with poor methylation.

Glucuronidation seems to be a kind of "backup" conjugation process that can mop up some of the toxic substances not dealt with by the others. It requires the presence of glucuronic acid, which is a metabolite of glucose. This may be linked in some way to the craving for sweet foods by patients and represent an intuitive attempt to address toxic overload as well as the sometimes linked symptom of fatigue.

The general consequences of poor conjugation will be toxic overload. Lazarides describes the symptoms in similar terms to Brian Wright:

> Once breakdown of the main pathways occurs as a result of pollutant overload, toxins are shunted to lesser pathways, eventually overloading them, and disturbing orderly nutrient metabolism. Chemical sensitivity may then occur, followed by nutrient

depletion and finally fixed-name disease. Depleted immunity is also a potential outcome of a toxic overload.

Some of the foods suggested by Lazarides to aid detoxification are as follows:

- Beet: to aid liver drainage
- Broccoli, cauliflower, and other cruciferous vegetables: to aid p450 action
- Radish and watercress: rich in sulfur

In general Lazarides's work demonstrates the complex and frequently misunderstood nature of liver dysfunction and consequent need for precise dietary adjustment and supplementation. This analysis also demonstrates that there is a scientific basis for many of the bewildering symptoms experienced by patients but denied by some doctors. Findings hint at the potential benefits of the following practices:

- Carefully managed diets to bring about heavy metal detoxification or a temporary reduction in the burden to the liver allowing the clearance of any accumulated toxins.
- Long-term dietary planning to reduce toxins and increase presence of nutrients that support detoxification.
- Amino acid, vitamin, and mineral supplementation (often including NAC, taurine, essential fatty acids); with this in-depth understanding of the importance of the presence of amino acids and the symptoms of specific deficiencies it should be practical to prescribe individual programs.
- The use of herbs such as silymarin, dandelion root, globe artichoke, and turmeric or Chinese herbal formulations to "protect" the liver.
- The identification and avoidance of environmental risk factors.

Food Combining and the Hay Diet

This is a long-standing and widely respected approach to digestive disease and wider health problems. Developed by Dr. William Hay in the early decades of the twentieth century it is rooted in the observation that the body uses acids to help digest proteins and alkalis to help digest starches. Hay concluded that mixing the two food types in one meal resulted in the digestive process being "confused" resulting in sluggish performance. Hay also thought that such food mixing could result in more serious health problems such as arthritis and impaired immune function.

As well as addressing serious health questions, Hay was also interested in promoting improvements in the well-being and energy of his patients. Thus the feelings of heaviness and lethargy that are quite common in hepatitis C patients and that often occur after eating are likely to fall within his diagnostic and prescriptive system.

The basis of the system is to eat a diet largely composed of foods that are alkali forming and to avoid mixing incompatible, "confusing" foods, generally proteins and starches.

The Alkali/Acid-Forming Balance Principle

The former concept is based upon the observation that the body excretes 4:1 alkali:acid and that it should therefore be fed foods in roughly the same ratio, in order to support this natural balance. Unbalanced diets will be more difficult to digest and require more energy. Hay concluded that certain specific conditions such as arthritis were commonly caused by a diet too rich in acid-forming foods. Followers of the Hay diet have claimed success in treating degenerative conditions such as arthritis by having patients adopt a predominantly alkali-forming diet. They also recommend drinking celery juice (strongly alkali forming) and abstaining from vinegar, tea, coffee, and alcohol (*Food Combining for Health,* Thorsons).

Examples of alkali-forming foods are apples, apricots, bananas, dates, figs, eggplant, avocados, beet, broccoli, cabbage, carrots, grapes, lemons, mangoes, melons, peaches, pears, raisins, strawberries, almonds, hazelnuts, millet, cauliflower, celery, chives, dandelion leaves, lettuce, squash, mushrooms, onions, peppers, potatoes in skins, radishes, tomatoes, spinach, watercress.

Examples of acid-forming foods are: meats, fish, poultry, bread, cheese, eggs, all grains (rice, oats, barley, etc.) except millet, breakfast cereals, flour, sugar, beans, legumes (lentils, chickpeas, peanuts, etc.), tea, coffee, alcohol, milk, yogurt, cream.

In addition there are some neutral foods: sunflower, sesame, and pumpkin seeds.

The central tenet of the Hay System is that starches and sugars must not be eaten with proteins and acid fruits at the same meal. An interval of at least four and a half hours must elapse between incompatible meals. Incompatible foods are usually classified into lists for convenience.

The usual table is composed of three columns. The foods in column I must not be mixed with those in column III; foods from column II can be mixed with foods in either column I or column III (refer to the table on pages 383–384).

Bear in mind that following the table should automatically maintain a healthy alkali/acid-forming balance. Check out books on the subject of food combining for updates and specific recipes.

Table of Compatible Foods
(Columns I and III are incompatible)

I for Protein Meals	II Neutral Foods (can be combined with either Column I or Column III)	III for Starch Meals
Proteins: meat of all kinds, including beef, lamb, pork, venison; poultry, including chicken, duck, goose, turkey; game, including pheasant, partridge, grouse, rabbit; fish of all kinds, including shellfish; eggs; cheese; milk (combines best with fruit and not to be served at a meat meal); yogurt	**Nuts:** all, except peanuts	**Cereals:** whole-grain: wheat, barley, corn, oats, millet, rice (brown, unpolished), rye; bread: 100% whole-wheat; flour: 100% or 85%; oatmeal: medium
	Fats: butter, cream, eggyolks, olive oil (virgin), sunflower seed oil, sesame seed oil (cold pressed)	**Sweet fruits:** bananas (ripe), dates, figs (fresh and dried), grapes if extra sweet, papaya if very ripe, pears if very sweet and ripe, currants, raisins, sultanas
Fruits: Apples, apricots (fresh and dried), blackberries, blueberries, cherries, currants, (black, red, or white if ripe), gooseberries (if ripe), grapefruit, grapes, kiwis, lemons, limes, loganberries, mangoes, melon (best eaten alone as a fruit meal), nectarines, oranges, papayas, pears, pineapples, prunes (for occasional use), raspberries, satsumas, tangerines	**Herbs and flavorings:** chives, mint, parsley, sage, tarragon, thyme, grated lemon rind, grated orange rind	
	Seeds: sunflower, sesame, pumpkin	
	Bran: Wheat or oat bran, wheatgerm	

(continued on page 384)

Table of Compatible Foods (continued)
(Columns I and III are incompatible)

I for Protein Meals	II Neutral Foods	III for Starch Meals
For vegetarians: legumes, lentils, soybeans, kidney beans, chickpeas (garbanzo beans), lima beans, pinto beans	**Vegetables:** all green and root vegetables (except potatoes and Jerusalem artichokes), including asparagus, beans (all fresh green beans), beets, broccoli, Brussels sprouts, cabbage, calabrese, carrots, cauliflower, celery, celeriac, eggplant, kohlrabi, leeks, mushrooms, onions, parsnips, peas, spinach, squash, turnips, zucchini	**Vegetables:** potatoes and Jerusalem artichokes
Salad dressings: French dressing made with oil and lemon juice or apple cider vinegar, cream dressing, mayonnaise (home-made)	**Miscellaneous ingredients:** avocados, corn salad, cucumber, endive, fennel, garlic, green onions, lettuce, mustard and cress, peppers, red and green radishes, scallions, sprouts, tomatoes (uncooked), watercress,	**Salad dressings:** sweet or sour cream, olive oil or cold-pressed seed oils, fresh tomato juice with oil and seasoning
Sugar substitute: diluted frozen orange juice	**Sugar substitute:** raisins and raisin juice, honey, maple syrup	**Sugar substitute:** Barbados sugar, honey (in strict moderation)
Alcohol: Dry red and white wines, dry cider	**Alcohol:** whiskey, gin	**Alcohol:** ale, beer

Homeopathic Dietary Advice

The first homeopath interviewed for this book suggested that hepatitis C patients "should move to the country and live off brown rice and organic vegetables." This suggestion was symptomatic of the general approach of homeopaths to chronic hepatitis. They will often stipulate very strict regimes that exclude many standard items. The following is typical of the advice given to patients with suspected liver malfunction.[8]

Avoid	Eat in Unlimited Quantities
Meat, fowl, fried food	Fish (white preferred)
	Pulses—beans, peas
Eggs	Tofu
Refined bread and sweetened cereals	Whole-grain bread, unsweetened cereals, whole-grain brown rice, whole-wheat pasta (avoid bread and pasta with gluten allergy)
Sugar, syrup, treacle	Molasses, unsweetened jams, marmite
Cow's milk, goat's milk, cheese	Soya milk
Tomatoes, citrus fruits	Vegetables, pineapples, grapes, melons, suitable fruits canned in natural juice
Bananas, avocados	
Nuts (except almonds)	Almonds, sunflower and sesame seeds
Coffee, alcohol, cocoa	Grain coffees, herb teas, suitable unsweetened fruit juice
Only 2 cups of tea per day	Rooibosch and Maté teas
Chocolate	Carob powder

Restricted Foods: Berries (strawberries, raspberries, gooseberries, etc.), apricots, peaches, sultanas, raisins, and dates can be eaten twice a week in unlimited quantities. Less than ⅛ teaspoonful of salt per day.

David Curtin, a homeopathic practitioner at the Hale Clinic in central London, has a number of patients with hepatitis C. He had the following to say with regard to diet:

> It varies from person to person, but the main thing is for the diet to be of high quality with a minimum of junk and a maximum of fresh foods, particularly fruit and vegetables.

For cirrhotic patients he said he might recommend the complete elimination of fats and would consider the use of fasting, vegetable juices, and a raw vegetable meal every day. It is interesting to note that this is the polar opposite of current conventional practice.

So far as supporting the immune system is concerned, he stressed that the application of homeopathic remedies should achieve this, but that the addition of nutritional supplements also has a role to play. These would usually comprise echinacea, astralagus, and Siberian ginseng in the form of capsules containing the powdered herbs. In addition he said he would also prescribe vitamins and minerals (see chapters 16 and 18).

Patient's Experience of Homeopathic Diet: Clare

> I'd had a really appalling diet in the past—junk food, booze, drugs, coffee—and I'd realized that I couldn't go on after the diagnosis and talking to some other people with hep C. I was suffering from severe indigestion and fatigue. My work was suffering and I had no energy left for a social life. A friend recommended a homeopath, so I went to see her. I was given a really strict diet as well as the homeopathic remedy.
>
> I found it was quite easy to cut out the red meat and chicken—I'd already decided to become vegetarian so that was fine. I've had to work quite hard on learning to cook vegetarian meals with the right protein mix. I found it was more difficult when I went out—there aren't very many convenience

foods that fit the bill and not all restaurants cater for this diet. It was more difficult to cut out the coffee—no one told me you got withdrawals from caffeine. I substituted dandelion coffee and that really helped. When I feel run down I take a course of multivitamins, and that definitely helps.

I haven't completely cut out the sugar—I still eat pastries and cakes from time to time. I regularly ignore the advice on citrus fruits and bananas ("forbidden fruits")—I find them a particularly good source of fast energy. I do my best with this diet and don't beat myself up if I eat something on the "avoid" list.

I feel generally better for trying this system. It hasn't cured the hep, but it has diminished the symptoms. In some ways it helped to confirm my instincts. For instance fatty foods were causing me severe digestive problems. However, because no one told me that I was ill, I expected to be able to carry on eating them and would blame myself for feeling sick. Although it was a shock to have a hep C diagnosis, it was a relief to get treatment which acknowledged my experience. The doctors at the hospital didn't want to know about indigestion. I can lead a normal life although it's still a bloody nuisance having this.

Naturopathic Diet

Naturopaths are likely to recommend a daily diet similar to the homeopathic one listed above, although many practitioners will be vegetarians or vegans and would therefore exclude the fish. Balance is a feature of naturopathic dietary advice, both in terms of food content and the changing needs of the body through the day.

An interesting and sensible suggestion is to think about *when* as well as what to eat. Some naturopaths recommend the following pattern of foods throughout the day.

Breakfast should be substantial and consist of all the essential elements of diet, particularly protein. If the temperature is cold at this time of day, then the meal should be warm.

Lunch should be cooler, maybe containing raw vegetables (e.g., salad) and plenty of protein.

Supper should be light and does not have to contain protein.

Energy crises, which are common with HCV patients, may be alleviated by increasing the protein content of the diet, particularly at breakfast, and cutting out caffeine and sugar.

Beans, pulses, and their derivatives, such as tofu, should be the main source of protein. Whole grains such as brown rice should form the basis of the diet in combination with the proteins.

Fruits, meat, and dairy products should be consumed in smaller quantities with the above.

This is a simple, undisruptive approach that has benefited a number of patients.

Most dieticians stress the importance of vegetarians adopting the correct food-mixing techniques to ensure adequate supply of amino acids. For HCV patients with identified liver disease this is vital, particularly in the light of information indicating deficiencies in patients. It would be wise for vegetarians to consider taking supplements, particularly those containing amino acids such as chlorella (see chapter 18).

Traditional Chinese Medicine and Diet

TCM practitioners regard chronic hepatitis as a "hot, heavy, and damp" condition, which overflows from the liver into other energy centers as the disease progresses. General dietary advice is therefore likely to recommend the following.

Exclude or reduce heavy, hot, and dampening foods:

- Spices such as chili, curries, alcohol, coffee, fatty foods—regarded as "hot"
- Sugar/confectionery, dairy products (except yogurt)—regarded as "damp"
- Most red meats such as beef and pork, eggs—regarded as "heavy"
- Bread and pastries—regarded as "heavy, damp, and hot"

Also reduce or exclude foods that are cause "obstruct" the liver and cause Qi stagnation:

- Processed foods

- Foods containing chemical additives
- Refined foods
- Fats

In general, foods to include are cooling, drying, and light: for instance, cucumber, melon, steamed white fish, tofu, apples, whole grains, rice, and green vegetables.

For Specific Liver Conditions

To relieve a stagnant, swollen liver (e.g., patients who feel bloated, have inflammation): Reduce the volume of food intake and avoid all of the "bad" foods listed above. Include watercress, onions, beets, strawberry, peach, cherry, cabbage, turnip, kohlrabi, cauliflower, Brussels sprouts, and broccoli. Include culinary herbs such as garlic, turmeric, basil, bay leaf, horseradish, mints, angelica root, and black pepper.

To stimulate liver Qi (e.g., patients who are fatigued): Include fresh sprouted grains, beans, fresh vegetables and fruit all eaten raw, and congee (rice porridge).

To "harmonize" the liver (e.g., patients who have mood swings): Include small amounts of sweet foods such as licorice root, honey, whole sugar cane, barley malt, molasses, and date sugar.

To detoxify and cool the liver (e.g., patients who feel toxic due to hep C, diet high in "bad" foods, drugs, or alcohol): Include mung beans (note that mung bean noodles are a good substitute for wheat-based pasta), seaweeds (kelp in particular), lettuce, watercress, tofu, millet, plum, chlorella and other chlorophyll-rich foods, mushrooms, rhubarb, and radish.

To build liver Yin and blood (e.g., patients who feel cold or weak): Include foods for stimulating, harmonizing, detoxifying, and cooling as well as dark grapes and berries, blackstrap molasses, unrefined cold-pressed flax oil.

To accelerate liver rejuvenation: Include all chlorophyll-rich foods, cereal grasses such as wheatgrass and juice, microalgae, parsley.

A good selection of Chinese herbs will support and enhance the benefits of these dietary adjustments.

Because the pattern of disharmony precipitated by hepatitis C causes problems in the liver, which almost always overflow into other organ centers, dietary prescription may also address the other organs. Typically this will correspond to the degree of disharmony between these organs and the liver and also to environmental factors such as the time of year.

Chinese herbalists will recommend various decoctions that, in part, aim to counteract the "hot and damp" tendency; the herbs are regarded as an extension of the diet and seen as containing "forgotten foods." TCM practitioners are also wary of fasting because it may weaken the Qi. This may be partly due to the frequent occurrence of famine in Chinese history.

The initial treatment of hepatitis patients usually aims to build up strength and energy as well as boosting the eliminative functions of the body, using herbs that stimulate hunger and boost digestive metabolism. Thus they tend to echo the "keep eating" approach of Western medicine to begin with. However, patients with hepatitis are treated as being at risk of developing symptoms such as fluid retention or steatorrhea even if they have not yet manifested; diet and herbs are adjusted to acknowledge this and prevent the occurrence of disease in the future, a key strategy throughout TCM. Patients with digestive problems may be encouraged to perform certain Qi Gong exercises that open the stomach, spleen, and liver meridians. This subject is covered in detail in chapter 15.

A further classical observation of TCM is that people with liver disease tend toward rigid behavior patterns, and that these need to be loosened in favor of a more relaxed and spontaneous approach to life. Thus patients may be advised not to be obsessive about diet and not worry too much about "lapses."

Fats

Almost everybody is aware that a lot of fat in the diet is unhealthy. Some know that fats can place a particularly heavy burden on the liver. Few people understand that there are differing types of fats, some of which can be very beneficial and others particularly hazardous if high levels are consumed over a lengthy period. Because our livers are already under threat, a good knowledge of this aspect of diet will pay dividends if we are able to adjust our eating and drinking patterns accordingly.

This section will outline and explain the different types of fat and their associated properties; by adjusting intakes we should be able to find an alternative to adopting a strict "fat-free" diet, which is extremely hard, very boring, and usually impractical.

Saturated Status

Fats are often classified according to their "saturated" status, and labeled "saturated," "monounsaturated," and "polyunsaturated."

Saturated fats are primarily derived from animal sources, though some plants such as peanuts and coconuts yield very high levels as well. They are considered to be "heavy" and are solid at room temperature. Saturated fats cause a tendency for cholesterol to accumulate, leading in some cases to cardiovascular and circulation problems, and also present the greatest problems to the liver.

Monounsaturated fats are usually derived from plants. They do not cause the accumulation of cholesterol and neither do they deplete the blood of high-density lipoproteins (HDL), which help to keep the arterial wall "clean" of cholesterol. They are liquid at room temperature (unless you live in a very cold climate!), but solidify in the refrigerator.

Polyunsaturated fats are also usually derived from plants and are liquid, even in the refrigerator. They decrease HDL and low-density lipoproteins (LDL), which cause cholesterol deposition in the arteries, resulting in an ambiguous net effect.

Thus a general conclusion is that monounsaturated fats are less likely to present problems than polyunsaturated fats, and that saturated fats are likely to present the most problems.

Essential Fats

Some types of fat are regarded as being "good." Chief among these are the **omega-3** and **omega-6 essential fatty acids** (EFA), which include linoleic acid and alpha-linolenic acid. In this case "essential" means that the body is unable to "manufacture" the EFA on its own. Linoleic acid is classified as an omega-6 essential fatty acid, while linoleic acid is an omega-3 EFA. They support healthy skin and hair, efficient thyroid function and adrenal activity, underpin immune function, provide energy, keep the arteries clear, and promote healthy blood and nervous system.

HCV patients who have symptoms that indicate possible EFA deficiency—scaly skin, poor liver function, irritability, weight loss, thyroid disease, fatigue—could try EFA supplementation or dietary adjustment to include more.

Some of the benefits of these EFAs are thought to be due to their conversion by the body into a class of substances known as the **prostaglandins** (PGs). PGs are thought to play an important role in the regulation of every cell and organ in the human body.

EFAs are found in foods and oils rich in polyunsaturated fat. Good sources are olives, almonds, flaxseed, hazelnuts, pecans, walnuts, avocados, and soybeans.

A potentially harmful EFA is **arachidonic acid** (AA). In human beings the presence of this EFA is primarily derived from the consumption of animal products. Symptoms of excess include excessive blood clotting, pain, and inflammation. This EFA also gives rise to the production of substances called leuktrienes, an excess of which is associated with dermatitis, psoriasis, and lupus, which are all conditions suspected of being abnormally common in HCV patients. Thus some knowledgeable nutritionists may advise patients with such symptoms to reduce or eliminate animal products except for fish from the diet.

Another beneficial fat is **gamma-linolenic acid** (GLA), commonly referred to by nutritionists. This fat is also converted into prostaglandins. In addition and of particular interest to hep C patients, it is thought to have the following properties:

- Alleviates Sjögren's syndrome as it manifests in the eye (Sjögren's also manifests in the mouth).

- Effective against arthritis and other inflammatory diseases, though not when taking anti-inflammatory drugs.

- Protects against vascular disease such as thrombosis, of which some patients are at additional risk.

- Regulates the production of insulin, which is a factor in blood sugar disorders, and protects against damage to eyes, kidneys, heart, and nerves common in all forms of diabetes, which is clinically linked to HCV infection.

Rich sources of GLA include mother's milk, spirulina, and evening primrose, whose oil is widely available and has a good reputation as a safe and beneficial supplement.

Edible Oils and Fat Guidelines

- People with "sluggish" or "damp" conditions such as fatigue, candidiasis, and tumors should avoid all oils or keep consumption to a bare minimum, except for small amounts of omega-3 and GLA oils.

- In general, oils must be carefully scrutinized not just for their origin but also their method of extraction and production. Careful label reading is important!

- When cooking keep temperatures as low as possible or use an oil-water sauté technique.

- Avoid all refined oils. Such products are common on account of their long shelf life. These oils may be harmful to people with liver disease because of their extraction by solvents and their extreme heating during production. The heating process generates "trans fatty acids," which prevent the transformation of fats in the body into immunity-building fatty acids. Most vegetable oils on supermarket shelves will be refined and are characterized by a bland taste and an unclouded appearance.

- Avoid all polyunsaturated margarine that contains hydrogenated polyunsaturated vegetable oils. Hydrogenation leads to a buildup of trans fatty acids that inhibit immune function.

- Avoid peanut oil on account of its potential for containing aflatoxins.

- In general, try to avoid commonly available polyunsaturated oils such as safflower, corn, sunflower, linseed, and walnut unless they have been recently pressed. Safflower is regarded as unhealthy in Ayurvedic medicine and often has rancidity problems.

- Olive oil is the healthiest option for general use. Typically it contains 82% monounsaturated fat, 8% polyunsaturated, and 10% saturated. Buy only unrefined cold-pressed olive oil; those produced by other "modern" methods will be subject to the same hazards as other refined oils. Extra-virgin olive oil will have a lower acidity content than later pressings.

- Other unrefined oils high in monounsaturates include almond, canola, and apricot kernel; however, it is difficult to find unrefined products.

- Recently pressed flaxseed, pumpkin seed, and chia seed oils are good sources of omega-3 EFAs.

- Oleic and omega-rich oils made from various sources (sunflower, flax, linseed, walnut) are good sources of EFAs. Some of these oils should not be used for cooking and may be expensive.

- Butter is very rich in saturated fats, but not subject to suspect production techniques as are many brands of margarine.

- Clarified butter, also known as ghee, has had all milk solids removed and is regarded as being beneficial to health in Ayurvedic medicine. Ghee can be used in cooking. It contains butyric acid, thought to play a role in combating cancer and raising levels of interferon production!

- Generally try to reduce fat intake.

- Generally reduce saturated fats in favor of monounsaturated and polyunsaturated fats.

- Generally try to eat less or eliminate heavy fatty red meats such as beef, lamb, pork, duck, and chicken with the skin on it.

- Be wary of processed food products such as hamburgers, meat pies, and pre-prepared meals.

- Read food labels very carefully. Scrutinize "low fat" foods, particularly for hydrogenated fat and refined oil content.

The Organic Food Question

The debate about the real safety of the foods that are on sale is complex and heated. It is questionable as to whether or not government food safety policies are really geared to serve the interests of consumers; many accuse their governments of being more keen to serve the interests of producers. It is also sometimes apparent that the regulations that are in place are often not strictly enforced.[9] Certainly policies vary dramatically throughout the world, and what is deemed to be safe in the U.S. might be banned in Germany. The debate also extends to the safety of tap water and air quality.

There is no room to enter into that debate here. Individuals need to make up their own minds about which foods to purchase, what to drink, and where to live. It is a question of to what lengths you are prepared to go. There is a continuous stream of information that suggests that some pesticides are indeed very damaging, particularly when consumed continuously over a long period.[10] The presence of nitrates in the water supply appears to be positively correlated to the incidence of non-Hodgkin's lymphoma.[11]

There is also evidence that the heavy metals that are becoming present in increasing concentrations in modern man[12] seriously impair immune function[13] and tend to accumulate in the liver.

Since the symptoms of such damage include chronic fatigue and impaired immune function, two symptoms of HCV, many patients examine their diets for potential irritants. What is certain is that anything that you put into your body has to be processed by the liver and that the environment you live in will have an effect on your health.

Dietary Advice for Hepatitis C Patients from the U.K. National Acupuncture Detoxification Association Manual on Hepatitis C

Foods Harmful to the Liver

- **Fried foods:** These produce extra work for the liver.
- **Dairy foods** (milk, cheese, eggs): Should be reduced to a bare minimum.

- **Meat:** Digestion of meat produces nitrogenous waste products, which must be neutralized by the liver before they damage the body. This is hard work for the liver, so meat consumption should be minimal.

- **Margarine** and **non-cold-pressed oils:** Should be avoided, as these will probably contain chemical residues from their processing.

- **Sugar:** Should be cut from the diet wherever possible because it produces oxalic acid in the intestines, and this has to be neutralized by the liver. A little molasses, honey, or muscovado sugar may be used.

- **All chemicals** (i.e., artificial colorings and additives): Should be avoided.

- **Tea** and **coffee:** Best reduced to a bare minimum because of the stimulating effects they have on the nervous system and liver.

Foods Beneficial to the Liver

- **Carrots:** Eat two or three organic raw carrots daily, either as they are, or grated/chopped in salads or side salads. Alternatively, 1 pint of carrot juice can be drunk daily; this can be freshly juiced or can be obtained bottled. (Carrot juice in aluminum-lined cartons should be avoided because of the dangers of aluminum contamination.) Organic vegetables are readily available in most large supermarkets, good health food stores, and direct from wholesalers. Organic carrots are grown without chemical fertilizers, and so the liver does not have the extra work of detoxifying any chemical residues. Try to eat only organic vegetables and fruit.

- Most fruits benefit the liver. **Lemons** are particularly good, in that they relieve congestion and cleanse the liver. The juice of half a lemon can be added to a cup of hot water to make a refreshing, healthy drink. This also aids digestion, taken half an hour before meals. Use lemon juice to replace vinegar in all salad dressings and seasonings.

- **Artichokes** are particularly good for the liver, as they help with the detoxification of poisons.

- **Beet, asparagus, chicory, celery, radishes, leeks, onions, garlic, cabbage,** and **dandelion** are also of great benefit. In the spring, dandelion leaves can be obtained from young plants and added to salad. Later in the year these become more bitter—but can still be used.

- In addition to the foods to be avoided and those to be encouraged, a **good whole-food diet** is best used, including cereals (wheat, barley, brown rice, millet, rye, oats, whole-wheat noodles, sprouted seeds, and pulses) alfalfa seeds, sunflower seeds, whole-wheat grains, radish seeds, and so on; cooked lentils and pulses and whole-grain pastry and bread in moderation; a little honey; an occasional egg from a free-range source.

- Drinks that especially benefit the liver include **thyme tea** (infuse a teaspoon in a cup of boiling water for ten minutes), **rosemary herb, chamomile,** and **meadowsweet teas**—this last is particularly good for liver problems if they are nerve related.

Food Outline

A. Beneficial Foods

Fruits	Cleansing, antiseptic, alkaline, easy to digest
Vegetables	Healing, higher-value protein, alkaline
Whole grains and beans	Good source of protein, oils, acid
Nuts and seeds	Protein, oils, acid
Soured dairy products (yogurt, etc.)	Protein, easy to digest, opposes harmful bacteria alkaline, increased B and K vitamins (from bacteria)
Special foods	Sprouts, tofu, garlic
Supplements and vitamins	Yeast, fish liver oil, E, lecithin, C, bioflavanoids, minerals (bone meal, dolomite, zinc)
Juice fast	Alkaline, increased "microelectric" energy, promotes self-healing

B. Dangers from Improper Eating

Sugar	Acid, leach enzymes, vitamins and minerals, psyche changes, adrenal fatigue, hypoglycemia and diabetes

Refined flour	Acid, leach enzymes, vitamins and minerals, no bulk
Rancid fats	Destroys fat vitamins, acid, irritate digestion, cancer, involved with high blood pressure
Salt, mustard, hot sauces, vinegar, pepper, pickles	Irritate stomach and kidney, high blood pressure
Additives and poisons	Many kinds of damage from hyperactivity in children to cancer
High proteins	Acid, toxic, residue, stops body cleansing, causes excess mucus, strains kidney, mixes poorly with other foods, uric acid, arthritis, penetrates thick mucus
Meat	High fat, putrefaction, animal waste, hormones
Thick mucus	Especially from chronic high-protein (meat and acid dairy) diet, blocks digestion and most organ function
Overacidity	From refined flour and sugar and high protein, causes fatigue, aches and pains, fevers, shallow breathing
Putrefaction	High protein, poor mixing, constipation, absorbed into blood, mucus-coated tongue, destroys good bacteria
Cooking	Kills all enzymes, denatures most proteins, destroys vitamins
Fast eating	Inadequate chewing and salivation, tense poor breathing
Poor mixing	Drink only water with meal, eat most fruits alone, don't mix fruits and vegetables, eat concentrated proteins alone and/or at start of meal (with other Yang foods), aim for one-food meals, vegetables and grains mix best

Alcohol

If you have HCV, then anything other than moderate consumption or complete abstinence is likely to be harmful. The words "very moderate" mean about 4–6 alcohol units per week—that's 2–3 pints of beer or 4–6 glasses of wine. This should be consumed only with food. The Roche booklet is cautionary on alcohol:

> If you are a carrier of the virus it would be wise to try and limit your alcohol consumption to the occasional glass of beer or wine at the most, as cirrhosis is most likely to develop in moderately heavy drinkers.

The term "moderately heavy" is ambiguous and conveys a certain reluctance to state the facts. Numerous studies have shown that HCV patients with histories of heavy drinking have significantly poorer prognoses. For instance:

> New mechanisms of injury have been appreciated, most prominently the association between hepatitis C infection and alcoholic liver disease, and the formation of protein-acetaldehyde adducts in the liver of alcohol-fed subjects....[14]

Dr. David Mutimer, consultant hepatologist at the Queen Elizabeth Hospital in Birmingham, stated:

> We believe that alcohol may be synergistic with hepatitis C virus in causing liver damage.... Viral hepatitis and alcohol are the main conditions which give rise to cirrhosis.[15]

Epidemiological research has also demonstrated that HCV infection rates are higher in alcoholics than in the general population. Patients with a history of heavy drinking may need to abstain completely; a positive HCV diagnosis can be the last nail in the coffin of some people's drinking careers. Many patients without a history of drinking problems choose to err on the side of caution and avoid it altogether.

It is suspected that alcohol can have a triple adverse effect on patients: it puts stress on the liver, causing direct damage in higher quantities; it compromises the local immune response to HCV; it weakens the overall immunity of the body, thus giving rise to higher levels of the virus, which finds it easier to attack a liver with weakened defenses.

The necessary research into the consequences of moderate alcohol consumption in HCV patients has not yet been completed. Currently Dr. Leonie Grellier of the Royal Free Hospital in London is trying to establish whether moderate alcohol consumption leads to an increase in the viral load of HCV in the blood. If this is the case, then all HCV patients should abstain completely because higher viral loads are a clear indicator of poorer prognosis.

Complete abstinence from alcohol is stipulated by most natural health practitioners, particularly during treatment. For patients with a history of heavy alcohol consumption, abstinence is highly advisable; the latest research demonstrates the association between alcohol consumption, HCV, and liver cancer. The following quote is typical of current thinking:

> It appears that chronic hepatitis may act as a cofactor for the development of HCC in patients with alcoholic liver disease. In a case controlled study by Yamauchi et al.,[16] HCC developed in 81% of anti HCV+ patients with alcoholic cirrhosis at ten years [after diagnosis of cirrhosis], compared to only 19% for anti HCV negative patients with alcoholic liver disease and 57% for cases of HCV infection without alcoholic liver disease. These figures suggest a synergistic effect of both risk factors, an observation confirmed by others.[17]

If you have HCV and cannot stop drinking too much, then it is advisable to seek help. In the meantime some think that certain supplements such as N-acetyl cysteine or silymarin may help to minimize any harm.

Patient's Experience: Paul

I loved drinking. Going to the pub and sinking a few beers with my mates was my main pleasure in life. About two years ago I started to have real difficulties—it must have been about that time that the hep started to kick in. I couldn't get up and go to work as I had in the past, even if I'd only had two or three pints. I knew something was wrong but I had no idea what it was. I stopped for periods of time and things got better. But whenever I drank, even small amounts, I would take days to recover.

Getting the diagnosis and going to the support group has

put me in the picture, but I sure as hell miss it. I really wanted someone to say, "Yeah alcohol, it's the best thing for hep C; drink as much as you like—the more the better in fact." Unfortunately that didn't happen, and it's not going to either. I find that accepting that I cannot drink is the most difficult thing about having hepatitis C.

Other Drugs

All drugs exert strain on the liver and have immunosuppressive qualities, making them doubly hazardous. Taken in conjunction with alcohol over a long period of time, they often prove extremely debilitating, if not fatal. Research into the life-spans of active drug users with HCV reveals a very high likelihood of early death, much higher than theoretically clinically worse-off patients such as hemophiliacs with high viral loads. Impaired liver function and other symptoms of HCV may contribute towards the likelihood of drug overdose, although this has yet to be properly investigated.

Faced with the facts about drugs and HCV, it is difficult to avoid the conclusion that "clean living" has to be a priority. Damage limitation is another option—for example, eating hashish instead of injecting heroin. Eating well and taking high-power vitamins often help. If exercise doesn't sound like too absurd an idea, then try it, particularly something that works up a good sweat.

If you want to stop and can't, then remember that help may be available—twelve-step programs such as Narcotics Anonymous and Alcoholics Anonymous are a good place to start, and their telephone numbers will be listed.

Opiates—Heroin, Morphine, Codeine, and Methadone

Although it has previously been claimed that pure heroin is not directly hepatotoxic and therefore "safe," and that maintenance doses of methadone do not harm hepatitis C patients, it is now clear that this advice is based on a poor understanding of the pathogenesis of HCV and the pharmacological impact of opiates.

It is now clear that a healthy immune system, particularly the local response to HCV in the liver, is of vital importance in countering progressive viral damage. Opiates of all descriptions are now recognized as having immunosuppressive qualities; their ingestion therefore contributes to the pathogenesis of HCV. The following quotes outline the facts:

> There is an increasing body of evidence obtained both in vitro and in vivo showing that exogenous opioids have a variety of effects on cells in the immune system. They suppress cell mediated immunity, as reflected by depressed T dependent antibody production by B lymphocytes, altered T lymphocyte functions and decreased killer cell activity. The macrophage oxidative burst and phagocytosis are also impaired.... Data shows that morphine increases susceptibility to bacterial and viral infections, the latter effect possibly being related to a depressive effect of opioids on gamma interferon levels.[18]

> Previously it has been demonstrated that morphine suppresses hepatic and splenic phagocytic activity through an opiate receptor mediated pathway that involves the release of corticosterone. It would appear that methadone plays a similar role in the suppression of hepatic and splenic phagocytosis.[19]

> Our results suggest that the inhibition of macrophage defensive functions caused by drugs may be an important cofactor in the pathogenesis of infectious diseases.[20]

Since phagocytosis, described in the "Outline of the Immune System" notes in part 5, is vital in the prevention of liver damage, it is not surprising that patients on methadone complain of severe symptoms over and above those experienced by HCV-negative methadone users. It seems likely that the presence of opiates in the bloodstream leads directly to an accelerated rate of liver damage.

Further unambiguous evidence comes from a recent French report:

> In the presence of morphine, cultured monocytes showed an increase in the fluidity of their membranes as well as an inhibition in their capacity to differentiate into macrophages. Furthermore, the response of the cells to interferon gamma was significantly decreased and the release of superoxide anions was

altered. Finally the production of interferon-alpha and of prostaglandin E2 induced by stimulation of the cells with endotoxin (LPS) was diminished. We conclude that morphine decreases the functions of monocytes that are essential for their antiviral defense and inhibits their response to activating stimuli, which may explain the increased multiplication of HIV in morphine treated monocytes.[21]

Impurities in street heroin also contribute to myriad problems in the livers of intravenous drug users (IVDUs). For instance, talcum powder, a common adulterant, can be found in the livers of ex-IVDUs and is sometimes used by doctors to assess the likelihood of HCV infection via that route, particularly if they suspect a patient is not being truthful about previous IV drug use.

Another problem is that the addictive use of opiates means that the liver never gets a chance to reassemble its defenses. Occasional light use of drugs or alcohol does at least give this stressed organ a chance to recover during subsequent abstinence.

A Note about Methadone

Patients on methadone maintenance often complain of devastating symptoms despite being reassured by their doctors that it is "perfectly safe." It certainly seems that such complaints have a rational biochemical basis; not only does methadone exert the immunosuppressive effects listed above, the linctus form also contains known liver poisons. The long-term mass prescription of medicines containing ethanol and chloroform, albeit in small amounts, to patients with liver disease would seem to be extraordinary.

Since a significant proportion of methadone clients are likely to have HCV, there would be a sizeable market for a "liver friendly" version of this drug. The pharmaceutical company Schering-Plough appears to be considering introducing a new form of methadone. These circumstances would also combine to support the case for the adoption of diamorphine prescription policy, which is thought by some to be safer and more humane. The continued prescription of methadone linctus to HCV+ addicts would seem to be unnecessarily punitive and ethically questionable.

Cocaine, Amphetamines, and Other Stimulants

These are directly hepatotoxic and immunosuppressive, and are also particularly likely to have adverse consequences on mental health, especially if crack cocaine is used. Appetite suppression associated with stimulant use is also likely to lead to important nutritional deficiencies developing. Since these are linked to fibrogenesis (the development of cirrhosis) and oncogenesis (the development of cancer), it would seem to be very hazardous to take anything likely to reduce nutrient intake or storage capacity.

Benzodiazepines, Barbiturates, Sleeping Pills, Antidepressants, and Other Prescribed Stress Management Medications

These will all place additional stress on the liver and are "middleweight" toxins. Although they may present little or no risk to healthy people, they could accentuate liver damage in hepatitis C patients. The extent to which this is likely to occur varies. Patients with symptoms of faulty detoxification would be advised to steer well clear of benzodiazepines and barbiturates; as pointed out earlier, poor liver function may lead to the natural formation of similar substances, and these may be linked to symptoms of apathy and fatigue. If drugs to assist sleep are required, a sedating tricyclic like amitryptiline may be safer. Tricyclic drugs are used to treat depression and are safest in low doses. (Note that poor sleep quality is a noted symptom of liver disease in both conventional and traditional Chinese medicine—herbal treatments can sometimes help.)

Because so many patients encounter depression, antidepressants are sometimes necessary. Many patients on antidepressants such as Prozac complain of additional liver pain, although documented evidence of hepatic damage is difficult to obtain. There are a number of different serotonin reuptake inhibitors available apart from Prozac—ask your doctor for one that is gentle on the liver. Some reports suggest that Lustral may be relatively safe, while Seroxat may be associated with a number of disturbing side effects, particularly when discontinued. Some doctors suggest that Manerix, also known as Moclobemide, may be a more suitable antidepressant drug where fatigue is also present. However, this drug is classed as an MAO inhibitor and should therefore be avoided by patients with an impaired ability to process amines according to Lazarides; symptoms of hypertension or chemical sensitivity may be signs of problems in this area. Note that hypericin, the St. John's wort extract with antidepressant qualities, may also work through MAO inhibition, and therefore the same caution would apply.

The effects of these drugs on the livers and immune systems of patients have not been sufficiently well researched to be able to categorically state that they are all safe for hepatitis C patients. It is still wise to investigate other approaches to depression and sleeplessness as well. If you are prescribed these drugs, then try to monitor their effect on you, and trust your own experience. Also refer to the "Environmental Cofactors and Hepatitis C" section; some people believe that many such medicines contain ingredients that may act as cofactors in liver disease progression.

There are many drugs that can be toxic to people with liver disease under certain circumstances. You should always run prescriptions past your specialist. Some examples of drugs that can cause problems include acebutolol, phenylbutazone, allopurinol, phenytoin, atenolol, piroxicam, carbamazepine, probenecid, cimetidine, pyrazinamide, contraceptives, corticosteroids, dantrolene, quinidine, diclofenac, flurazepam, flutamide, ibuprofen, indomethacin, halothane, naproxen, antidepressant tricyclics, penicillins, and quinine.

Drugs that may be capable of causing liver tumors include anabolic steroids, danazol, oral contraceptives, and testosterone.

For details refer to *The Essential Guide to Prescription Drugs* by James Long and James Rybacki.

Marihuana and Hashish

Not thought to be directly hepatotoxic. However, smoking is carcinogenic, and therefore to be avoided if possible. Eating them may be less unhealthy than smoking.

Many recent research "findings" appear to have been inspired by particular views on the wider political debate regarding "The Drug War." The overall impact of these drugs is still not properly understood. In the absence of in-depth pharmacological understanding a common-sense-based approach may be advisable. For example, it is reasonable to conclude that the soporific qualities of these drugs will not help with fatigue or mental function.

Cigarettes and Nicotine

As mentioned above smoking is carcinogenic and may be a cofactor in the development of liver cancer as well as a proven cause of other cancers, particularly in the lungs and throat. Acetaldehyde, one of the toxic substances found in cigarette smoke, is known to destroy vitamins B_1, B_6, and C. Some researchers suggest that supplements of these vitamins plus cysteine and N-acetyl cysteine may help to counteract these effects.

Nicotine also presents particular problems to a compromised liver, which cannot metabolize the toxin as effectively as normal. This is obviously likely to contribute to compounded nicotine-related problems throughout the body.[22]

Many patients have poor blood circulation and related disorders; smoking will certainly contribute to the severity of these conditions. Depression is thought by some to be caused by poor cerebral blood circulation; therefore giving up smoking may help to alleviate depression in these patients.

The health of the lungs is linked to the health of protective Qi in Traditional Chinese Medicine. Western researchers have also linked lung health to levels of vital immunological substances such as glutathione and interferons. Some doctors believe that the development of cancerous tumors is enabled by immunological dysfunction.

Cigarette smoking is thought to be most damaging in combination with other unhealthy activities, particularly alcohol consumption. Many patients regard giving up cigarettes as a lower priority than giving up drugs or alcohol.

Hallucinogens: Magic Mushrooms, LSD, Ecstasy/MDMA, "Designer Drugs"

Some magic mushrooms place a heavy strain on the liver, particularly the fly agaric. Peyote is also suspect, and they will both have an adverse impact on the digestive system. LSD, ecstasy, and other designer drugs present risks through the presence of adulterants.

Long "trips" are likely to leave patients feeling particularly exhausted.

Aspirin, Disprin, Paracetamol/Acetaminophen, and Ibuprofen

All of these will have some impact on liver function. Occasional light use of aspirin and disprin may be safe for most patients. However, those with impaired liver function and associated blood clotting disorders must avoid these two products altogether; both of these reduce the ability of blood to clot. Persistent long-term use is contraindicated for hepatitis C patients. Paracetamol can be highly liver toxic when taken in excess—no more than 4X 500 mg should be taken in one day. Overdose leads to death, unless treated immediately with N-acetyl cysteine (see chapter 18). Until recently ibuprofen was often recommended to patients as being the safest option; however, recent studies suggest that this has an adverse impact on liver function and should therefore also be used with caution. Because information is still emerging, it is a good idea to consult your specialist for advice on what is the safest pain relief treatment.

If you do get persistent recurrent headaches, then take a close look at chapters 15, 16, and 18 and the "Diet and Digestion" section of this chapter.

Amyl Nitrate

Severely toxic to the immune system. Places stress on the cardiovascular system and the liver.

Environmental Cofactors and Hepatitis C

This section examines hepatitis C from the perspective of the cofactor theory; the central concept in this idea is that significant progression of HCV is enabled by exposure to particular environmental and dietary cofactors. It is suggested that progression can be limited or even arrested by the strict avoidance of these identified cofactors.

This is a radical perspective that owes much to a naturopathic view of health and the world in general. However, the logic is coherent, and many people coming to terms with hep C will find something of practical use in this approach; it may not be necessary for you to go "all the way." Because these "cofactors" are so deeply infiltrated into our environment and other aspects of life, the radical changes necessary to action all of these insights will be impractical for most people. An example of somebody who has taken extreme measures follows.

E.P. is a long term hepatitis C patient who was also diagnosed with aplastic anemia in the mid-1980s; this is a very serious condition that features the failure of the bone marrow to produce the blood cells necessary for life. (It has been suggested that this condition may be linked to HCV infection.) E.P. wrote to the hepatitis C support group in England to share his views on the virus, causes of progression, and his recovery from this condition, which in his case involved moving to the French countryside to avoid risk cofactors:

> Fortunately for me the information necessary for survival for aplastic anemia (avoidance of drugs, chemicals, and radiation), is exactly the same as necessary for hepatitis C.... Most prescribed drugs can cause serious liver damage—benzene, fluorine, chlorine, etc., in many drugs are very toxic to the liver and bone marrow causing a large percentage of all cancers. Virus and genetics are red herrings as causes of cancer, being only secondary contributory causes.

E.P. went on to expound the theory in a number of articles and letters to various U.K. newspaper editors; for example in an article entitled "Hepatitis C does not have to be fatal" in the *Halifax Evening Courier,* January 8, 1997, he wrote:

> Since August 24, 1989, when the story first broke, many reports have appeared in the Press which suggest that a high percentage of those infected with hepatitis C will eventually die of cirrhosis or cancer of the liver in following years.
>
> As one infected with the virus in 1986 through a blood transfusion given for severe aplastic anemia I was suffering from at that time, I have looked at the problem of long-term fatal liver conditions developing from the infection, and I am convinced that victims can do quite a lot to help themselves prevent a fatal outcome.

The government and medical profession, as well as the media, are guilty of not giving victims information that is vital for their survival or recovery.

As far back as 1986 I was taking measures to treat the disorder, which was showing up as chronic liver malfunction.

The first obvious thing to do with a liver disorder is to avoid all the things that are toxic to the liver which can cause fatal liver disease.

Avoiding alcohol as much as possible is essential, and also if at all possible avoid all the many prescribed drugs which should only be taken by hepatitis C sufferers when not taking the drug might prove fatal. All the drugs taken for depression and anxiety can be toxic to the liver and should also be avoided.

In addition to drugs and alcohol, there are many environmental chemicals which can be very toxic to the liver and can be easily avoided. These include solvents, paints, dry cleaning fluids, and all other petroleum-based chemicals. In addition, tap water should be avoided as the halogen chemicals added could be toxic to the liver. I refer to chlorine and also to fluoride, which in some areas are added to the water.

It is a pity that the Government, the medical profession, and the media have terrified so many victims of hepatitis C by leading them to believe that they will probably die of a fatal disease in the long term and denying them information which is vital for their survival.

E.P. went on to point out that his letter had been slightly censored with respect to the need for a low-fat diet and also cited the chemical content of Prozac (2-benzene 3-fluoride) as being a known liver toxin, and therefore a likely cofactor in disease progression.

Environmental pollutants that are theoretically capable of contributing to liver disease progression and the development of cancers include the following:

Benzene:

A genotoxin, hematoxin, and carcinogen. Chronic exposure causes aplastic anemia in humans and animals and is associated with increased incidence of leukemia in humans and lymphomas and certain solid tumors in rodents. Bioactivation of benzene is required for toxicity. In the liver, the major site of benzene metabolism, benzene is converted by a cytochrome p450-mediated pathway to phenol, the major metabolite.... Phenol is metabolized in the marrow cells ultimately to quinones, the putative toxic metabolites.[23]

Benzene has been a suspect in a number of epidemiological studies looking at the incidence of cancers. For instance one Swedish study linked its presence in air to leukemia:

Benzene is an established cause of leukemia in adults, especially acute non-lymphocytic leukemia (ANLL). A few studies have indicated that exposure to gasoline is a cause of childhood leukemia.[24]

It is reasonable to presume that benzene is processed less effectively in a compromised liver, leading to a greater possibility of a vicious cycle of toxicity setting in (refer to Linda Lazarides's work earlier in this chapter for more information on the liver and toxins). Benzene is present in unleaded gasoline (the supposedly "green" fuel), paints, thinners, varnishes, solvents, pesticides, herbicides, solvent adhesives, correcting fluid, and all petroleum products. It is thought to be doubly carcinogenic in conjunction with other suspect substances such as fluorine and fluoride.

Fluorine and **fluoride:** Fluorine is also present in unleaded gasoline; a form of both of these chemicals is present in Prozac and many other antidepressant drugs. In many areas water is treated with fluoride as well as chlorine.

Chlorine: Another agent cited by E.P. as being a known cause of cancers and anemia. Often used to treat tap water.

Radiation in all forms, including X-rays and long-term exposure to VDU emissions. Some people believe that proximity to electric pylons can cause increased rates of cancer and blood abnormalities. Obviously avoid atomic and nuclear explosions!

A Summary of Steps Patients Could Take to Avoid or Minimize Risks from Environmental Cofactors

- Avoid or reduce exposure to air pollution, particularly traffic related.

- Avoid or reduce exposure to all petroleum-based products.

- Avoid all pharmaceutical medicines containing cofactors unless not taking them will have severe consequences.

- Drink bottled spring water if possible.

- Otherwise drink filtered and purified water, avoiding or reducing chlorine, fluoride, and nitrates.

- Avoid or reduce exposure to radiation, including low-level sources.

Further Reading on Diet

Nutritional Health Bible. Linda Lazarides. Thorsons.
Healing with Whole Foods: Oriental Traditions and Modern Nutrition. Paul Pitchford. North Atlantic Books, 1993.
A Real "Hep" Cookbook. Ramona Jones CNC and Vonah Stanfield. Published by Nature's Response, $12.95 plus $3 shipping in the U.S.; phone (800) 216-5195 in the U.S.
Food Combining for Health. Doris Grant and Jean Joice.
Fit for Life Diet. Harvey and Marilyn Diamond.
Chinese System of Food Cures. Heng C. Lu.
The Tao of Nutrition. Mao Shig Ni.
Prince Wen Hui's Cook Book. Bob Flaws.
Staying Healthy with Nutrition. Elson Haas. Celestial Arts Publishing, 1992.

References

1. *Hepatitis C Patient Information Booklet.* Dr. JP Watson and Dr. MF Bassendine. PP 10. Produced by Roche Products Ltd.

2. *Liverlink* (Royal free liver support newsletter). May 1995.

3. Oltipraz chemoprevention trial in Qidong, People's Republic of China:

modulation of serum aflatoxin albumin adduct biomarkers. Kensler TW et al. *Cancer Epidemiol Biomarkers Prev,* 7(2):127–134, Feb 1998. Contact Department of Environmental Health Sciences, Johns Hopkins School of Hygiene and Public Health, Baltimore, Maryland 21205, U.S., for further information.

4. Positive Health. Brian Wright. July/August 1996.

5. Considering wheat, rye, and barley proteins as aids to carcinogens. Hoggan R. *Medical Hypotheses,* 49(3):285–8, Sept 1997.

6. *Probiotics.* Chaitow L et al. Thorsons, 1990.

7. Oral citrus seed extract in atopic eczema. Ionescu et al. *J. Orthomolecular Medicine,* 1990.

8. *The Family Guide to Homeopathy.* Dr. Andrew Lockie. Hamish Hamilton.

9. For example: Survey of pesticide residues in food. British Association of public analysts, 1983. Also see *This Poisoned Earth.* Nigel Dudley. Piatkus Books, 1987.

10. For example: *Immunologic Considerations in Toxicology, Volume 1.* Sharma RP. CRC Press, Baton Rouge, Florida, 1981.

11. Drinking water nitrate and the risk of non-Hodgkin's lymphoma. Ward MH, Mark SD, Cantor KP, Weisenburger DD, Correa-Villasenor A, Zahm SH. *Epidemiology,* 7(5):465–71, Sept 1996.

12. New dimensions in calcium metabolism. *Osteopathic Annals,* 11, 38–59, 1983.

13. Single nutrients and immunity. Beisel WR. *Am J. Clin Nutr,* 35, 417–468, 1982.

14. Recent developments in alcoholism: the liver. *Alcoholism,* 11: 207–30, 1993.

15. Letter. October 6, 1994.

16. Prevalence of HCC in patients with alcoholic cirrhosis and prior exposure to hepatitis C. *Am J Gastroenterol,* 88: 39–43, 1993.

17. Viral hepatitis and hepatocellular carcinoma. Sallie R et al. *Gastroenterology Clinics of N America,* 23(3), Sept 1994.

18. Opiates and immune function consequences. Rouveux B. *Therapie,* 47(6):503–12, Nov 1992 (France).

19. Study by Levier DG et al. *Fundamental and Applied Toxicology,* 24(2):275–84, Feb 1995.

20. Macrophage functions in drugs of abuse treated mice. Pacifici R et al. *International Journal of Immunopharmacology,* 15(6):7 6–11, Aug 1993.

21. Effects of morphine on purified human blood monocytes. Modifications of properties involved in antiviral defenses. Stoll-Keller F et al. *Int*

J Immunopharmacol, 19(2):95–100, Feb 1997.

22. Nicotine metabolism in liver microsomes from rats with acute hepatitis or cirrhosis. Nakajima M, Iwata K, Yamamoto T, Funae Y, Yoshida T, Kuroiwa Y. *Drug Metab Dispos,* 26(1):36–41, Jan 1, 1998. Clinical Pharmacy, School of Pharmaceutical Sciences, Showa University.

23. Recent advances in the metabolism and toxicity of Benzene. Kalf GF. *Crit Rev Toxicol,* 18(2):141–59, 1987.

24. Environmental exposure to gasoline and leukemia in children and young adults—an ecology study. Nordlinder R, Jarvholm B. *International Archives of Occupational and Environmental Health,* 70(1):57–60, 1997.

23

Exercise, Yoga, and Qi Gong

DRAMATICALLY CONTRASTING and contradictory advice is often given to hepatitis patients with regard to exercise. This confusion sometimes arises out of the differing disposition of people with acute and chronic conditions. Since hepatitis C is overwhelmingly a chronic, long-term condition, patients should disregard the cautionary advice given to acute-phase sufferers unless they are a part of the small minority who suffer an acute phase in the first instance. During the acute phase, characterized by symptoms such as jaundice and severe liver inflammation, patients should heed advice to relax completely and undertake no physically demanding tasks whatsoever.

Advisory booklets on chronic hepatitis often advocate exercise for patients. HCV+ people that I have talked to report that regular exercise has helped to counteract some symptoms and has contributed to a more positive outlook and a greater sense of well-being. It seems that exercise can be a good coping mechanism and may contribute to improved prognosis and reduced debilitation. Exercise is also a great method of monitoring one's health; the benefits of any particular therapy or lifestyle change can be assessed by checking the impact on regularly performed exercises.

Broadly speaking there are two types of approaches to exercise: the first involves what can be termed "conventional" activities like running, playing football, swimming, tennis, and so on; the second involves activities like yoga and Qi Gong that can be described as "alternative."

Conventional Exercise

Almost all patients who have taken up regular exercise report that they think it has been of benefit; some regard it as a vital component in their management of hepatitis C. The benefits of taking conventional exercise have not yet been adequately studied in chronic hepatitis. The following benefits are therefore largely speculative.

Increased blood circulation may help to prevent the development of cirrhosis or to slow its progression; keeping the blood vessels open and regularly flushed may counteract the scarring process, which is associated with stagnant blood flow as well as viral infection. The chances of developing cardiovascular problems may be reduced.

However, patients with portal hypertension may find that their clinical situation deteriorates or is antagonized by taking such exercise.

Increased fitness and physical stamina may help to alleviate chronic fatigue, although it will not address energy problems related to the glycogen cycle that are caused by organ malfunction or diet. Higher levels of fitness and a body weight close to what would be expected for a patient's height and build are associated with better responses to antiviral therapy. Good blood access to infected organs such as the liver may be also be a factor in response rates.

Sweating is a very important part of the waste elimination system, whose efficiency is regarded as being of central importance in hepatitis C patients by many complementary medical practitioners. It is also a recognized part of the immune system; regular sweating will help to take to take the strain off the rest of the body's defenses. Obviously swimming and other water sports do not provoke sweating. Less energetic patients could consider visiting Turkish baths.

Taking exercise and being reasonably fit has been strongly linked to improved immune function. Studies of obese people have shown decreased neutrophil activity. Improved self-esteem and increased strength can help patients feel that they are fighting back effectively; this positive change may contribute to revitalized immune function. The health of the lungs is linked to the production of important antibodies in both conventional and some traditional medicinal models.

Exercise counteracts stress, which is associated with decreased immunological efficiency and increased production of adrenaline and other immune suppressants. The feeling of relaxation that follows exercise is a healthy sign.

Exercise may help to prevent lymphoma; however, if lymphoma has been diagnosed, it is advisable to abstain because it is thought that cancerous cells will be spread throughout the body, perhaps assisting the development of secondary cancers in other sites.

A Note of Caution

If you are out of condition and want to start to take some exercise, it is a good idea to start slowly and adopt a patient ('scuse the pun) approach. So far as something like running is concerned, it is a good idea to just try to keep going for a period of time, rather than complete a given distance in a set time. If you live in the city, try to find somewhere away from the exhaust fumes, as these will not do you any good at all. After a few weeks of doing this every other day or so, you will begin to get an idea of your capacity.

Overexercise or compulsive exercising is dangerous and is associated with reduced immune function and increased susceptibility to a range of illnesses. Top athletes are constantly going down with viral infections.

It is important to eat well, particularly proteins and carbohydrates. If you sweat a lot, remember to replace these fluids, preferably with purified water.

If you are doubtful about your ability to exercise safely, check it out with your doctor, or consider the alternatives listed below.

Alternative Exercise: Yoga, Qi Gong, Tai Qi, and So On

Almost everybody can take up these disciplines—some patients use them as a form of treatment. In general, these practices aim to open up the internal energy channels and chakras, whose condition is associated with health in Eastern models of well-being. They all embrace mental and emotional balance together with improved physical strength and vitality. The impact is often subtle and may be slow to materialize at the beginning. It usually takes a while to reap the rewards of practice, so perseverance is necessary.

The emphasis is on the health of internal organs rather than muscular strength in these systems. They all have sets of movements or stances that are designed to improve the health of the liver and increase overall energy levels. They also help with relaxation and may therefore be expected to benefit the immune system. Qi Gong can be regarded as a complete health system in its own right (it is discussed in chapter 15, pages 260–264).

It is important to get a good teacher—experience counts for a lot in these practices. They are particularly suitable for older patients and those who have debilitating secondary symptoms such as arthritis. Some patients take up both conventional and alternative exercise—they are not mutually exclusive.

24

Stress

IT IS THE OPINION of many patients and a number of medical practitioners that the physical, mental, and emotional symptoms of hepatitis C are all accentuated either by high levels of stress or by unhealthy methods of coping. Many think that the onset of stress precedes an "attack" of symptoms, particularly fatigue; this experience echoes that of M.E. patients. One patient interviewed for this book keeps a chart of liver function test results that she claims correlate with stressful episodes in her life, such as tumultuous love affairs or business pressures.

Removing unnecessary sources of stress, developing healthy ways of responding to the inevitable levels of stress inherent in being alive, and learning how to relax are therefore key issues for patients. It is also likely that stress reduction and the use of effective relaxation techniques will improve prognosis; although this would be nearly impossible to prove statistically, it is a logical conclusion based upon what is known about the various effects of mental and emotional stress on human physiology and the pathogenesis of hepatitis C. In other words, the onus should be on skeptics to disprove the assertion that measures to counteract stress improve health and long-term prognosis, rather than on those who suggest that this approach is likely to be beneficial to prove their case.

The Physiological Impact of Stress

The nervous system responds to stress in much the same way as the immune system responds to an antigen. Stress has been defined as any perceived or actual demand upon the body to adapt or readjust. Research undertaken as long ago as the 1930s, by doctors such as Hans Selye, demonstrated a pattern of physiological response that includes the following clinical conditions: enlargement of the adrenal cortex; intense atrophy of the thymus, spleen, and lymph nodes; and bleeding stomach and duodenal ulcers. The process appears to start with the hypothalamus triggering the pituitary gland to produce hormones that regulate the endocrine system, which in turn "asks" the adrenal glands to release corticosteroids and adrenalin, both hormones. It is a surge in the level of adrenalin that causes the hypervigilant sensation we feel when under threat.

These potent hormones have a powerful impact on the body, which can be particularly damaging if they are frequently present in large quantities over a long period of time. Unrelieved stress or a prolonged response to a perception of being threatened gives rise to elevated levels of cortisol in the blood. Diseases associated with chronic high levels of cortisol include depression, cancer, alcoholism, drug addiction, hypertension, ulcers, diabetes, arthritis, stroke, and multiple sclerosis. These chemicals will also indirectly affect the liver, which has to deal with the overall chemical balance of the body. Many practitioners believe that the liver is intimately connected with emotion; it is seen as the seat of anger in many traditional health systems. It does seem probable that there is a link between the biochemistry of stress, negative emotion, and the physical state of the liver.

It therefore seems that patients need to be concerned not only with the chemical makeup of the substances that are consumed, but also the chemicals that are produced inside the body. Cortisol is an immunosuppressant. It destroys lymphoid tissues, particularly in the vital thymus gland, reduces the number of T helper cells, and blocks the production of natural killer cells and interferon. Thus it will undermine the body's defense against HCV, particularly in the liver region, where the immune process is so important in the prevention of HCV pathogenesis.

Chronic high levels of cortisol are also thought to damage certain parts of the brain, particularly those dealing with memory. Research undertaken at the University of California by Robert Sapolsky suggests that damage is compounded by high levels of alcohol intake, another symptom of stress. These findings indicate yet another potential cause of the mental dysfunction commonly reported by patients.

Studies of students comparing their status prior to exams and after them have shown reduced levels of natural killer cells and higher levels of antibodies to Epstein Barr and herpes viruses when the stress level was high before the exam.[1] Other studies have appeared to demonstrate that happy emotional states such as love or feeling safe produce healthy immunological profiles. Some health professionals go on to suggest that people who repress their emotions are less likely to have healthy immune systems and are quite literally "dis-eased.'

Unhealthy Stress Responses

Doctors do not really know why some HCV patients progress rapidly and others very slowly, particularly when factors such as active alcoholism have been excluded. It may be the case that chronic unhealthy response to stress explains at least some of these cases of accelerated progression and why some patients do not progress. A number of doctors have also linked autoimmune diseases with stress and the emotions of anger and anxiety in particular. Michael Weiner, author of *Maximum Immunity,* has noted that autoimmune disease tends to cluster in people who have difficulty in expressing negative emotion, particularly women who find it difficult to express anger:

> People with autoimmune diseases seem to show a pronounced tendency to suppress anger and other negative emotions. Traditionally it has been women in our society who have been discouraged from expressing anger, and this may help to account for the high incidence of autoimmune diseases in women.

It seems that some people have permanently high levels of stress response regardless of the presence or absence of threatening stimuli. This state is often called the "flight or fight" state. Much has been written about this, and a common observation is that such people are often unable to express emotion, that they bottle up feelings and therefore fail to clear the biochemical response to trauma. It is this state of undischarged emotion that is associated with chronic high levels of cortisol and its associated illnesses. It is going to be very difficult to attain a satisfactory state of health while this state persists regardless of whether it actually influences disease progression or not.

Solutions

If it is true that the physiological consequences of feeling stressed contribute to the progression of hepatitis C, then it should be possible to favorably influence the outcome by adopting effective relaxation techniques and appropriate lifestyle changes.

The book *AIDS and the Healer Within* (Amethyst Books), by Nick Bamforth, is an excellent account of the relationship between emotional and physical health and examines both the causes of chronic stress and ways in which it can be addressed. The book's view of health and its conclusions are remarkably similar to those of yoga and Qi Gong teachers. Although it is obviously aimed at HIV patients, everything he says applies equally to hepatitis C, if not more so.

Yoga, meditation, and Qi Gong will be effective methods of relieving stress for many patients, and for some may provide a method of more profound change towards a less stressful lifestyle or a different attitude to life.

Psychotherapy or twelve-step programs may also help patients to come to terms with deep-rooted causes of chronic stress.

Autogenic training, which is based on yoga techniques, has a good reputation for promoting relaxation. It has been used extensively in Germany to treat people at risk from stress-related heart disease.

Exercise is known to be a good stress reliever and management tool. Vigorous exercise can be an excellent way of discharging anger, as well as having wider benefits for patients.

There are a wide range of therapies aimed at stress relief, such as biofeedback, hypnosis, deep breathing, and visualization.

Taking Power Back: Disempowering Hepatitis C

It is possible to give hepatitis C too much power in your life. Fear of the implications of having this virus can be a real source of stress in itself. Assimilating all of the material in this book may have had the effect of making this virus appear overwhelmingly threatening. In fact it is well within the bounds of possibility that most patients will be able to live with HCV without diminished life expectancy. This is particularly true for those who have been diagnosed early or in whom the disease has not yet progressed.

The ability to change and adapt to the facts so far as they are known is key to the disempowerment of HCV. It seems possible that patients may effectively but unwittingly give permission to the virus to progress by not making positive changes. This is understandable given the fact that the virus is only now beginning to be understood, and that the links of lifestyle and attitude to prognosis are slowly becoming apparent. Unexpressed, undischarged emotions exert power over our lives and our health. It seems quite likely that in addressing these emotional issues we will be effectively treating hepatitis C as well.

It is a common experience that people who begin to unravel the causes of chronic stress often start to find it easier to make other, apparently unrelated positive changes. This virus thrives on alcohol and drug abuse, indolence, apathy, depression, stagnation, emotional repression, junk food, isolation, and ignorance. All of these attitudes and behaviors help to empower HCV; replacing them with abstinence, moderation, exercise, positivity, dynamism, free expression of feelings, a healthy diet, communication with other patients, and an understanding of the virus disempowers hepatitis C and constitutes a basis for genuine health in conjunction with appropriate treatment.

The essential purpose of this book is to highlight what HCV actually is, how it can manifest itself, what gives the virus power, and what gives patients the power to regain authority over their lives. Having found out what works for you, what genuinely makes you feel free of a sense of stress and "dis-ease," you can put this book on the shelf and concentrate on living your life as fully and rewardingly as you care to.

Reference

1. Stressor exposure and immunological response in man; interferon producing capacity and phagocytosis. Palamblad et al. *Psychosomatic Res,* 20, 193–199, 1976.

Part

5

Notes, Afterword, Resources, and Index

Notes:
An Outline of the Immune System
and Its Key Components

It is now widely thought that the immune response to HCV is vital to understanding pathogenesis and defining treatment strategy. Many doctors think that this is largely an immune-mediated condition. This means that the extent to which it progresses in an individual patient, clinical disease profile, symptoms, and treatment strategy can all be largely defined and understood in terms of immunology. This is now accepted by many in the conventional, complementary, and alternative medical establishments. For instance, the conclusions of two recent studies read as follows:

> In acute hepatitis C infection viral elimination depends on a HCV specific CD4+ T cell response.... Our results indicate that a virus specific CD4+ T cell response which eliminates the virus during the acute phase of the disease has to be maintained in order to persistently control the virus. These results may contribute to therapeutic approaches, which should aim at an induction of virus specific CD4+ T cells in patients with chronic HCV to achieve viral elimination.[1]

> Expansion of B lymphocytes and antibody production to virtually any HCV protein can be detected in most infected patients. However, observations suggest that HCV infection does not induce protective immunity and reinfection can be readily demonstrated. Nevertheless the immune system may gain partial control over HCV even in patients with chronic infection, as HCV infection in severely immunocompromised patients runs a particular cholestatic course which may rapidly lead to death from liver failure.

Cytotoxic CD8+ T lymphocyte responses to HCV proteins have been characterized in peripheral blood and liver tissue and were found to be remarkably polyclonal and multispecific. The HCV core and NS4 proteins appear to be most immunogenic for peripheral blood lymphocytes and NS4 specific CD4+ lymphocytes are preferentially compartmentalized to the liver.

However, there is an inverse relationship between CD4+ lymphocyte responses and antibody levels in infected patients. Furthermore a strong cellular response to the HCV core protein apparently favors a benign course of infection. Alternatively this virus may have found devices that can disturb immunoregulation in infected patients.[2]

The function of the human immune system is to protect the body from attack by foreign agents, or antigens, and to eliminate toxins and other damaging or superfluous substances; seen from the immune system's point of view, the world is full of pernicious bodies trying to cross its boundaries. Antigens are usually recognized, intercepted, and neutralized in a variety of ways before they can get established.

Until recently it was thought that about 50% of those exposed to HCV managed to either clear the virus or confine its presence to undetectable levels in the blood; in other words the immune system did its job.[1] This figure was often cited to reassure both patients and the general public. It is now known that a much lower percentage actually clear the virus, at most 20%; it is possible that no one who has gone on to develop HCV infection gets rid of the virus without treatment. Inaccuracies in early antibody and PCR tests and the soothing approach of public health officials contributed to this misconception.

The high rates of chronic disease and the persistence of the virus may be explained by the fact that the immune system fails to generate effective neutralizing antibodies. It appears that HCV has a variable genetic identity that enables it to change its appearance to killer cells. Killer cells cannot neutralize HCV unless they have the correct description. This does not mean that other arms of the immune system stop trying to fight the virus; however, the interception of HCV seems to occur at a later stage in its pathogenesis. (It may be the case that a depressed immune system at the time of infection contributes to allowing HCV to get established; this may be linked to lifestyle. Mode of transmission also contributes to the likelihood of chronic infection; transfused patients usually receive a higher viral load. It has also been suggested that HCV somehow eludes detection and is therefore not properly intercepted.) As the virus becomes more established in obscure parts of the body, it becomes more difficult to dislodge. Even if it can be temporarily eliminated from the blood, "reservoirs" of the virus persist in other parts of the body.

Some HCV patients seem to develop an overactive immune system or a kind of faulty functioning that means that the body starts to attack itself; this leads to autoimmune diseases such as those listed in the "Nature and Characteristics of the Hepatitis C Virus" section of chapter 1. It appears that hepatitis C is not properly engaged by the immune system, which leads many practitioners to believe that a long-term cure for HCV is most likely to be found by trying to effect a 100% healthy immune response over a considerable period of time.

The drug interferon alpha reflects this line of thought. Many practitioners of natural medicine also feel that therapy should aim to optimize immune function; in their case the technique is different, consisting of tactics like dietary change, herbs, exercise, meditation, vitamins, and so on. While the health of the liver is very important, the key to a cure or long-term survival without debility is thought by many to be closely linked to the healthy functioning of the immune system.

It is now clear that the human immune system is extremely complex. Doctors do not yet possess a fully accurate model of its functioning. The behavior of many viruses when they are introduced into the human body is still unpredictable, indicating that the model is faulty or incomplete. It has become apparent that many "immune stimulants" actually have quite complex actions on the various components. For instance, interferon alpha may enhance intracellular immune response, but it depresses other parts, such as white blood cells. The same goes for many herbs, which can both activate and depress different parts of the immune response. Many so-called immune supplements could more accurately be described as retuning the immune system.

The Key Components of the Immune System

The following is a brief outline of the components of the human immune system as they are currently understood.

The **lymphatic system** can be seen as the body's command and control network for immune response. It is a complete circulatory system independent of the blood vessels; it contains lymph, a yellowish thin fluid that contains the lymphocytes, one type of white blood cell. Lymph nodes are situated throughout the body, including on the sides of the neck. When the system is more active than usual these nodes may swell, causing the classic swollen appearance of the flu patient, for instance.

Because HCV inhabits the lymphatic system, its health needs to be closely monitored. It is also arguable that HCV is an immunosuppressive virus in the sense that it inhibits the overall effectiveness of this vital system, even though it does not directly attack particular immune cells like HIV.

Lymphocytes are programmed to recognize a particular antigen. They are clones of an original parent cell that was initially created in response to a particular antigen, either from a prenatal genetic code or exposure during the organism's lifetime. There are estimated to be a million billion lymphocytes in circulation containing information on up to 10 million different infections.

Phagocytes are very important destroyers of antigens (they came up frequently while I was researching this book). The liver biopsy reports of HCV patients frequently refer to the presence of phagocytes surrounding infected tissue. The process of phagocytosis is a vital component of the liver's self-defense mechanism against HCV pathogenesis. There are two main types.

Macrophages are unusually large white blood cells that actually engulf antigens. They are sometimes visualized as being like "Pac-Men." Once an antigen has been recognized and marked these cells gobble them up (scientifically this is known as *phagocytosis*). Sites of chronic infection are often surrounded by macrophages, which can survive for long periods of time. They are also capable of consuming protozoa and are thought to attack cancer cells.

Granulocytes are the other type. They comprise three categories of much smaller, shorter-lived white cells. They are thought to help in the process of cleaning up infected sites.

Cytokines are chemical messengers secreted by infected cells. They alert other parts of the body, both locally and remotely, that something is wrong, and help to reset the immune system. Interferons and interleukins are both cytokines.

The **spleen** is a secondary lymphatic organ located on the left side of the abdomen below the ribs. This organ helps to regulate the balance between the various immune cells. A chronically swollen spleen indicates ongoing immune problems. The appendix and the tonsils are also important sites in the lymphatic drainage system.

The **bone marrow** is where B and T cells are first produced. B cells mature here, while T cells migrate to the thymus. It is also the site of phagocyte and red blood cell production.

T cells deal with antigens that have penetrated into cells; this area of the system is known as "cell-mediated immunity." They also combat bacteria, fungi, and parasites. They develop into different types.

T helper cells/CD4 cells influence neighboring cells, apparently alerting them that something is wrong, and setting the immune response in motion. They activate the B cells, which release the antibodies. It is these cells that are supposed to release interferons and interleukins, which activate macrophages and cytotoxic T cells.

It is the behavior of these cells that are thought to be the primary indicator of who is likely to clear the virus upon infection and who is not. Researchers at the Institute of Liver Studies, Kings College Hospital, London, have shown that "a strong and multispecific CD4+ lymphocyte response to HCV proteins is only present in HCV infected patients who successfully clear the virus.... Of particular interest is the maintenance of the CD4+ lymphocyte response for many years after initial exposure to HCV."

There are thought to be two types of CD4 cells, TH1 and TH2. TH1 cells govern cellular immunity, and TH2 cells govern antibody production. In the case of HCV a few patients seem to cease to produce antibodies, indicating a weakened or even a discontinued response (see chapter 6 for reports).

T cytotoxic cells/CD8 cells, also known as killer cells or natural killer cells, are able to infiltrate body tissue. They kill infected cells, although the mechanism by which they achieve this is still not properly understood. It is thought that CD4 cells target infected cells for CD8s to destroy. They may also produce substances that inhibit viral replication. Long-term survivors of HIV tend to have high levels of cytotoxic CD8 cells. The activity level of this "cell-mediated immunity" is thought to be key in the process of viral clearance.

T suppressor cells help to regulate the immune system by "turning off" certain functions in adjacent cells. They are like helper cells in reverse.

The thymus gland lies at the center of this network. Situated in the center of the upper chest, it is here that the vital T cells mature. The gland governs the release of T cells into the system. The thymus gland shrinks in later life, and this may be linked to less efficient response.

White blood cells, sometimes known as leucocytes, comprise a small fraction of overall blood cells—99% are red. There are a number of types: polymorphonuclear neutrophil leucocytes (the most numerous), lymphocytes, monocytes, basophils, eosinophils.

Antibodies are also known as immunoglobulins, or IGs. Produced by B cells, they fight antigens by combining with the specific antigen that stimulated their production; they disable bacteria from producing toxins, coat antigens for consumption by scavenger cells, and block viruses from entering body cells. They are ineffective as single agents and seem to function by enabling cytotoxic T cells to attack their targets.

B cells form a large component of the lymphocytes. The "B" means that they originated in the bone marrow. B cells actually produce the antibodies that help to neutralize antigens. It is these cells that produce the antibodies that are detected in the ELISA and RIBA tests. Some B cells are thought to play a role in the "memory" of the immune system, reflecting a history of previous exposure to antigens, and are able to trigger a rapid immune response upon reinfection.

References

1. The role of hepatitis C virus specific CD4+ T lymphocytes in acute and chronic hepatitis C. Diepolder HM et al. *Journal of Molecular Medicine,* 74(10):583–8, Oct 1996.

2. Immune responses in hepatitis C infection. Spengler U et al. *J Hepatol,* 24:2 Suppl 20–5, 1996.

Notes:
Models of Viral Persistence

Some researchers have attempted to create models of how and why certain viruses are so difficult to treat successfully. These frameworks have been used to speculate about how future treatments should be adapted and how long they might need to be applied in order to clear the pathogen in question.

Little work has been done on the dynamics of the struggle between HCV and the immune system. However, it may be the case that the "indolence" of hepatitis C is due to the fact that it is constantly being intercepted by the immune system. Although it is not being completely eradicated, the virus is being countered. The common symptom of tiredness may be caused in part by this extra stress on body defenses and the effects of this struggle.

Dr. David Ho, a famous HIV virology specialist based in New York, recently concluded that HIV was indeed being engaged by the immune system, with millions of virions being destroyed every day (known as "turnover"); the trouble, he suggested, was that the rate of viral reproduction was faster than that of its destruction by the immune system. As the immune system becomes more compromised, the deficit gets larger, leading to a greater viral load in the blood, which, in turn, leads to a worse prognosis. It was previously assumed that the immune system was "missing" HIV or only engaging it in a half-hearted manner. Early speculation about HCV reached similar conclusions and may be similarly mistaken.

A second vital conclusion of Ho's is that antiviral drug treatment for HIV needs to be sustained for at least three years, despite the fact that the virus may become undetectable in the blood following only a few weeks' treatment.[1] This is due to the fact that it "lurks" in "reservoirs" within the body such as lymph glands and the liver. From these "compartments," whose infected cells live longer than lymphocytes, the virus can replicate and diffuse into the blood, although the primary infection of blood cells may have been curtailed. Thus the rate of decline of the viral load in the blood decreases. Ho has speculated that it would take three years for these antiviral drugs to eradicate the virus from these reservoirs. This is significant because this drug combination—a proteinase inhibitor + two nucleoside analogues—is extremely expensive and causes serious side effects in many patients.

It is worth noting that herbal treatments have also achieved considerable success with newly diagnosed patients. Austrian research suggests that a similar result can be achieved using antiviral herbs; however, there is an interesting difference in the profile of the decline in the viral load. Herbal treatment appears to achieve a slower but steadier decline in the viral load, indicating that it is penetrating into the "compartments," and neutralizing the virus in longer lived cells; in other words, "it reaches the parts that antiviral drugs cannot reach." This is consistent with the idea often put forward by herbalists that plant products are able to achieve an effect within living cells that drugs cannot. This suggests that certain herbs can act synergistically with cell-mediated immunity and do not necessarily have to be in direct contact with these cells to achieve this effect.

By comparison, research into the efficacy of HCV antiviral treatments is in its infancy. HCV is theoretically easier to treat than HIV because it is not a retrovirus. However, the results to date are very disappointing. Interferon alpha treatment may only achieve a sustained PCR negative response in about 18% of trial patients overall, while that figure may rise when it is used in combination with other drugs like the nucleoside analogue ribavirin.

Ho's theories may help to explain why the sustained response rate of HCV patients is so low, particularly among the 50% or so of trialists who initially go PCR negative. It seems probable that HCV has its own "compartments" whence it is more difficult to eliminate them using antiviral drugs. The fact that patients with cirrhosis have the worst response rate might be linked to the fact that the blood supply containing the antiviral drug doesn't come into proper contact with infected cells. HCV is also known to inhabit certain white blood cells, known as peripheral mononuclear blood cells (PMBCs). Even when the virus is eliminated from other regions, it often persists in the lymphatic system. The longer HCV is present or the larger the amounts of the virus, the more likely it is to infect obscure body parts, longer-lived cells, and cause damage.

This implies that treatment for some patients needs to go on for longer or that a different strategy needs to be considered. Money is not currently forthcoming for systematic research into herbal treatments for HCV, although this may be the best way forward for some patients if it is true that they can influence cell-mediated immunity. There is also much evidence to suggest that acupuncture can improve T cell ratios and the activity of leucocytes as a whole.[2]

References

1. Much publicized triple therapy treatment of newly infected HIV cases in New York showed that the virus could be reduced to undetectable levels in the blood after a few weeks. However, virus can still be found in infected organs and declines at a much slower rate.

2. Clinical report. Yang C. Sansi acupuncture symposium, 1959.

Research talk by Dr. Novera Spector at the First International Workshop on Immunomodulation, Washington DC, 1984.

Notes:
A Technical Description of HCV

(For informed or brave readers!)

HCV is a positive-sense, single-stranded RNA virus that is related to the family of flaviviridae. HCV is not a retrovirus. It is difficult to categorize as either cytopathic or immunopathic; it causes injury by both mechanisms.

It is small, 30–38 nm in diameter with a lipoid envelope. The genome consists of one large open-reading frame of 9379–9481 nucleotides. At the 5' end there is a terminal region of 329–341 nucleotides with a 92% homology among different HCV types. This region probably has a function in translation of the viral genome, and its highly conserved character renders it suitable for diagnostic detection of viral nucleic acid with PCR amplification. Further downstream in the genome one finds the encoding region of the putative HCV core, p22, two regions (E1 and E2) that encode for the envelope glycoproteins (gp33 and gp70) and four nonstructural regions. The nonstructural regions have a role in virus replication and encode for proteases (NS2, NS3, glycoproteins p23 and p70), helicase (NS3), and an RNA-dependent RNA polymerase (NS5). Finally the 3' terminal regions show considerable variations, both in length and sequence. In some isolates there is a poly-(rU) tail and in others a poly-(rA) tail. Several HCV isolates have now been cloned revealing wide sequence variation. This sequence heterogeneity is not evenly sequenced over the genome but differs between the regions. Apart from the conserved 5' terminal region, the putative core and NS3 regions are relatively well conserved, and antigens from these regions are used in anti-HCV antibody assays. Hypervariable domains have described in the N-terminal part of the E2 envelope region. Sequential mutations in this region probably have a role in viral escape from the host immune response. HCV is classified as a separate genus to the flaviviridae. There are at least six HCV genotypes, according to one proposed classification system based on 5' terminal region and NS5 sequence analysis. Other researchers have described twelve genotypes based on E1 sequence analysis, and more data may be needed before a formal classification system can be achieved.[1]

HCV is exceptionally small, at 30–38 nm (nanometers, equal to one billionth of a meter) in diameter. The influenza virus measures 80 nm in diameter. By comparison staphylococcus, a typical bacterium, measures 1,000 nm.

A further description of HCV and explanation of the dynamics of its replication has been provided by Brendan Duffy, BSc, a patient who holds a PhD in molecular genetics:

> If you could magnify a picture of an HCV viral particle it would look somewhat like a weird soccer ball. This "soccer ball" is comprised of a protein shell with external glycoproteins (a protein with sugars bound onto it), all organized into a spheroid shape to form a protective envelope, which surrounds and protects the precious RNA message kept inside. This envelope must be very strong, as it is the only barrier between the RNA and the pressures of the outside world. It must also be able to withstand the rigors of its human host's immune system if it is to survive. To this end, some of these external glycoproteins are variable. This means that within a population of HCV particles, all of the same genotype and all derived from the same infection event, there will be a wide range of differences in their external shape and constitution due to these variable glycoproteins on the outside. Often this fools the human immune system into not recognizing and destroying the virus particles in question. In this manner, an HCV infection may evade detection by the immune system through evolving these so-called

"escape" mutants, and a continuing "chronic" infection results.

Inside the envelope is the HCV RNA genome. A "genome" is all of the coded instructions required to reproduce a copy of the organism. As this information is encoded in a genetic form, it is also all of the heritable material possessed by the individual that will be passed on to its offspring, or progeny. It could be said that the genome defines the individual or species because it encodes all of its possible characteristics. The HCV uses RNA as a medium to encode its genome. RNA is a long, linear molecule that contains coded genetic information. This information generally comes in the form of "genes," which are coded linear instructions of how to build particular proteins. These RNA genes are "translated" into proteins, and these proteins are what HCV is made from (and by). As RNA is a linear molecule it has a start and a finish. The start is the 5 prime end, or 5', while the finish is 3 prime, or 3'.

Although the HCV genome is similar to most flaviviridae, it differs from the standard flavivirus enough to cause some researchers to believe that it is a member of a new virus family, recently diverged from flaviviridae. It consists of the 5'UTR (UTR means untranslated region), 3 structural genes, 6+ nonstructural genes, and the 3'UTR. The structural genes code for the proteins that comprise the envelope, while the nonstructural genes encode the enzymes that replicate the RNA genome (that will go inside the envelope) and put the whole thing together. The two untranslated regions contain messages of what to do with these genes, and how to do it. The HCV genome contains all the information it needs to fully replicate itself into a new viral particle, just like its parent particle, but it can't do this on its own. The virus lacks the machinery to do it with. HCV particles are so small they cannot possibly contain the incredibly complex apparatus that is required for reproduction. It takes a (relatively) huge autonomous cellular organism to do this. This is where we come in. It invades our cells and appropriates our cellular machinery for its sinister purposes of reproduction.

Once inside the host cell the HCV RNA leaves its envelope

and travels to one of the many ribosomes. These are the cell's "factories," the places where our cells manufacture proteins from RNA. This process is called "translation." Our DNA, locked far away in the nucleus of the cell, is too precious, and way too huge and cumbersome to travel to a ribosome, so it reads off and synthesizes a small RNA copy of the desired gene and sends that "messenger" RNA to the ribosome to be translated into protein. Once made, the protein is transported to its encoded destination to do what it has to do. The HCV RNA fools the cellular machinery by mimicking this process. It presents itself to the ribosome, pretending to be a normal piece of RNA (too bad about the deadly message it carries), and the ribosome starts translating it!

Below is a diagram of the HCV +RNA genome, genes not to scale. Please remember that over the course of investigation there have been various name changes of the genome's constituents.

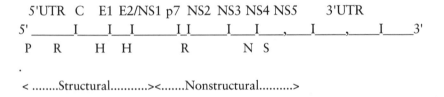

P = promotor, R = internal ribosome entry site (translation start)
H = hypervariable region, S = translation stop signal
N = interferon sensitivity determining region
C = core, E = envelope, NS = nonstructural

The first section of the HCV RNA genome is the 5' UTR. As a UTR it is not translated into a protein. Its function is that of organization. At the start of the 5'UTR there is a "promoter" motif, which is recognized only by the HCV "replicase" enzyme, which synthesizes new RNA strands. The replicase enzyme is encoded by the NS gene, and once translated and processed it rapidly moves along the RNA strand until it finds its specific recognition site (the replicase promoter). At this point it attaches to the RNA and begins to synthesize a new strand of RNA using the existing strand as a template. At the end of the UTR there is an IRES (internal ribosome entry site) motif, which allows the ribosome (cellular factory for translating RNA message to protein) to enter the RNA molecule here and translate the subsequent ten genes into one big polyprotein precursor, which is later processed into the smaller individual functional proteins by protease (a protein enzyme that cleaves bigger proteins into smaller ones) encoded by NS and also by cellular proteases.

Other functions for the 5'UTR I can only guess at as I haven't read that many of the references and science may not know. Guesses are stabilizing the whole 3D structure of the RNA so it can be packaged properly, protection from cellular exonucleases (enzymes that would eat away at the ends of the RNA), and possibly a transportation message that enables it to get from the cell membrane to the ribosome.

The three structural genes are for making proteins that will form the viral structure, or envelope that the RNA will be carried in. These genes are C (core), E1 (envelope 1), E2/NS1 (envelope 2/non-structural 1; when they named the protein the general arrangement of the flaviviridae family indicated that there should have been separate E2 and NS1 proteins). The most variable regions of the HCV genome are found here.

There are two HVRs (hypervariable regions), which are in the front end of E2/NS1 and also (somewhere) in E2. When different HCV strains from different people all over the world are sequenced, the most variability is found in these two regions. Variation was even found when the same test case was sampled three years later.

The variation occurs when the replicase is synthesizing a new RNA strand from the template. It appears to make deliberate copy errors in areas such as the HVRs (other errors may just be normal mistakes) in order to increase its genetic variation, which in turn causes changes in the structural protein and thus immunogenic variation. These errors remain in the RNA and affect the translation process so that different E2 proteins are produced that may escape immune detection. It appears that the envelope is comprised of core proteins that fix E1 and E2/NS1 proteins to the outside, forming the "soccer ball," with the HVR regions projected to the outside. This is how the immune system is fooled; the only contact with the immune system is a part that is never constant for very long.

The core protein is one of the first proteins released from the newly translated polyprotein precursor. A cellular protease cleaves the C protein away from the huge precursor, and some travels to the cell's nucleus where it interacts with cellular mechanisms. The C protein found in the nucleus is different from that found in mature virus particles. It carries a small segment (the "anchor") attached to the "carboxy terminus" (the end). It appears that this interactive C protein is the first protein created, by cleavage with a cellular protease. Some travels to the nucleus of the cell to deliver the message, while some remains and is processed further (the anchor is removed), by viral protease, to become the structural protein for the envelope.

The mechanism that the anchor C protein interferes with is apoptosis, or cellular suicide. When a cell realizes that it has been virally infected, it will normally undergo apoptosis. This is where the cell systematically starts closing down, shredding its nuclear material, destroying its cellular organelles (machinery), and finally, lysis, where the cell pops and withers, releasing its contents. Part of this process is to release a type of interferon to its external environment. This is a form of cellular communication, as the interferon acts as a messenger telling the neighboring cells that this cell has been virally infected and is committing suicide, and that they should all do likewise. The benefit of this is to ensure that high yields of viral progeny are not created within the cell, and that those viral particles that do escape before cell death only infect cells that are in the process of apoptosis anyway. This appears to be such a successful viral defense mechanism that most viruses have evolved opposing strategies to evade or delay apoptosis. It appears that the HCV anchor C protein can control the stages of apoptosis, inhibiting cell death, so viral progeny can build up to a maximum level inside the cell, evading the host's immune responses, and then it rapidly induces apoptosis, releasing them to the neighboring cells quickly and efficiently.

The nonstructural genes perform such a complex array of functions that as yet little is known (or published). Also, adding to the confusion is the phenomena of pleiotropy, where a gene, or protein, has more than one function, as seen with the C protein. Some of these NS proteins were found to have many abilities, and no single function could be assigned to them. In fact, NS4 and 5 had to be split into NS4A and NS4B and NS5A and NS5B. Don't ask what p7 is. Some basic functions known for these proteins are for making proteases that cleave the huge polyprotein precursor into its smaller functional units, enzymes to assemble the structural proteins into the finished viral envelope, a helicase to unwind RNA, and a replicase to replicate more copies of the RNA molecule.

The function of NS2 is as yet undefined, but one function appears to be to form a complex with NS3 to create a metalloprotease, that is an enzyme that uses metal ions as cofactors to cleave the HCV polyprotein precursor at specific places. Remember that the HCV +RNA is translated into one big linear protein comprised of all the genes in order. Most of these have to be processed, or cleaved into their individual units to form working proteins. It should be noted that further processing may also be necessary. This big blob of polyprotein is pretty cumbersome and useless as it is. It appears that one cellular and three(?) viral proteases do this job. One of the new generation of HCV drugs is an antiprotease, designed to interfere with proteases, so that the polyprotein precursor cannot be processed and remains useless.

The NS3 protein has a few different domains. The start, or "amino terminal region" of the protein, has a protease ability. It can form a complex with the NS2 protein to become a metalloprotease, or on its own it is a serine protease with the possible ability to cleave the polyprotein at the end, or carboxy terminus of NS4A, NS4B, NS5A, and NS5B. Also, this section of the NS3 protein can bind to the NS4A protein to form the protease complex required to cleave the NS4B/NS5A junction.

A central domain has the typical structure of a helicase, and as such it unwinds RNA. Another domain is for the metabolism of cellular energy, which it probably uses to drive these processes.

The NS4 protein is also mainly undefined, except for the role mentioned above. There is another IRES here, located at the start of NS4, allowing this section to be translated first, without having to wait for the whole polyprotein precursor to be processed into its individual constituents. This allows for the rapid production of NS4 and NS5 proteins, allowing them to function as soon as possible.

The NS5A protein is a protein kinase, which may modify the viral proteins once they have been cleaved from the polyprotein precursor. However, the major function of this protein is to inhibit the cellular viral response, which involves the above-mentioned interferon mechanism. This protein disrupts the workings of the interferon viral defense mechanism (still reading this stuff).

NS5B is believed to be an RNA-dependent RNA replicase, which will synthesize a complementary (or mirror image) RNA strand from an RNA template. As such, it would synthesize a negative strand of RNA from the original infecting positive RNA. Positive RNA codes for genes and can have negative strands copied from it by a replicase. Negative strands code for garbage and can't be read due to not having an IRES site, but they are used as templates to synthesize more positive strands. Replicase can speedily find the specific binding site in the 5'UTR and start transcribing negative RNA copies of the HCV genome, using the +ve genome as a template. These same replicases will then in the same way transcribe many, many +ve RNA copies of the HCV RNA genome by using these new -ve strands as templates. The new +ve RNA strands will be packaged into the finished envelopes to create finished HCV viral particles.

The start of the 3'UTR contains a stop signal, which tells the ribosome to stop translating. The RNA is now free to be translated again by a ribosome, or to be used as a template so the newly synthesized replicase enzyme can transcribe a -ve RNA strand. Both can occur at once, and typically there will be as many enzymes on this RNA strand as can fit, all transcribing RNA copies or translating the polyprotein precursor.

This goes on and on, over and over, and the whole thing cascades exponentially, because each new strand is synthesized very rapidly, and, of course, they're reusable. Transcription increases the number of negative strands. Each -ve strand can make more and more positive strands.

Positive strands can transcribe more negative or can be translated to make the polyprotein precursor. While a +ve strand is being translated by a ribosome, another ribosome will enter the IRES at NS4 to make more replicase! While this is happening, the polyprotein precursors are building up and being processed into working proteins, MORE replicases, and so on, and the viral envelopes are assembled. The cell becomes overloaded and cannot perform its designated function anymore. It just makes more and more HCV particles. The finished product builds up to a maximum yield. The cell is eventually overcome and succumbs to the pressures placed upon it.

Further Reading

Molecular virology of hepatitis C virus. Berwyn Clarke. *Journal of General virology,* 78, 2397–2410, 1997.

Characterization of the hepatitis C virus encoded serine proteinase: determination of proteinase dependent polyprotein cleavage sites. Grakoui A et al. *Journal of Virology,* 2832–2843, May 1993.

Mutational analysis of the hepatitis C virus RNA helicase. Kim JL et al. *Journal of Virology,* 9400–9409, Dec 1997.

Direct interaction of hepatitis C virus core protein with the cellular lymphotoxin-B receptor modulates the signal pathway of the lymphotoxin-B receptor. Chen et al. *Journal of Virology,* 9417–9426, Dec 1997.

Structure and organization of the hepatitis C virus genome isolated from human carriers. Takamizawa A et al. *Journal of Virology,* 1105–1113, Mar 1991.

Genetic organization and diversity of the hepatitis C virus. Choo Q-L et al. *Proc. Natl. Acad. Sci,* 88, 2451–2455, Mar 1991.

Evidence that hepatitis C virus resistance to interferon is mediated through repression of the PKR protein kinase by the nonstructural 5A protein. Gale MJ et al. *Virology,* 230, 217–227, 1997.

Characterization of the terminal regions of the hepatitis C viral RNA: identification of conserved sequences in the 5' untranslated region and poly(A) tails at the 3' end. Han JH et al. *Proc. Natl. Acad. Sci,* 88, 1711–1715, Mar 1991.

Internal ribosome entry site within hepatitis C virus RNA. Kyoko et al. *Journal of Virology,* 1476–1483, Mar 1992.

Gene mapping the putative structural region of the hepatitis C virus genome by in vitro processing analysis. Hijikata M et al. *Proc. Natl. Acad. Sci,* 88, 5547–5551, Jul 1991.

Full-length sequence of a hepatitis C virus genome having poor homology to reported isolates: comparative study of four distinct genotypes. Okamoto H et al. *Virology,* 188, 331–341, 1992.

Genetic drift of hepatitis C virus during an 8.2 year infection in a chimpanzee: variability and stability. Okamoto et al. *Virology,* 190, 894–899, 1992.

Reference

1. Hepatitis C virus 6 years on. Cees van der Poel L et al. *The Lancet,* Vol 344, Nov 26, 1994.

Glossary of Key Terms

Acupuncture: Ancient medical treatment involving insertion of fine needles.

Acute: Used to describe a disease with short and severe symptoms.

Alpha interferon: Main focus of drug treatments for HCV.

Amantadine: Antiflu drug found to have some value in HCV treatment.

Amino acids: The ultimate products of protein digestion and the source of body proteins. Impaired liver function can adversely affect their metabolism. Supplements may be necessary.

Antibody: Substances in the blood that destroy foreign substances.

Antigen: A substance that causes the formation of an antibody.

Apoptosis: Programmed cell death, associated with liver disease.

Ascites: Accumulation of fluid in the abdomen.

Autoimmunity: A reaction to one's own tissues.

Ayurveda: Traditional (Asian) Indian medical system.

Biopsy: Removal of tissue sample from living body for diagnostic purposes.

Cancer: A malignant tumor. Cancer cells demonstrate lower differentiation than normal cells, disorganization, and a faster proliferation rate.

Chronic: Used to describe persistent or recurring disease.

Cirrhosis: State where normal tissue is replaced by scarred tissue.

Cytopathic: Destructive to cells.

Depression: State of mind characterized by apathy, disinterest in life, anxiety, guilt, and poor concentration that can lead to suicidal thoughts. Common in HCV patients.

Fibrogenesis: Process of forming scar tissue, associated with cirrhosis.

Genotype: A virus strain with a distinct genetic makeup.

Glutathione: An amino acid normally manufactured in the body, it has been found to be deficient in HCV patients. It plays a vital role in keeping cells healthy.

Glycogen: Carbohydrate stored in liver prior to conversion into glucose.

Healing crisis: Term used by naturopaths to describe the process of detoxification or clearance where the patient temporarily feels extremely ill.

Hepatologist: Doctor specializing in liver disease.

Heterogeneity: The degree to which a group of virions vary from one another in terms of their genetic makeup.

Histology: The study of microscopic cellular states.

HLA system: Refers to human leucocyte antigen, a genetically determined regulator of immune response. HLA type has been found to influence the likelihood of patients clearing HCV and also influences susceptibility to other diseases.

Homeopathy: System of medicine based on "treat like with like."

Immunopathic: Causes destruction by triggering destructive immune response.

Infectivity: The ease with which a pathogen can be transmitted from a carrier to a new host.

Interferons: Glycoproteins released in response to presence of antigens, they inhibit the proliferation of viruses and host cells. Now synthesized and used to treat HCV, the drug was originally developed to treat cancer.

Lysis: In the context of liver disease, loosening of cell adhesion.

M.E.: Myalgic encephalomyelitis. British term embracing debilitated conditions such as chronic fatigue syndrome postviral fatigue syndrome. Diagnosis is common in HCV patients.

Milk thistle: Powerful herb used to detoxify the liver.

NAC: N-acetyl cysteine. A powerful glutathione precursor with liver protective and antiviral properties. Used with interferon in Spain. Despite promising results not widely offered to patients.

NANB: Non-A non-B hepatitis.

Necrosis: Death of a limited portion of tissue or a few cells.

Oncogenesis: Cancer development, or cell changes characteristic of cancer.

PCR: Polymerase chain reaction. A type of test used to detect extremely low quantities of any given organic material. This is the "gold standard" used to assess HCV positivity.

Phagocytosis: Process by which foreign bodies are neutralized.

Qi: Basic concept of energy in TCM. Similar to "vital force."

Quasi species: Substrains of HCV that have mutated so far from the original infecting type that they can be classified as a new type.

Recovery: Process of arresting drug or alcohol abuse, reviewing the individual causes making behavioral and attitudinal changes. Usually associated with Alcoholics Anonymous or Narcotics Anonymous, although the term also extends to other forms of compulsive behavior.

Spleen: Site of lymphocyte production. In TCM the spleen is not just the organ, but seen as the purifier of all body fluids.

Symptoms: Evidence of disease.

TCM: Traditional Chinese Medicine.

Varices: Distended blood vessels associated with cirrhosis.

Viability: The ability of an organism to survive on its own.

Viral load: A measure of the amount of virus present (see **PCR**).

Virions: Individual virus elements.

Virulence: The degree to which a virus causes disease and death.

Vitamins: Essential nutrients stored in the liver. Impaired liver function may mean that supplements are necessary.

Afterword

This afterword is based upon my own assessment of the current situation. It contains some ideas about possible ways forward and represents my personal view only.

It is clear that many questions about hepatitis C have not yet been satisfactorily answered. A recurrent theme in this book is that much more research needs to be instigated into the many poorly understood aspects of this condition and its treatment.

What is clear is that HCV can cause an array of chronic systemic illnesses; it is not merely a liver disease, as the word "hepatitis" suggests. Pathogenesis is complex, with some conditions apparently arising as a result of a series of "knock on" effects. Many common, debilitating, but clinically obscure symptoms, such as fatigue and cognitive dysfunction, cannot be easily linked to specific cytopathic viral disruption. They can only be properly understood by viewing the whole body of a patient as a system, with ongoing tendencies toward disequilibrium. Thus hepatitis C needs to be redefined in the minds of patients and practitioners.

A broader scope for symptom identification and validation might be expected to lead to improved patient-doctor relationships and may make patients feel less misunderstood. Doctors who are prepared to depart from their specific specialization and even their own medical tradition will necessarily have an advantage when deciding upon treatment strategy. Given that any one of the existing systems lacks a satisfactory solution on their own, it must be the case that a wider search is more likely to yield practical solutions to patients. Doctors who have been listening to their patients are already supportive of a broad approach provided it is well thought through and safe.

A cool analysis of the current treatment system and the varied needs of patients reveals that a coherent strategy can already be assembled with currently available options. Patient profiles lend themselves to particular treatment priorities and methodologies. A single treatment for everyone with HCV is impractical. The following is a crude breakdown of patient groupings and associated priorities, and represents a possible basis of a rational systematic approach. The various medical traditions are regarded as competing paradigms, and each is suggested on the basis of their practical ability to address the needs of patients.

Patients who present with drug and alcohol problems need these addressed first as the top priority. Available evidence suggests that chemical dependency is a highly influential cofactor that accelerates disease progression and may precipitate early mortality through a range of mechanisms. Drug and alcohol dependency is also a contraindicator for the major treatments.

Patients who have been successfully treated and those who present without chemical dependency in the first place can then be offered a range of symptom alleviation treatments and advised in detail on lifestyle adjustments. Systematic and heavily screened Chinese herbal formulations specifically addressed to the varying needs of HCV patients are now becoming available. These will help patients to feel better and, where secondary clinical conditions, such as depression, are linked to HCV, these will offer an option for a practical way forward. These treatments may help to level the playing field for patients in recovery from chemical dependency, who sometimes feel ill despite stopping taking drugs or drinking alcohol. They can also address the needs of cirrhotic patients, who are often advised not to take drug therapy. Patients might also be briefed on other secondary options such as relaxation, amino acid supplementation, acupuncture, aromatherapy, lymphatic drainage, and so on.

Because the practice of TCM is so varied, these consistent formulations can be viewed even by conventional doctors as a useful option and might be offered as an option to patients. Symptoms such as fatigue, poor digestion, bloating, and malaise are particularly responsive to these treatments. Emerging clinical evidence supports the subjective improvements reported by patients consuming these products. Safety and tolerability compares extremely well to chemotherapy.

Patients can then be offered antiviral drug therapy and given a fair appraisal of the current situation with regard to efficacy and side effects. It is reasonable to expect that patients who have already achieved a degree of symptom alleviation and functional improvement are more likely to last the course and are perhaps even more likely to respond.

Patients who are in a critical condition due to imminent organ failure can be referred to transplant facilities. Because of the relative youth of many HCV patients, successful transplantation can be argued to provide great benefit in terms of improved life expectancy compared to other groups needing transplant.

At all times the patients' "psychological autonomy" should be respected. The best way of achieving this is to give them a balanced and accurate diet of information about hepatitis C and treatment options. This book may help to serve that purpose and also help doctors not to have to take responsibility for treatment decisions that may have adverse consequences.

Research into treatments for hepatitis C is ongoing but not particularly balanced, being almost exclusively carried out only where there is the prospect of a patent drug being validated. This is not necessarily in the interests of the overall health of patients. While more combination drug therapies are being researched, they tend to suggest that those patients who are not contraindicated will have to face the prospect of even more arduous courses of chemotherapy with additional side effects. Despite the fact that at least 50% of patients will be either clinically or behaviorally contraindicated for interferon-based therapy, or choose to reject this option as unacceptable, or have already failed or not responded, most new drugs appear to be lined up as interferon combinations. This is irrational. Other avenues need to be explored as well.

On the positive side there are distinct signs that nonchemotherapeutic medicines may be developed for availability from within the mainstream medical system. Changes in patenting and quality control technology mean that some plant-based medicines may become available in the near future. Adjunct therapies based on plant ingredients are also being developed and proposed for testing.

Given the scale of the HCV pandemic and the powerful adverse impact on overall levels of health, with the damaging economic and social consequences, the level of research into HCV treatment is woefully inadequate. A commercially disinterested source of research funding may be necessary to instigate urgently required research.

For instance, it would surely not be particularly difficult to arrange an analysis of the vitamin, mineral, and amino acid profiles of broad groups of the patient population. Such research would be immensely useful in providing an informed basis for supplementation strategies and would not be expensive. Such a study could include profiles of those consuming alcohol and drugs, and lead to a greater understanding of factors that may contribute to disease progression and the use of biochemical harm reduction agents for this group of patients.

The validation of treatment efficacy also needs to be reviewed. Pre- and posttreatment assessment should be expanded to include qualitative questioning of trialists and functional testing; this would be particularly appropriate for symptoms such as fatigue, digestion, cognitive dysfunction, and depression. These are very important elements in overall health. Surely patients have the right to "mark" their treatment in terms of the benefits it has actually delivered to them, as well as doctors assessing clinical impact. Given the fact that hepatitis C is a highly complex condition, such a triangulation of criteria may generate a more meaningful assessment, giving patients the ability to make better-informed treatment decisions.

Health delivery systems may need to be reformed in order to meet the needs of patients. Certainly the unique Gateway clinic provides an example of how large numbers of patients, particularly those who present with chemical dependency, can be given treatment combined with their other needs, such as ear acupuncture, effectively and economically. Indeed this model may be the only economically viable option for hard-pressed public health services; hepatitis C has the theoretical capacity to bankrupt every health funding system in the Western world as they are currently structured.

The epidemiological data clearly shows that HCV poses a serious global threat to public health. Current rates of infection are very high within the IVDU communities in affluent countries. Yet workable and economic measures that could be reasonably expected to retard rates of transmission are not being taken, usually for political reasons.

These are just some of the relevant issues and questions. Not everyone will agree with this assessment; a debate on the matter might yield more concrete changes. Hepatitis C is not discussed enough and does not attract the attention that it deserves, given its massive prevalence and serious impact. I hope that this book acts as a catalyst to the process of discussion and policy making. If you have any comments, suggestions, or contributions, please write to Catalyst Press, P.O. Box 13036, London NW1 3WG, U.K.; or email Jason McClure at one of the following:

JasonMcClure@compuserve.com
JasonMcClure@focusonhepc.com
HCVNEWS@focusonhepc.com

Resources

For further information about this book, and issues arising, visit: http://www.hepchandbook.com.

U.S.

American Liver Foundation
1425 Pompton Ave
Cedar Grove, NJ 07009-1000
(800) GO-LIVER (465-4837)
(888) 4-HEP-ABC (443-7222)
http://www.liverfoundation.org

Cooley's Anemia Foundation Inc.
Gina Cioffi, National Executive Director
129/09 26th Avenue, Suite 203
Flushing, N Y 11354
(800) 522-7222 or (718) 321-CURE
Fax: (718) 321-3340

HCV Global Foundation
2807 Swan Way
Fairfield, CA 94533
(707) 425-5343
Fax: (510) 569-3743
Contact Ron Duffy, president and founder for information
email: vironn@aol.com

The Hep C Connection
1741 Gaylord St.

Denver, CO
(303) 393-9395
HepC Hotline: (800) 522-HEPC.
Hepatitis Help Line: (800) 390-1202
http://www.hepc-connection.org
hepc-connection@worldnet.att.net

The Hepatitis C Foundation
1502 Russett Drive
Warminster, PA 18974
(800) 324-7305 or (215) 672-2606
http://www.hepcfoundation.org

United Liver Association
11646 West Pico Blvd.
Los Angeles, CA 90064
(310) 914-8252

Hepatitis Education Project
P.O. Box 95162
Seattle, WA 98145
Email: graham@phoenix.artsci.washington.edu

For information on harm reduction in the U.S. and on range of other related subjects, call the **Lindesmith Center** in New York City at (212) 548-0695 or in San Francisco at (415) 921-4987.

Or visit their Website: http://www.lindesmith.org

For information on support groups in the San Francisco Bay Area, call: (415) 676-4888.

Government Agencies

Centers for Disease Control and Prevention (CDC)
Hepatitis Branch, Mailstop G37
Division of Viral and Rickettsial Diseases
National Center for Infectious Diseases
Atlanta, GA 3033
CDC Hepatitis Hotline: (404) 332-4555
CDC Public Inquires: (800) 311-3435

The National Institutes for Health (NIH)

This is the largest biomedical research center in the world. It's the research arm of the Public Health Service, U.S. Dept. of Health and Human Services. Among its institutes that conduct and support research on hepatitis viruses are the National Institute of Allergy and Infectious Diseases (NIAAID) and the National Institute of Diabetes and Digestive and Kidney Diseases (NIDDK).

NIAID Office of Communications

Building 31, Room 7A50
Bethesda, MD 20892
(301) 496-5717
Press releases, fact sheets, and other materials are available on the Internet via the NIAID Website: http://www.niaid.nih.gov

National Institute of Diabetes and Digestive and Kidney Diseases (NIDDK)

For a packet of materials on hepatitis C, write to
National Digestive Diseases Information Clearinghouse (NIDDK),
2 Information Way
Bethesda, MD 20892-3570
http://www.niddk.nih.gov
nddic@aerie.com

Transplant Organizations and Agencies

Transplant Recipient International Organization

Nationwide support group for patients and families.
1735 Eye St. NW, Suite 917
Washington, DC 20006
(202) 293-0980

United Network for Organ Sharing (UNOS)

1100 Boulders Parkway, Suite 500
P.O. Box 13770
Richmond, VA 23225-8770
(804) 330-8500
Patient information: (888) 894-6361
http://www.unos.org

U.S. Department of Health and Human Services
Division of Transplantation
5600 Fishers Lane, Room 7–29
Rockville, MD 20857
(301) 443-7577

Canada

Hep C British Columbia
http://www.geocities.com/HotSprings/5670
Email: hepcbc@iforward.com

British Columbia Hepatitis Foundation
P.O. Box 21058
Penticton, B.C. V2A 8V9
(250) 490-9054. Fax: (250) 490-0620
Email: bchepc@bc.sympatico.ca

Hepatitis C Society of Canada, Victoria Chapter
1611 Quadra St.
Victoria, BC V8W 2L5
Tel. (250) 388-4311
hepcvic@pacificcoast.net
http://www.pacificcoast.net/~hepcvic/hepcvic~1.htm

Hepatitis C Society of Canada
National Office
383 Huron Street
Toronto, Ontario, M5G 2S5
(800) 652-Hepc (4372)
(416) 979-5855. Fax: (416) 979-5856
hecsc@idirect.com
http://web.idirect.com/~hepc

Parksville/Qualicum support group
305-335 Hirst Street West
Parksville, BC.
(205) 248-5551
Email: dbamford@island.net

Cowichan Valley Hepatitis C Support Services Group
464 Trans Canada Highway, Duncan, BC
Contact Debbie at (250) 748-5450 or Leah at (250) 748-3432

For Parents with Children That Have HCV
Cindy Makarenko (250) 767-2026
Email: magenta@okanagan.net

Manitoba
Claude Jones and Dawn Lawson joneslawson@techplus.com

U.K. and Ireland

The HCV Group maintains a Hep C Support Network list and runs support meetings. Write to P.O. Box 13036, London NW1 3WG for details; if you are starting a new meeting in the U.K., fax details to 0171 916 7942.

The HCV Group is currently applying for national charitable status and aims to be the first U.K. national charity run for and by hepatitis C patients. Contributions and practical help will always be appreciated.

The British Liver Trust keeps a list of private support contacts and may help you to set up a support group. Call Sue Kent at 01473 276326.

The Mainliners Agency is a long-term supporter of hepatitis C related activities. It has a "how to set up a hep C support group" pack and hosts regular support groups meetings, seminars, and conferences. Their telephone number is: 0171 582 3338; ask to speak to Leena or Monique.

The Hemophilia Society produces information packs and organizes a range of supportive activities. Their number is 0171 380 0600 and the contact is Lucy McGrath.

The Irish Hemophilia Society can be contacted in Dublin at 01872 4466.

The Yuan Centre is a new medical resource to be located in central

London. It will specialize in the treatment of hepatitis C as well as a number of other chronic diseases.

The treatment director will be John Tindall. It is intended that it will be a center of excellence for the development of treatment expertise, facilitate research, and act as a focal point for exchange of experience, ideas, and information between varied medical traditions. The center will have a charitable arm. For information send an A4 stamp-addressed envelope to: P.O. Box 13036, London NW1 3WG.

Or visit their Website: http://www.yuancentre.com

A Selection of Resources and Support Group Meetings

The South London HCV support group meets at the Mainliners Agency, 38–40 Kennington Park Road at 7 pm on the first Tuesday of each month. Also newcomers meetings. Call 0171 582 3338 to confirm details.

The Gateway Clinic, Old SW Hospital, Landor Road, Stockwell; call 0171 346 5451.

Bath: 109 New Bridge Road, Bath BA1 3HG
Call Jim Phillips at 01225 445337.

Border and other contacts in **Scotland:**
Write to Feyona, P.O. Box 14466, Glenrothes, Fife, KY7 6WA.

Glasgow: Hepatitis C Glasgow;
contact Jimmy 01389 603286.

Kent: Preston Hall Hospital, Maidstone ME20 7NJ.
Call Nigel Hughes 01622 713088.

Sussex: Second Wednesday of the month;
call Pamela Spalding at 01444 415827.

For Professional Training Courses

Call **Christine Beveridge** at 44 (0)171 209 0993; she can also arrange talks by Matthew Dolan. Courses can be run overseas.

For Information on Standardized, Tableted Chinese Herbal Formulae for Hep C

Call **East West Herbs** at 44 (0)1608 658941 or visit their shop in Neals Yard, Covent Garden, London 44 (0)171 379 1312.

Australia and New Zealand

A much more comprehensive list will appear in the Australasian edition.

Hepatitis C Councils (Australia)
New South Wales Tel: 1-800-803 990
Queensland Tel: 1-800-648 491
Victoria Tel: 1-800-703-003

Hepatitis C Support Group (New Zealand)
Tel: 0800 224 372

Internet Resources

Quantum Media and Jason McClure's Websites
http://www.focusonhepc.com
http://pages.prodigy.com/hepc

Emailing Lists—A Source of Information and Support
Send an email to majordomo@lists.vossnet.co.u.k. including the message **subscribe HEPC** in the main body of the text.
Queries to crina@vossnet.co.uk.

Ask Emaliss—Hep C Info and Support Magazine
This is a free monthly online magazine which provides a venue for submitting and receiving personal questions.
http://soli.inav.net~webbsite//
Emaliss@aol.com

Hep-C ALERT! is a dynamic and quickly growing nonprofit hepatitis advocacy organization. http://www.hep-c-alert.org/

The St. Johns University Hepatitis Support Group
To subscribe send an email message to listserve@maelstrom.stjohns.edu. In the body of the email, type only **Subscribe hepV-L First name, Last name**

The Hepatitis Webring
Contains links to about 80 sites. http://www.hepring.org

Peppermint Patti's Junk Drawer
http://members.bellatlantic.net/~clotho/

HCV Global Foundation is an international HCV only non profit organization which combines a blend of HCV patients and members of the medical community in order to provide education and support programs, research priorities, create awareness, find the best treatment opinions and cure for hepatitis C.
Contact Ron Duffy: vironn@aol.com
Or visit their Website:
   http://members.aol.com/chapfest/SoCAhepfestHP.htm

Transplants Pre and Post
http://pages.prodigy.com/Transplant/transpnp.htm

HepNet—The Hepatitis Information Network
HepNet is designed for both medical professionals and patients who are looking for current information on viral hepatitis A to G.
http://www.hepnet.com

Political Action/Education Community (PAEC) Email Discussion List
Contact Beau Hooker: beauh@roanoke.infi.net.

Nashville Hepatitis C Coalition
Dedicated to providing information and support to hepatitis C patients, families, and friends.
http://members.aol.com/HEPPER/NashvilleHepC.html

The Hepatitis and Liver Disease Referral Network
A listing of prominent hepatologists
http://arens.com/hepnet

Hepatitis C Got You Down? Get Hip to Hep
Site focuses on hepatitis C, links to other hepatitis sites, as well as alternative healing methods, government sites, drug sites, and conventional medicine sites. Fun things to come . . .
http://www.geocites.com/hotsprings/villa/4883/
http://www.geocities.com/hotsprings/5633

My Liver Transplant
This is a story of two liver transplants in two years due to hepatitis C.
http://www.geocities.com/Heartland/Flats/6652/transplant.html

America Online
Sponsors a hepatitis C support group "chat" every Wednesday night from 8–9 p.m. EST. You must be subscribed to America Online to join.

Alternative Therapies

Ask Dr. Weil
Dr. Weil takes questions on alternative medicine.
http://cgi.pathfinder.com/drweil/

East West Herbs (U.S.)
http://www.eastwestherbs.com/
ewherbs@hooked.net

Ed's Guide to Alternative Therapies
http://worldmall.com/erf/altermed.htm
Ed Friedlander, MD
Email to: erf@alum.uhs.edu

Nature's Response
An Oklahoma-based company that provides vitamins, herbs, other nutritional supplements, and homeopathic remedies. Its owner is a certified nutritional counselor who provides consultations.
To request a catalog, call (800) 216-5195 or fax: (888) 842-8168.

Natural Medicine and More
Anthony G. Payne, M.D.
AOL Alternative Medicine Board Community Leader (AltM DocP).
http://members.aol.com/DrAGPayne/index.html

DAAIR has been suggested as a good source of food supplements:
Direct Aids Alternative Information Resources
31 East 30th Street, Suite 2A
New York, NY 10016
Email: info@daair.org
Website: http://www.immunet.org/daair
Phone toll-free outside NYC: (888) 951-LIFE (5433)
Phone inside NYC: (212) 725-6994
Fax: (212) 689-6471

Vitamin Research Products Inc.
3579 Hwy. 50 East
Carson City, NV 89701
(800) 877-2447. Fax: (800) 877-3292
Website: http://www.vrp.com

Drug Therapy

Amgen's Safety Net Program
This program is for people who are unable to pay for Infergen (interferon formula). (888) 508-8088

Schering-Plough's Commitment to Care Program
This program is based on a sliding scale. (800) 521-7157 ext. 147

Roche Biocare's financial assistance line
(800) 443-6676

Glaxo Wellcome Inc.
Tel: (919) 248-2100. Fax: (919) 248-2381
Website: http://www.imgw.com/forms/GWcoform.html

Finance, Disability, and Insurance

Checkup on Health Insurance Choices. Tel: 1-800-358-9265
National Committee for Quality Assurance. Tel: 1-800-839-6487
Disability Information. Tel: 1-800-232-9675
Social Security. Tel: 1-800-772-1213

Index